KU-003-949

A Guide to Psychiatry in Primary Care

Third Edition

P/O NO:
ACCESSION NO: KH04158
SHELFMARK: 616.85225

HSE South Kerry General Hospital
Library

KH04158

For my husband

A Guide to Psychiatry in Primary Care

Third Edition

PATRICIA R. CASEY

Professor of Psychiatry, University College Dublin and
Consultant Psychiatrist, Mater Misericordiae Hospital, Dublin

WRIGHTSON BIOMEDICAL PUBLISHING
A Division of Judy Wrightson Design Ltd
Petersfield, UK and New York, USA

Copyright © 2005 by Wrightson Biomedical Publishing
(A Division of Judy Wrightson Design Ltd)

All rights reserved

No part of this book may be reproduced by any means
or transmitted, or translated into machine language
without the written permission of the publisher.

Editorial Office:
Wrightson Biomedical Pulishing
Ash Barn House, Winchester Road,
Petersfield, Hampshire GU32 3PN, UK
Telephone: 01730 265647
Fax: 01730 260368
Email: wrightson.biomed@virgin.net

British Library Cataloguing in Publication Data
Casey, Patricia R.
   A guide to psychiatry in primary care. – 3rd ed.
   1. Psychiatry 2. Primary care (Medicine)
   I. Title
   616.8'9

Library of Congress Cataloging in Publication Data
A catalog record for this book is available from the
Library of Congress

ISBN 1 871816 50 5

Composition by Scribe Design Ltd, Ashford, Kent, UK
Printed in Great Britain by Biddles Ltd, King's Lynn, UK

Contents

Preface

The bulk of psychiatric practice is now firmly rooted in general practice. The involvement of general practitioners in the diagnosis and management of those with mental health problems has spawned large volumes of research, published in prestigious peer reviewed journals and there is at least one journal in Britain devoted exclusively to this. The World Health Organisation has recognised explicitly the importance of primary care as the therapeutic environment in which most mental health problems present by developing a classification of psychiatric disorders exclusively for use in this setting. Against this background the publication of the third edition of *A Guide to Psychiatry in Primary Care* hardly needs explanation or justification.

This latest edition addresses many of the complex problems seen in primary care, many of which receive little attention in the standard psychiatric textbooks. One such condition is premenstrual dysphoric disorder, a disorder that overwhelmingly is managed by general practitioners and rarely by psychiatrists. The aetiology of and evidence base for the effective management of this condition is addressed. Similarly, chronic fatigue syndrome, a condition that has generated a significant amount of controversy, is covered in detail since this too is predominantly managed in primary care. Other more difficult areas are considered, including the usefulness or otherwise of screening for depression and the management of attention deficit hyperactivity disorder in adults. Newer terminologies such as generalised anxiety disorder, somatoform disorder and bipolar II disorders are introduced to familiarise the general practitioner with the changing and evolving concepts in psychiatric classification. The increasing recognition of child sexual abuse and of its devastating consequences manifesting themselves in adulthood has warranted an expanded section on this topic.

Since the publication of the last edition of this book there have been a number of developments that affect general practice psychiatry directly. The beginning of the third millennium has witnessed the development of a range of new pharmacological treatments including antidepressants that go beyond the SSRIs and a number of atypical antipsychotic agents. Their ultimate place in psychiatric treatment has yet to be established but their current status must nevertheless be considered as it applies in general practice. A further dilemma for general practitioners is to know the appropriate response to the increasing numbers who opt for alternative treatments instead of conventional remedies, and information on the efficacy of some of these is presented in a new chapter on herbal remedies.

Psychiatry has also been the subject of controversy and the most public has been the, at times, stormy debate concerning the possible link between the SSRI antidepressants and suicidal behaviour. At the time of writing it is on the threshold of resolution with the imminent publication of the National Institute for Clinical Excellence (NICE) guidelines on the treatment of depression. This issue is discussed to assist general practitioners in responding to the concerns that patients may raise with them about antidepressants and suicidal behaviour.

Globalisation is associated with greater access to information. The internet is now ubiquitous and has the capacity to exert an enormous influence on our perspective and knowledge about mental health matters as it does in every other sphere. However, there is also a danger that much misinformation will be conveyed through this medium and to enable both doctor and patient the author has scrutinised a large number of websites for accuracy and usefulness and provided relevant addresses at the end of each chapter.

In spite of additions and expansions in most of the chapters, much about the new edition is also familiar including the continuing use of case vignettes, the provision of addresses for self-help and other useful organisations and a list of suggested reading material for doctors and patients.

As ever I am deeply indebted to Judy Wrightson of Wrightson Biomedical Publishing who more than 12 years ago had the intuition and foresight to publish the first edition of the book. Without her belief in and commitment to it, *A Guide to Psychiatry in Primary Care* would not have withstood the test of time to now be available in a third edition. As ever I am very grateful to those many general practitioners who have read this book and whose interest and commitment to dealing with mental health problems has stimulated this newest edition. Finally, my family deserve special mention for their forebearance during the months when I worked on this new edition of *A Guide to Psychiatry in Primary Care.*

PATRICIA CASEY
January 2005

1

Prevalence of Psychiatric Disorder

It is now accepted that the bulk of psychiatric disturbance is seen not by psychiatrists but by general practitioners. Furthermore, a sizeable proportion of those with psychological problems are not identified but remain undetected in the community. The factors determining which patients are identified and which are not are collectively referred to as 'filters' (Goldberg and Huxley, 1980) and will be described in more detail in Chapter 2. To begin, it is useful to consider the prevalence of psychiatric disorder amongst different clinical populations of relevance to general practice. These populations or levels, as they are referred to in Goldberg and Huxley's model (1980), are illustrated in Table 1.1 although recently it has been amplified by the addition of a sixth level identified as the forensic services, who accept referrals from the courts and the psychiatric services (Commander *et al.*, 1997). The addition of management by other agencies, such as the voluntary sector or traditional healers prior to consultation with the general practitioner has also been suggested (Bhui and Bhugra, 2002) in recognition of the more complex route that some groups, such as ethnic minorities, have into care. Notwithstanding these proposed modifications, the original model remains a very useful way of conceptualising the mental health care pathway.

LEVEL I

This refers to the total psychiatric morbidity in the community and can only be ascertained by screening whole communities or random samples from them. Despite some efforts in the early part of the 20th century, it was not until recently that interest realistically focused on psychiatric epidemiology. In 1956 the first such survey was conducted when a community sample in Sweden was interviewed to determine the distribution of both personality disorder and psychiatric disorder using predetermined criteria. Of that population, 8.5% had evidence of definite psychiatric disorder and a further 45% possible or probable psychiatric disorder. Personality disorder and the neuroses predominated.

After a lull, the early 1960s ushered in a number of epidemiological studies, mainly from the United States. These found that between 45% and 81% of the

Table 1.1. The pathway to psychiatric care: five levels and four filters.

	The community		Primary medical care				Specialist psychiatric services	
	Level 1	First filter	Level 2	Second filter	Level 3	Third filter	Level 4	Fourth filter	Level 5
	Morbidity in random community samples		Total psychiatric morbidity, primary care		Conspicuous psychiatric morbidity		Total psychiatric patients		Psychiatric inpatients only
One year period prevalence, median estimates	250 →		230 →		140 →		17 →		6 (per 1000 at risk per year)
Characteristics of the four filters		Illness behaviour		Detection of disorder		Referral to psychiatrists		Admission to psychiatric beds	
Key individual		The patient		Primary care physician		Primary care physician		Psychiatrist	
Factors operating on key individual		Severity and type of symptoms; psychosocial stress. Learned patterns of illness behaviour		Interview techniques. Personality factors. Training and attitudes		Confidence in own ability to manage. Availability and quality of psychiatric services. Attitudes towards psychiatrists		Availability of beds. Availability of adequate community psychiatric services	
Other factors		Attitudes of relatives. Availability of medical services. Ability to pay for treatment		Presenting symptom pattern. Sociodemographic characteristics of patient		Symptom pattern of patient. Attitudes of patient and family		Symptom pattern of patient, risk to self or others. Attitudes of patient and family. Delay in social worker arriving	

(Reproduced with permission, from Goldberg and Huxley, 1980.)

population had psychological problems, ludicrously suggesting that psychological dysfunction was the norm! These early attempts, whilst well meaning in their intentions, were widely criticised for the broadness of their concepts of psychological dysfunction and for their failure to use diagnostic labels.

A number of techniques were used to address the shortcomings including the use of screening schedules and the adoption of cut-off scores to define the threshold for psychiatric disturbance. This was the approach utilised by the General Health Questionnaire (GHQ). Developed by Goldberg and his colleagues in the 1970s, it was used initially in a random community sample. The GHQ does not provide a definitive diagnosis but gives an indication of those likely to be ill and in need of a full psychiatric assessment. Of those interviewed, 11% had scores in the range suggestive of illness and were mainly women (Goldberg *et al.*, 1976). Others using this schedule have found slightly higher figures.

A further development in the detection of psychiatric illness was the use of the structured interview, which both standardised the interview, thereby improving reliability, and provided a diagnosis. Inevitably this increase in sophistication also led to greater complexity in the interview and to the necessity for training in the use of these schedules. This was the approach adopted in the monumental study of Robins (1984). Known as the Epidemiological Catchment Area (ECA) study, it measured psychiatric disturbance at five sites scattered throughout the US according to DSM III criteria (see Chapter 4). A one-year prevalence ranging from 13.7–15.2% and a lifetime prevalence from 23–25.2% were found, with major depression, substance abuse and phobias predominating. Substance abuse and antisocial personality occurred principally in men whilst affective disorders and panic disorder were significantly more common in women. Overall, the rates were twice as high in the under 45s as in those over 45.

One of the few studies in Britain in the early 1980s to investigate psychiatric illness in the community was that of Casey and Tyrer (1986) in which they attempted to measure the prevalence of all psychiatric disorders including personality disorder and social functioning: 8% met the criteria for psychiatric disorder and depressive illness predominated; 13% of those interviewed also had personality disorder independent of illness and explosive type was the most common. Although the sample size was small, this study emphasised the need to assess underlying personality in addition to illness.

Recent studies have continued the trends of large-scale epidemiological investigations in the general population similar to the ECA study. The National Co-Morbidity Survey (NCS) (Kessler *et al.*, 1994) conducted among 8000 adults dispersed throughout all the states in the US used lay interviewers to examine the lifetime and one-year period prevalence of psychiatric disorders. Using a structured interview an extraordinarily high lifetime rate of almost 50% for any psychiatric disorder was found and the rate for one year was 30%. Moreover, the investigators found that major depression, alcohol dependence, social phobia and simple phobias were the most common disorders and that fewer than 40% with a lifetime disorder had received professional help, whilst less than 20% with a recent disorder had been on drug treatment. Major depression and anxiety were more common among women and the reverse applied to substance use disorders and antisocial personality disorder. All disorders decreased with increasing age and with increasing social class. However, these data were re-analysed using criteria incorporating information on the impact of symptoms on functioning and relationships and using this more stringent methodology the one-year rate for any disorder dropped to 18.5%. Subsequent examination of the disorders by severity found that 16% were rated as mild and the rest moderate, serious and severe although all four categories carried the risk of an adverse outcome suggesting that a mild disorder may still be in need of treatment.

In Britain the National Psychiatric Morbidity Surveys (Jenkins *et al.*, 1997) selected 13 000 adults aged between 16–65 for interview. Over 10 000 were assessed by lay interviewers for the presence of neurotic disorders as well as alcohol and drug dependence. Psychiatrists evaluated the presence of psychotic disorders. In both instances, the interview schedules were lengthy and required training in their use. Overall, 16% of subjects scored above the cut-off for any neurotic disorder. Men had a one-week period prevalence of 12.3% and women of 19.5%. Those who were married and those in social class 1 had the lowest rates and urban dwellers the highest. All disorders were significantly more common in women with the exception of panic disorder, which was equally prevalent in both. Surprisingly generalised anxiety was more common than depressive episode (3.1% v. 2.1%), followed by obsessive–compulsive disorder (1.2%) and phobias (1.1%). For psychotic disorders the one-year prevalence was 0.4%, being equally common in both sexes, and for alcohol and drug dependence the prevalence was 4.7% and 2.2%, respectively, with a large male preponderance in each.

Although the overall prevalence of disorder was similar in both studies, after re-analysis of the NCS data, the pattern of diagnoses differed from the Jenkins study (1997), pointing to the problems of generalising from data obtained in one country to another with a very different culture.

LEVEL 2

Epidemiological studies in the community are useful in developing our understanding of the nature and natural history of psychiatric illness. However, their applicability is limited and so the investigation of psychiatric morbidity in general practice consulters is more relevant to the education of family doctors and to planning psychiatric services. Level 2 in this model refers to general practice attendees and studies at this level include all consulting patients.

Goldberg and Blackwell (1970) assessed 553 consecutive attendees at a general practitioner's surgery using the GHQ to measure the extent to which psychological factors contributed to the consultation. Some degree of psychiatric disturbance was found in 24.4%, but only 7.8% had entirely psychiatric illness. Over a quarter had mild or subclinical disturbances. A similar study in 1976 (Goldberg *et al.*) showed that 33% of consecutive attendees at a surgery had scores on the GHQ suggestive of psychiatric disturbance and that 12% of attendees were not so identified. When interpreting these high figures it must be borne in mind that the GHQ is a screening rather than a diagnostic instrument. Despite these misgivings this study does point to the magnitude of the problem of psychological distress and morbidity in the primary care setting and to the need for further research in this area.

The failure to identify those with significant emotional disturbance as suggested by the above study shifted the focus from the clinical interview to the use of screening instruments to improve the identification of these disorders among consulters. Recent studies compared the impact of screening upon doctors' propensity to make a diagnosis of depression or anxiety. Using the GHQ Hoeper *et al.* (1984) found that 28% of a screened population screened positive, but whether feedback was provided or not did not impact upon the proportion who were diagnosed by the general practitioner (16% and 16.8%, respectively). The failure of screening to improve the detection of psychiatric disorder by general practitioners has been confirmed by a recent meta-analysis (Gilbody *et al.*, 2001) and the authors conclude that the routine use of a screening questionnaire to improve diagnosis is not supported. One of the possible reasons for this is that only about 50% of screened positive patients have clinically important emotional disorder and it may be that general practitioners intuitively recognise this having taken account of the context of the symptoms. Moreover, the detection of those with depression does not make any difference to outcome at 12 months (Dowrick and Buchan, 1995). However, a recent study (Arroll *et al.*, 2003) has suggested that asking two simple questions may be superior to a questionnaire: 'During the past month have you often been bothered by feeling down, depressed or hopeless?' and 'During the past month have you often been bothered by little interest or pleasure in doing things?'. In this study however the negative predictive value was over 95% showing that those who respond negatively to the questions do not have depression; on the other hand the positive predictive value (the proportion scoring positive on screening who actually had depression) was very low at 18%, demonstrating that much more detailed questioning is required and that over 80% will not have the condition even when screened positive.

LEVEL 3

This refers to morbidity as identified by the general practitioner (conspicuous morbidity). Studies in this context are often criticised for not measuring the 'true' prevalence of morbidity. This argument is specious since studies of this type are a reflection of the practices of general practitioners and of the service needs as defined by them. This is an important principle since the general practitioner is the principal agent of referral. The difference between the prevalence at levels 2 and 3 is referred to as hidden or undetected morbidity and the magnitude of this is a measure of the educational needs of practitioners in terms of psychiatric identification.

Using case note identification in a single practice, Kessel (1960) found that 9% of the sample had psychiatric illness and a further 5% had personality abnormalities independent of illness. Both were more common in women than men and consisted of anxiety states, hypochondriacal and depressive reactions. Only 10% were referred to the specialist services. In attempting to address the unrepresentativeness of single practice studies a number of multi-practice studies were conducted, of which that by Shepherd *et al.* (1966) is the most oft quoted. A random sample of case notes was selected from 12 London practices and the GP identified the reason for consultation in the subsequent year. In addition, each patient was classified into one of the major diagnostic categories. The overall results can be seen in Table 1.2.

Formal psychiatric illness represented about 70% of the reported morbidity, the neuroses predominated and the overall rate in females was double that in men. However there was a nine-fold inter-practice variation in reported morbidity. Although the broad diagnostic categories of illness were identified, no attempt at a more specific classification was made. It can be said that this study was more an investigation into perceived reasons for consultation than a measure of psychiatric

Table 1.2. Patient consulting rates per 1000 at risk for psychiatric morbidity, by sex and diagnostic group.

Diagnostic group	Male	Female	Both sexes
Psychoses	2.7	8.6	5.9
Mental subnormality	1.6	2.9	2.3
Dementia	1.2	1.6	1.4
Neuroses	55.7	116.6	88.5
Personality disorder	7.2	4.0	5.5
Formal psychiatric illness[a]	67.2	131.9	102.1
Psychosomatic conditions	24.5	34.5	29.9
Organic illness with psychiatric overlay	13.1	16.6	15.0
Psychosocial problems	4.6	10.0	7.5
Psychiatric-associated conditions[a]	38.6	57.2	48.6
Total psychiatric morbidity[a]	97.9	175.0	139.4
Number of patients at risk	6783	7914	14 697

[a]These totals cannot be obtained by adding the rates for relevant diagnostic groups because while a patient may be included in more than one diagnostic group, he will be included only once in the total.
(Reproduced with permission, from Shepherd *et al.*, 1966.)

morbidity. The broad findings of Shepherd and his colleagues have been replicated since then.

In 1969 Cooper and colleagues carried out a longitudinal study over 7 years of
the prevalence of psychiatric disorders in a single London practice. The mean
annual prevalence was 60/1000 for men and 172/1000 for women. There was a
peak of disturbance in the middle-aged and considerable variation in the rates
between years. Depression and anxiety were the principal disorders.

Others have identified a psychiatric component in 40% of the consulting population (Skuse and Williams, 1984) and correcting for the fact that only a subsample
was seen, a prevalence of 26% for depression and of 8% for other diagnoses was
estimated. Casey and colleagues (1984, 1990) investigated the diagnostic breakdown of those with conspicuous morbidity, initially in an inner city practice and
subsequently in a rural one. Assessments were made clinically and using structured
interviews. This study was unusual in that it was the first of its kind to assess
personality independent of illness. Using the general practitioner to screen for
psychiatric disorder, a prevalence of 5% was found and 33% of those classified as
having psychological disturbance also had personality disorders. Depressive illness
predominated followed by anxiety states and adjustment reactions. A large-scale
study of the prevalence of psychiatric illness in primary care under the aegis of the
World Health Organisation was carried out among 15 international centres
(Sartorius *et al.*, 1993). Almost 26 000 subjects were screened using a structured
interview schedule and 243 per 1000 of the sample were diagnosed with at least
one of depressive illness, anxiety or alcohol related disorders.

In the USA equivalent studies are difficult to assess because of the differing
health care delivery systems. One such study in a very large practice in California
(Olfson *et al.*, 1997) found that the overall prevalence for any disorder was 19.8%
and that anxiety disorders were the most common at 11.6% followed by affective
disorder (8%). Substance abuse was the diagnosis in 6.3%. Surprisingly nobody
was diagnosed with adjustment disorder. A possible reason for the high prevalence
of anxiety disorders is the failure to use a hierarchical approach to diagnosis,
instead including as a substantive diagnosis those who met criteria for both major
depression and anxiety, even when the latter might be integral to the depressive
disorder as is commonly observed in practice.

DOES THE SEVERITY OF ILLNESS VARY IN DIFFERENT POPULATIONS?

It is recognised that individual general practitioners see fewer psychotic patients
than the psychiatrist. Even when this group with the most serious illnesses are
excluded, those seen and treated in general practice are different from those seen
in the specialist services. This view represents a change from the earlier position

that there was little to distinguish those treated in these settings with respect to severity of disorder. It was the belief that many with psychiatric disorder, especially depression, not identified as such in general practice, nevertheless experienced significant suffering and incapacity, both social and personal. Hence, there was a move to improve detection rates using educational packages and screening instruments. However, recent evidence points to the fallacy of this view and suggests that there is a difference in the severity of depression treated in primary and secondary care settings. For example suicide has been shown to be more common in those with depression treated as in-patients, followed by out-patient care, then primary care and lowest in those diagnosed but not given any treatment by their general practitioners (Simon and Von Korff, 1998). Similarly, deliberate self-harm is more common among those being treated by psychiatrists, pointing to the greater disturbance among this group (see also level 2 above).

SUMMARY

1. The prevalence of psychiatric illness varies in different populations, being highest in community samples and lowest when hospital populations are examined.
2. The broader the concept of illness the higher the prevalence, and screening schedules arrive at higher prevalence rates than diagnostic instruments.
3. Psychiatric disorder predominates in women, both in the general population and in general practice patients.
4. The principal diagnosis in both populations consists of affective disorders and anxiety disorders. A sizeable proportion have personality disorder independent of illness.
5. Psychiatric illness in general practice patients is probably less severe than among those referred to the secondary services.

REFERENCES

Arroll, B., Khin, N. and Kerse, N. (2003). Screening for depression in primary care with two verbally asked questions: cross sectional study. *British Medical Journal*, **327**, 1144–1146.
Bhui, K. and Bhugra, D. (2002). Mental illness in Black and Asian ethnic minorities: pathways to care and outcomes. *Advances in Psychiatric Treatment*, **8**, 26–33.
Casey, P.R. and Tyrer, P.J. (1986). Personality, functioning and symptomatology. *Journal of Psychiatric Research*, **20**, 363–374.
Casey, P.R. and Tyrer, P. (1990). Personality disorder and psychiatric illness in general practice. *British Journal of Psychiatry*, **156**, 261–265.

Casey, P.R., Dillon, J. and Tyrer. P. (1984). The diagnostic status of patients with conspicuous psychiatric morbidity in general practice. *Psychological Medicine*, **14**, 673–682.

Commander, M.J., Dharan, S.P.S., Odell, S.M. *et al.* (1997). Access to mental health care in an inner-city health district. I: Pathways into and within specialist psychiatric services. *British Journal of Psychiatry*, **170**, 312–316.

Cooper, B., Fry, J. and Kalton, G. (1969). A longitudinal study of psychiatric morbidity in a general practice population. *British Journal of Preventive and Social Medicine*, **23**, 210–217.

Dowrick, C. and Buchan, I. (1995). Twelve month outcome of depression in general practice: does detection or disclosure make a difference? *British Medical Journal*, **311**, 1274–1276.

Gilbody, S.M., House, A.O. and Sheldon, T.A. (2001). Routinely administered questionnaires for depression and anxiety: systematic review. *British Medical Journal*, **322**, 404–406.

Goldberg, D. and Blackwell, B. (1970). Psychiatric illness in general practice. A detailed study using a new method of case identification. *British Medical Journal*, **2**, 439–443.

Goldberg, D. and Huxley, P. (1980). *Mental Illness in the Community. The Pathway to Psychiatric Care*. Tavistock Publications, London.

Goldberg, D., Kay, C. and Thompson, L. (1976). Psychiatric morbidity in general practice and the community. *Psychological Medicine*, **6**, 565–569.

Hoeper, E.W., Nycz, G.R., Kessler, J.D. and Pierce, W.E. (1984). The usefulness of screening for mental illness. *Lancet*, **1**, 33–35.

Jenkins, R., Lewis, G., Bebbington, P. *et al.* (1997). The National Psychiatric Morbidity Surveys of Great Britain – initial findings from the Household Survey. *Psychological Medicine*, **27**, 775–789.

Kessel, N. (1960). Psychiatric morbidity in a London general practice. *British Journal of Social and Preventive Medicine*, **14**, 16–22.

Kessler, R.C., McGonagle, K.A., Zhao, S. *et al.* (1994). Lifetime and twelve-month prevalence of DSM-III-R psychiatric disorders in the United States. *Archives of General Psychiatry*, **51**, 8–19.

Olfson, M., Fireman, B., Weissman, M. *et al.* (1997). Mental Disorders and disability among patients in a primary care group practice. *American Journal of Psychiatry*, **154**, 1734–1740.

Robins, L.N., Helzer, J.E., Weissman, M.M. *et al.* (1984). Lifetime prevalence of specific psychiatric disorders in three sites. *Archives of General Psychiatry*, **41**, 949–958.

Sartorius, N., Ustun, T.B., Costa e Silva, J.A. *et al.* (1993). An international study of psychological problems in primary care. Preliminary report from the World Health Organisation Collaborative Project on 'Psychological Problems in General Health Care'. *Archives of General Psychiatry*, **50**, 819–824.

Shepherd, M., Cooper, B., Brown, A.C. and Kalton, G.W. (1966). *Psychiatric Illness in General Practice*. Oxford University Press, Oxford.

Simon, G.E. and von Korff, M. (1998). Suicide mortality among patients treated for depression in an insured population. *American Journal of Epidemiology*, **147**, 155–160.

Skuse, D. and Williams, P. (1984). Screening for psychiatric disorder in general practice. *Psychological Medicine*, **14**, 365–377.

FURTHER READING

Bhui, K. and Bhugra, D. (2002). Mental illness in Black and Asian ethnic minorities: pathways to care and outcomes. *Advances in Psychiatric Treatment*, **8**, 26–33.

2

Consultation, Detection and Referral

The process determining which patients decide to consult their doctors, which are labelled as ill and which are referred for specialist assessment is not just a haphazard chain of events but is governed by a set of 'rules' which have been the subject of much investigation by those interested in human behaviour. These serve to eliminate some and to include other patients at each stage of the process. The first, second and third stages or levels have been described in Chapter 1 and refer to the totality of psychiatric dysfunction in the community, among all general practice consulters and among those identified as psychiatrically unwell by their family practitioners. The fourth and fifth stages describe the disorders seen among psychiatric out-patients and among in-patients. Between each stage there is a shortfall of patients so that the total number identified in the community is not the same as the total number seen in hospital settings. The variables, which affect this process, are known as filters and are described in detail below.

THE FIRST FILTER – THE DECISION TO CONSULT

The relationship between symptom frequency and the likelihood of consultation is not a direct one to one association but has many intervening variables which underpin the decision to seek medical advice. Symptom surveys have shown that more than two-thirds of people surveyed believed themselves to have a health problem, yet only a small proportion consulted with this. The issue is complex since some seek advice for trivial symptoms while others belong in what is called the 'iceberg' category that despite serious symptoms do not seek medical help. The behaviour shown by the symptomatic population is termed 'illness behaviour' (Mechanic, 1962) and has been investigated in detail since first described.

It is undoubtedly true that symptom severity is one factor which prompts consultation although many others are involved also. The influence of symptom severity upon help-seeking behaviour is most apparent where depression or anxiety are the presenting symptoms and epidemiological studies of depression have shown that up to 60% of those with depressive illness have sought help, even in communities which are relatively deprived. This finding has been partly confirmed by the Defeat Depression Campaign of the Royal Colleges of Psychiatrists and General Practitioners in the finding that 60% of those surveyed said they would consult their general practitioner first before any other individual. It is indeed surprising and heartening that the proportion is so high. The presence of stress as measured by life events in the 3 months prior to consultation also increases the propensity to seek help and for those with physical symptoms the likelihood of consultation is increased by the presence of concomitant psychological symptoms.

In addition to symptom severity, the degree of subjective distress and the extent of dysfunction also impinge upon this process. There is often an incongruity between the severity of symptoms and the degree of social disruption and where the latter is high, help is more likely to be sought. It is hardly surprising that the sufferer whose usual activities are disrupted or whose subjective level of distress is high will seek help promptly. A number of other features relating to symptoms also contribute to the process: thus symptoms of insidious onset are more often tolerated without treatment than those of acute onset, and those that are generally believed to be common are unlikely to prompt a visit to the doctor. Interestingly attitudes to illness and to consultations follow clear trends within families across generations and have been shown to account for a significant proportion of the variance in predicting consultation. The importance of sociodemographic factors may not at first seem relevant but have indeed emerged as exerting an influence on this complex process. A consistent finding is that women have more contact with their family doctors than men and that consultation increases with increasing age. Whether this is due to an excess of symptoms and illness in women or whether they are more willing to acknowledge them is as yet unresolved. Also unresolved is the influence social class may have on consultation rates. It is not surprising that the lonely seek help more frequently than those who are in close, confiding relationships – the consultation will not only provide reassurance but is also a source of human contact. This has been verified by the repeated finding that the separated, single and widowed as well as those in relationships of conflict consult more frequently than their married counterparts.

THE SECOND FILTER – THE DETECTION OF PSYCHIATRIC ILLNESS

It is apparent from Chapter 1 that a proportion of patients with psychological disturbance are not identified when consultation with the family practitioner takes place. This has been referred to as hidden psychiatric morbidity. Some studies have in fact found a nine-fold variation in the perceived prevalence of psychiatric disorder among general practitioners while comparative figures using screening schedules demonstrate much less variability between practices. A number of variables contribute to the recognition and non-recognition of psychiatric disorders in primary care.

Patient variables

It is well known that many patients describe only physical symptoms even though their primary pathology may be psychological and this may lead to a mistaken diagnosis of a physical disorder. First, up to 25% of those with psychiatric disorder present to their general practitioner with physical symptoms of that disorder (Weich *et al.*, 1995); for example in depression, symptoms such as palpitations, aches and pains, etc., suggest a physical cause and make diagnosis difficult. Secondly, patients may feel their doctor only wants to hear of physical symptoms and thus avoid mention of those concerned with the emotions. Thirdly, some patients have a sense of guilt or stigma about feelings such as gloom and sadness when 'there is nothing to be depressed about' or when such complaints are viewed as evidence of weakness. Fourthly, the patient may consult with some other more major symptom such as haemoptysis and neglect to mention psychological symptoms, or the doctor may diagnose some major organic pathology and feel the psychological sequelae are understandable in the circumstances, even where the two may be unrelated. Finally, many patients, especially those who are not psychologically minded, those of low intelligence or those from other cultures, may not have a vocabulary for or a concept of emotional hurt.

In addition to the manner in which symptoms are presented, a number of demographic variables facilitate the identification of those with psychiatric disorder and vice versa. Thus, women, those in middle age, the unemployed, those of low socio-economic status and those who are separated, widowed or divorced are more likely to be correctly identified than their male counterparts. This is probably related to stereotyped views of those who constitute the psychiatric population in this setting which either heighten or diminish the doctor's vigilance for detecting these disorders.

GP variables

It is important to examine two aspects of the process of general practitioner diagnosis (Marks *et al.*, 1979). The first of these is referred to as 'bias' and is defined as the doctor's tendency to make, or to avoid making a psychiatric diagnosis, while the second is 'accuracy' and refers to the correctness of diagnosis either in terms of severity or of labelling. Since different factors influence each, they will be considered separately.

Bias towards making psychiatric diagnosis is determined by emphasis and interest in this area. It is reflected in interview style by questions with a psychiatric focus, by emphatic and psychotherapeutic comments and by an awareness of psychological factors in illness. The doctor will make enquiries about home and work and will identify the verbal and non-verbal cues that emotional problems exist. The style of questioning will commence with open questions and later proceed to closed and more focused enquiry. Finally, older doctors have a higher bias than their younger colleagues.

A doctor with a high bias towards diagnosing psychiatric illness may incorrectly label patients as being psychologically disturbed where in fact no such disturbance exists. The appropriateness of the psychological tag is described as *accuracy* and is governed both by the personality attributes of the doctor and by the style of interview he conducts. Thus self-assured doctors, those who are extrovert and who are aware of their own feelings, are more accurate than their counterparts. High academic ability and accurate concepts of illness also facilitate accuracy. In relation to interview style, dealing with over-talkativeness, clarifying symptoms, making eye contact and not reading notes during interview, all contribute to the accuracy with which psychiatric disturbance is diagnosed. In addition, asking questions that follow from what a patient has just said rather than from theory increases the number of verbal distress cues thus improving the likelihood of detection.

It is apparent that bias and accuracy are distinct from each other and determined by different variables: the latter by interview techniques, by the personality of the doctor and by his knowledge of the subject. On the other hand, bias is a measure of the doctor's interest in his subject and during the interview is reflected in his style of questioning. The implications for the training of GPs are obvious. A recent study of the impact of training GPs in the assessment and management of depression surprisingly did not have any impact on outcome although those practices that were less involved in teaching and research did demonstrate a benefit from such training (Gask *et al.*, 2004). This study confirms that encouragement to be aware of psychological aspects of their work, a sound knowledge of psychiatry and treatments as well as training in interviewing techniques are imperative for general practitioners. The latter is dealt with in detail in Chapter 3.

THE THIRD FILTER – REFERRAL TO THE PSYCHIATRIC SERVICES

Since only between 5 and 10% of those identified as psychiatric patients by their general practitioners are referred to the specialist services, it is apparent that the majority are managed by family practitioners themselves. Direct access to the psychiatric services is rare in Britain and Ireland and a number of obstacles have to be overcome before the patient reaches the psychiatrist. These form the components of the third filter as shown in Table 1.1.

The reasons for referral are various. A common feature of those referred is failure to respond to treatment from the primary care team. Implied in this is transfer of clinical responsibility to the specialist services. A further and obvious reason is the request for a specialist opinion on diagnosis and management, but this is not as frequently the reason for referral as perhaps desired by specialists. Up to a quarter are referred because they seek this themselves or because others request it on their behalf, particularly when behavioural disturbance becomes problematic.

Patient variables

There is some evidence that men are more likely to be referred than women, probably a reflection of the perceived impact of psychiatric illness upon the traditional breadwinner. The finding that younger patients pass this filter more easily than older patients has similar connotations since illness in the young is believed to be more socially restricting than in those who are retired. Those belonging to high socio-economic groups are over-represented among psychiatric clinic attendees partly because they seek referral themselves but also because many of the psychiatric problems in primary care are brief, short-lived reactions which do not necessitate specialist help and which are more common in those of low socio-economic status. The role of marital status is uncertain in this filter.

Illness variables

Those who are referred are generally more seriously ill than those who are not. In particular GPs tend to refer all those who are psychotic and those who are suicidal. Those who have behavioural disturbances pass this third filter easily as a result of the social mayhem they often generate. It is surprising that a higher proportion of those with depressive illness are not referred, especially those who have illnesses of moderate to severe intensity. This shortfall may be due to the nature of the illness itself which causes withdrawal rather than social disturbance. In view of the reasons for referral described above it is not surprising that established conditions rather than acute illnesses are more frequently referred.

Practitioner variables

In general older doctors have higher referral rates than their younger colleagues as do those in urban areas, the latter presumably due to ease of access for the patients to the services. A similar high referral rate has been noted among single-handed practitioners.

Service variables

There is evidence that the delay until first appointment does not generally deter referral. However, the type of facility does have an impact on the decision to refer and those areas which have community based facilities and are located in general hospitals are more acceptable to the practitioners. The excess in these settings however has been shown to be due to an increase in the proportion who are seriously ill rather than, as feared, a tendency to refer the 'worried well'. Furthermore, the personnel to whom patients are referred, excluding those with psychotic illnesses who are always referred to a psychiatrist, depends on the ready access that the general practitioner has to mental health professionals, e.g. those who have visiting social workers to their practices tend to refer their patients to them irrespective of the perceived problem or diagnosis (Verhaak, 1993).

THE FOURTH FILTER

This filter refers to the factors governing the decision to move from out-patient to in-patient care – a process that inevitably involves the psychiatrist but seldom the general practitioner. Surprisingly, not all patients referred to specialist services receive treatment. Among those offered help are patients with psychotic illnesses. However, contrary to expectation only selected suicidal patients are treated and selection is made especially where suicide risk is believed to be related to personality disorder or chronic alcohol abuse. Among neurotic patients referred to out-patient clinics there is no diagnostic difference between those offered further treatment and those returned to their general practitioner's care. A history of parasuicide, of alcohol abuse or personality disorder in addition to the main condition increases the likelihood of rapid discharge as does being elderly with a neurotic disorder. Thus, factors extraneous to the main clinical state may create a feeling and practice of therapeutic nihilism. The fourth filter will not be considered further since its operation is not related to general practice but to factors arising within the specialty of psychiatry itself.

THE FILTERS AND ETHNIC MINORITIES

Black patients have more complex pathways to specialist services than do white people (Bhui and Bhugra, 2002) and this route is not due to lack of help-seeking behaviour since almost half the black patients presenting for initial assessment with the psychiatric services have contacted a helping agency in the previous week compared with 2% of the general population. Black and Asian people are less likely to be registered and have lower attendance rates with their general practitioner, seeking help initially from traditional healers. Even when they attend they often present with physical symptoms rather than with psychological symptoms and are less likely to be diagnosed with a psychiatric disorder but having been diagnosed are more likely to be referred for specialist treatment if they are black but less so if

Asian (Commander *et al.*, 1997). Studies of the process of consultation show that black women are more distressed than white women, are less likely to know what they want from their doctor and instead make multiple requests. They are also less likely to be given a follow-up appointment, to be less satisfied with the consultation and are more likely to attend the emergency department for subsequent visits.

A further difficulty is that many of the 'symptoms' are culturally sanctioned and are not evidence of disorder especially those of religious or persecutory content. This is particularly true among those of African or West Indian origin. The police are also more likely to be involved in the admissions of both black and Asian patients and this is more likely to be done under the Mental Health Act than with white patients. A possible explanation may be that as general practitioners are less involved with these patients they present in crises, often with the emergency departments as the initial point of contact (Bhui *et al.*, 2003). However, since being single and lacking a close friend or relative are even more important determinants of compulsory admission it may be that the pattern among ethnic minorities is primarily a reflection of social isolation.

There is a clinical impression that those from ethnic minorities lose contact with the specialist services as time passes. However, studies vary in their findings with some services maintaining similar contact with white as with ethnic minority patients while others seem to have less follow-up. It is likely that service quality rather than ethnicity may be the factor that determines continuity of care.'

SUMMARY

1. Women and those who are isolated and unsupported are more likely to consult. Several variables relating to the illness govern this decision also. Up to two-thirds of those with psychological problems consult their doctors. These variables constitute the first filter.
2. The second filter identifies those factors which assist the GP in identifying the psychological component to the consultation. A number of social and demographic variables increase the GP's vigilance for detection as do attributes of the doctor himself.
3. Fewer than 10% of those with psychological disturbance are referred to the psychiatric services. Men and young patients pass this third filter more easily than women or the elderly as do those who are socially incapacitated, suicidal, psychotic or have chronic illness.
4. The fourth filter determines who becomes an in-patient and who remains an out-patient. This has little to do with the general practitioner but is related to the psychiatric services themselves.
5. Ethnic minorities have different mobility through the filters.

REFERENCES

Bhui, K. and Bhugra, D. (2002). Mental illness in Black and Asian ethnic minorities: pathways to care and outcomes. *Advances in Psychiatric Treatment*, **8**, 26–33.

Bhui, K., Stansfeld, S., Hull, S. *et al.* (2003). Ethnic variations in pathways to and use of specialist mental health services in the UK. Systematic review. *British Journal of Psychiatry*, **182**, 105–116.

Commander, M.J., Dharan, S.P.S., Odell, S.M. *et al.* (1997). Access to mental health care in an inner-city health district. I: Pathways into and within specialist psychiatric services. *British Journal of Psychiatry*, **170**, 312–316.

Gask, L., Dowrick, C., Dixon, C. *et al.* (2004). A pragmatic cluster randomized controlled trial of educational intervention for GPs in the assessment and management of depression. *Psychological Medicine*, **34**, 63–72.

Marks, J., Goldberg, D. and Hillier, V.F. (1979). Determinants of the ability of general practitioners to detect psychiatric illness. *Psychological Medicine*, **9**, 337–353.

Mechanic, D. (1962). The concept of illness behavior. *Journal of Chronic Diseases*, **15**, 189–194.

Verhaak, PF. (1993). Analysis of referrals of mental health problems by general practitioners. *British Journal of General Practice*, **43**, 203–208.

Weich, S., Lewis, G., Donmall, R. and Mann, A. (1995). Somatic presentation of psychiatric morbidity in general practice. *British Journal of General Practice*, **45**, 143–147.

FURTHER READING

Goldberg, D. and Huxley, P. (1980). *Mental Illness in the Community. The Pathway to Psychiatric Care.* Tavistock Publications, London.

3

History Taking

THE INTERVIEW

The interview should be conducted in a relaxed manner, with the practitioner giving the impression of having time to listen. This will elicit more information than if the doctor appears to be in haste (Goldberg *et al.*, 1993). The practitioner will have much information already from his previous knowledge of the patient and will therefore be able to concentrate, in most cases, on current symptomatology and precipitating stresses.

It is best to sit on a chair the same height as the patient's but this should not be behind a desk since this creates an atmosphere of distance. Having the desk by his side with the patient sitting opposite is probably the best position for an interview. The question of taking notes is problematic where a lot of information is being given. Ideally they should not be taken whilst the patient is with the doctor. However, this may be impractical, and unobtrusive writing may be acceptable as the interview progresses. The doctor should never begin with his pen in hand. The 'open' sitting position should be used – this refers to sitting with the hands resting on the lap and feet on the ground or legs crossed. On no account should the doctor sit with his arms folded or in a hunched position – this creates an impression of tension or defensiveness. Interruptions from the telephone make a psychiatric interview difficult and if possible telephone calls should not be taken.

It is best to begin the interview with open questions followed later by closed questions in order to clarify the presenting complaints. The doctor can begin the interview with an open question such as, 'How can I help you Mrs X?' or, 'Tell me about your problem'. Later in the interview clarification of symptoms will require closed questions, e.g. 'How do you sleep?'. This should only occur when the doctor has achieved an overall impression of the patient's difficulties. Some erroneously believe that there is no need to hone in on specific areas of dysfunction and that an unstructured approach is best. This is mistaken and there is much evidence to suggest that clarification of symptoms is an important factor in determining accuracy of diagnosis (see Chapter 2). The use of closed questions is particularly beneficial when used by those who are high identifiers of emotional disturbance and a hindrance in those who have a low bias since their inappropriate use stifles the freedom of the interview (Goldberg *et al.*, 1993). In addition to open and closed questions, other types include single, double, triple, etc. A single question, 'How is your appetite?', is preferable to 'How is your appetite and your concentration?' since double or larger questions confuse the patient who may choose to reply to either part. The habit of asking a question and also replying is common, e.g. 'I suppose you don't drink too heavily?', as is the tendency to frame vague questions, e.g. 'Do you ever have odd experiences?', when trying to elicit psychotic symptoms; both should be avoided.

In order to encourage the patient during the interview, techniques such as nodding, saying 'I see' and 'I understand' are useful. Expressions of sympathy, both verbal and non-verbal are particularly helpful when emotional information as distinct from factual information is being given. Repeating what the patient has said may also act as a prompt. The interviewer who is verbally active during the session (known as floorholding) and who interposes questions while the patient is speaking freely does not elicit any extra information. It is however important for the interview to be controlled if it is not to ramble and be nothing more than a social exchange. The doctor can gently guide the patient through the interview and where necessary return the patient to the area under discussion. Eye contact should be established early on in the interview.

Some patients are vague and circumstantial and the skill of the doctor in such interviews is of paramount importance if it is to be of clinical use. Controlling the responses is crucial and statements such as 'We will return to that later' or 'Perhaps we could concentrate on your panics for the moment' are useful when the patient is bringing up irrelevant material or not answering the questions which have been asked.

Further difficulties arise when a patient refuses to answer questions. A common sentiment is 'What does that have to do with how I feel now?'. This reluctance may represent a painful area for the patient and if so can be returned to at a later interview. In general, however, the reluctance of patients to answer questions is related to a lack of understanding about what the doctor is trying to achieve. Reassurance must be given that the interest is not prurient but that the aim is to understand the present difficulties. Failure to get the patient's co-operation may necessitate terminating the interview and offering the patient another appointment when he has considered the matter more fully.

SENSITIVE AREAS

The GP must be finely attuned to the sensibilities of the patient who may resent or be embarrassed by questions of a personal nature. In particular, questions about sexual abuse, sexual orientation and activity, previous abortions or criminal involvement and those dealing with spiritual matters should be handled with delicacy. Instead of asking directly about the frequency of sexual intercourse, the doctor can euphemistically enquire about 'the intimate side' of the relationship. Similarly, instead of asking directly about terminations of pregnancy, questions can be asked about previous pregnancies. Information can often be obtained about sexual orientation indirectly from the history of previous romantic relationships. In general it is difficult not to enquire directly about criminal activity, and spiritual matters will be clarified by simple enquiry about church attendance, prayer and involvement in religious organisations. This latter is not as irrelevant as many believe since it gives the therapist an insight into the patient's value system and into a potential area of support from which the patient may derive benefit. Questions relating to sexual abuse in childhood should rarely be broached at the first interview.

Some doctors are reluctant to enquire about suicide but failing to do so is potentially negligent. The subject can be broached by initially enquiring of the patient if he sees hope for the future followed by, 'Do you ever wish you went to sleep and didn't wake up?' and, 'Do you ever get so depressed you wish you were dead?'. If the patient answers positively the doctor may then ask, 'Do you ever think of harming yourself?' followed by questions about any such plans. In general it would be inappropriate to ask the patient directly if suicide has been thought of and the more circuitous approach described above is preferable.

THE PSYCHIATRIC HISTORY

There is a standard format for psychiatric history taking to which every psychiatrist adheres. However, the general practitioner because of his unique position in having a personal and long-term knowledge of the patient will not necessarily follow this regime unless the patient is new to him. Moreover, pressure of time will make it impossible to obtain all the information described below but in most instances this will not be necessary anyway since the GP will have prior knowledge of the patient and his background. The following areas are considered when taking a psychiatric history.

History of presenting complaint

This is a description in the patient's own words of the symptoms and problems which bring him to the doctor.

Family history

The family history includes information about siblings and parents especially information on any psychiatric history, including alcohol abuse and details of any psychiatric disturbance in more distant relatives, e.g. grandparents, etc.

Personal history

The personal history incorporates information on the patient's childhood and upbringing. Details of neurotic traits in childhood such as bed-wetting and night-mares are sometimes a clue to the development of future psychiatric difficulties. This part of the history should also include details of the patient's schooling and any difficulties with peers, teachers or education, generally followed by an employment history and finally a history of psychosexual relationships. For the married person this will include details of the relationship with their spouse at present and, for those who are not married or cohabiting, information on any current relationships. Those who claim not to have had any boyfriends/girlfriends should be questioned about reasons for this, especially shyness of the opposite sex, attraction to the same sex, lack of interest or over-protectiveness by their family. The GP's knowledge of the patient's family and the degree of support which they give to the patient should be included here. This is vital information frequently not available to the psychia-trist who has little contact with the patient's immediate family and social circum-stances. This is of more than theoretical interest since the adequacy of support is one of the factors determining the outcome of many psychiatric illnesses.

Past medical and psychiatric history

This includes disorders treated by the general practitioner, by counsellors or by psychiatrists. The diagnosis made during previous episodes of disorder should be noted along with response to treatment, if this information is available. This is particularly true where certain approaches to therapy, e.g. behaviour therapy, have failed or where certain pharmacological treatments have been successful or failed, e.g. ECT or certain groups of antidepressants.

Drug history

The drug history should include information on current prescribed as well as non-prescribed medication and in particular enquiries should be made about any tendency to use tranquillisers prescribed by others. This may sometimes be associ-ated with dependence on these drugs which the patient will not admit to unless specifically questioned. Where referral to a psychiatrist is being considered the duration of medication and its dosage should be noted as this will have a special bearing on the decision to prescribe or to change antidepressants.

Personality

The personality of the patient must be assessed and the GP is in a special position to do this in view of his knowledge of the patient over a long period of time and of the patient's response to previous stressors. The importance of distinguishing between long-term personality traits and current symptoms is emphasised in Chapter 11. Information about the person's alcohol consumption (if this is not the presenting complaint) should be provided in this part of the overall history.

This information is then followed by an assessment of the *mental state* which is the psychological equivalent of the physical examination and is considered under the following headings:

- Speech
- Behaviour
- Mood
- Perception
- Thought content
- Concentration
- Orientation
- Insight/motivation.

An attempt must next be made to *formulate a diagnosis* by first listing the most likely diagnosis then a differential diagnosis followed by a subsidary diagnosis if one is present. This last is a disturbance which is present but not the principal one, e.g. personality disorder. Thus the GP might describe the most likely main diagnosis as an anxiety state, depressive illness as the main differential diagnosis and a subsidiary diagnosis of personality disorder, passive dependent type. Then any social/environmental problems or precipitating stressors are described on axis 2, and on axis 3 the impact of the disorder on functioning is summarised. If DSM IV is being used then a somewhat different approach applies since the axes differ from those in ICD 10 (see page 29).

LETTER WRITING

The necessity to communicate is fundamental to the proper practice of medicine – hence the use of jargon specific to doctors. An area of communication between doctors which has received little attention is that of letter writing. This is often the only mode of communication used and consideration of ways to maximise its usefulness is therefore important. The habit of the ultra brief referral 'Depressed?' is to be deplored as is the tendency of the specialist to reply in a five-page letter. Somewhere between these two extremes lies a mutually acceptable compromise.

A number of key items required by psychiatrists in *referral letters* have been identified (Pullen and Yellowlees, 1985). These include family history, reasons for referral, past and current psychiatric history and medication prescribed so far. The knowledge that the family doctor has of the patient's personality and usual methods of coping are of great import, especially when considering the likely outcome, and should be included . There is no necessity to type the letter of referral but legibility is paramount.

In return general practitioners have expectations of the type of letter they should *receive from psychiatrists* (Yellowlees and Pullen, 1984). They should not be longer than one page and should include only the essential points about the patient's disorder and causation. Non-consultants tend to regurgitate the history exactly as taken at the clinic whereas consultants are more succinct. Some doctors have a tendency to utilise sub-headings in their letters but this is too rigid and is not favoured by most. A criticism of psychiatrists' letters is that they fail to mention prognosis, even after several consultations have taken place, and anticipated duration of treatment is seldom indicated. A further omission is that general practitioners are seldom informed of what details have been given to relatives about the disorder. This is pertinent in relation to psychotic and organic states. Some doctors may wish to receive an interim letter after initial in-patient assessments have been made but this may be an unrealistic request in all but the most well-staffed units. A large proportion of psychiatric case notes have been shown to contain pejorative remarks which could be expressed in a more acceptable manner and there is a danger that these would be conveyed also in letters, particularly those which are lengthy and written by junior doctors. This could be minimised by an ongoing hospital audit of letter writing (Shah and Pullen, 1995).

Letter writing does not stop with the initial letter following the patient's first appointment, but should continue while the patient is under the psychiatrist's care. Unfortunately, many GPs fail to receive any correspondence thereafter or alternatively receive a two-line letter after each visit. Neither is ideal and while it is important to update the family doctor on progress, there is no necessity to correspond following each and every visit, especially for those with protracted illnesses unless there is a change in the patient's condition or alterations are being made to treatment. A further problem arises with those who default from treatment and while most psychiatrists convey this information to the general practitioner when it involves new referrals, there is evidence that family doctors are not informed when those coming for follow-up fail to attend (Killaspy *et al.*, 1999). This is particularly relevant since this group is likely to be the most seriously ill.

In the UK, from April 2004, under Department of Health proposals (Department of Health, 2002), patients will be routinely sent copies of all correspondence between clinicians working in the NHS. Pilot schemes suggest that patients overwhelmingly value this but that doctors frequently omit information which they consider may distress the patient. (Murray *et al.*, 2002). It is likely that this innovation will impact considerably on the content of letters between doctors, and proper training and reassurance will be required to ensure its successful implementation. There are also concerns about security, especially for those patients who frequently change address.

The increasing use of computers might have been expected to produce a significant rise in this method of corresponding between psychiatrists and general practitioners. This does not seem to have occurred, largely due to fears about confidentiality. If this method is to find widespread use, adequate encryption will be essential.

SUMMARY

1. The interview should be conducted in a relaxed and informal atmosphere.
2. Frequent interruptions by the doctor and the use of closed questions are best avoided. Clarification of symptoms and problems may make closed questions necessary at the end of the interview.
3. The skilled interviewer takes control of the interview without appearing intrusive. Failure to achieve control will cause the patient to wander from the essential problems and a diagnosis may not be formulated.
4. The family doctor is in a position to provide information about the patient's past history and premorbid personality. In addition, details of the reason for referral, current medication and symptoms should be included in the letter of referral.
5. Psychiatrists frequently send excessively long letters to general practitioners but these should be no longer than one page and should include details of causation, treatment and its duration and prognosis. Information given to relatives should be mentioned also.
6. In the near future patients will receive copies of all correspondence between their doctors and adequate training must be provided to ensure its success.

REFERENCES

Department of Health. (2002). *The NHS Plan.* Stationery Office, London.

Goldberg, D.P., Jenkins, L., Millar, T. and Faragher, E.B. (1993). The ability of trainee general practitioners to identify psychological distress among their patients. *Psychological Medicine,* **23**, 185–193.

Killaspy, H., Banerjee, S., King, M. and Lloyd, M. (1999). Non-attendance at psychiatric out-patient clinics: communication and implications for primary care. *British Journal of General Practice.* **49**, 880–883.

Murray, G.K., Nandhra, H., Hymas, N. and Hunt, N. (2002). Doctors omit information from clinic letters when they know patients will be sent copies. *Student British Medical Journal* (Rapid responses), 13 November.

Pullen, I.M. and Yellowlees, A.J. (1985). Is communication improving between general practitioners and psychiatrists? *British Medical Journal,* **290**, 31–33.

Shah, P.J. and Pullen, I. (1995). The impact of a hospital audit on psychiatrists' letters to general practitioners. *Psychiatric Bulletin,* **19**, 544–547.

Yellowlees, A.J. and Pullen, I.M. (1984). Communication between psychiatrists and general practitioners. What sort of letters should psychiatrists write? *Health Bulletin*, **42**, 285–289.

FURTHER READING

Burnard, P. (1989). *Counselling Skills for Health Professionals.* Chapman and Hall, London.
Goldberg, D. (1997). *Maudsley Handbook of Practical Psychiatry.* Oxford Medical Publications, Oxford.

4

Classification of Psychiatric Disorders

In the United States psychiatric disorders are classified according to the system outlined in the Diagnostic and Statistical Manual, 4th edition (DSM IV), while the European approach is embodied in the International Classification of Diseases, l0th edition (ICD 10). There are some differences between these, centring largely on the specific categories which have been included. The principles underlying both are similar in that they are multi-axial (see page 29) and use operational definitions (see pages 30–31). In addition, ICD 10 has been extended for use in research by incorporating more rigid definitions that those of the clinical version.

Since primary care has special requirements and most psychological problems are seen in that setting, there is also a version of ICD10 for use there (International Classification of Diseases 10th edition Primary Care) (ICD 10PC). ICD 10PC consists of a brief description of the disorder and the diagnostic features and differential diagnoses. Definitions for 25 conditions are provided and a shorter version of six disorders for use by other primary care workers is also incorporated. Management guidelines incorporate information for the patient as well as details of medical, social and psychological interventions. Finally, assistance on when to refer for specialist treatment is provided. DSM IV also has a primary care version (DSM IVPC) that is similar to ICD 10PC, focusing on the most common disorders seen in primary care (anxiety, depression, substance abuse, etc.).

However, both of these classifications although developed for use in primary care do not assist the general practitioner in classifying the more nebulous social, behavioural and sub-syndromal problems that dominate their mental health consultations. To overcome this deficit the World Organisation of Family Doctors has developed its own classification – The International Classification of Primary Care (ICPC). It incorporates the reason for the consultation and the symptoms dominating the consultation. Thus it is possible to provide a symptom as well as a syndrome classification. Importantly, these various classifications are not in competition and there is a great deal of overlap between them.

Several studies have now examined the utility of these purpose-designed classifications, especially ICD 10PC, in diagnosing disorders in general practice, on the accuracy of diagnosis and on outcome (Ustun *et al.*, 1995). Unfortunately these studies suggest that although their use does significantly increase the numbers diagnosed with depression and with unexplained physical symptoms, they make little difference to diagnostic accuracy or to outcome (Croudace *et al.*, 2003).

WHY DIAGNOSE?

Psychiatric diagnosis, referred to cynically as labelling, has been the butt of criticism from disciplines as diverse as philosophy and statistics, sociology and psychiatry itself. The arguments against psychiatric diagnosis are typically varied, but the central theme is the dehumanising nature of labelling, the inadequacy of using single labels to describe human problems and the poor reliability of the specific diagnoses. The original diagnosis often changes from admission to admission and different psychiatrists may make different diagnoses on the same patient. The overall agreement for diagnosis between psychiatrists is poor and lies between 30% and 60%, being lowest for personality disorder and highest for the functional psychoses. Diagnosis does not predict treatment or outcome and the label gives a spurious notion of understanding. Many feel that using a label only serves to mystify rather than assist and hence confers power on doctors which they can abuse. It is argued that psychiatric illness does not exist and is a convenient epithet for the eccentric, the deviant or for those who society tries to scapegoat.

It is not the purpose of this chapter to enter in detail into this controversy which has been eloquently stated by Kendell (1975), but it is important to understand the need for diagnosis and classification. As with many controversies, there is an element of truth in some of the anti-psychiatry arguments. It is undoubtedly true that psychiatric labels have been given to those who were not ill but protesting and that these people have all too often been subjected to humiliation and degradation. However, to suggest, as many critics of psychiatry do, that schizophrenia or manic depression do not exist, but are chimeras in the minds of psychiatrists to perpetuate their own interests, is to ignore the distress and suffering that people so afflicted experience. It is also to ignore biological findings regarding the aetiology of these disorders.

The statistical arguments pointing to the low reliability of psychiatric diagnoses and the evidence that diagnosis does not have predictive value are also partly true. However, the call to abandon diagnosis because it is sloppy accedes to scientific nihilism. The plea should be for a more reliable diagnostic system and for the integration of diagnosis with treatment and prognosis. One approach to improving the reliability of psychiatric diagnosis is to define the criteria for making the diagnosis. Thus defined the diagnostic term can be applied more accurately. This is referred to as an operational definition and this technique underpins DSM IV and ICD 10.

Providing an operational definition, however, does not prove the existence of the condition defined. The next stage, proving its validity or existence, is to examine populations of patients so defined in terms of sydromes, course, response to specific treatments and common aetiological factors. It is this invidious task, i.e. identifying specific diseases, which makes operational definitions fundamental to further progress.

In psychiatry no less than in general medicine, it is necessary to label and classify patients so that features common to them can be examined. If this were not possible then not only would we be unable to distinguish illness from health but treatment would also be impossible since there would be no commonality. Each person would have a specific treatment tailored to him without reference to similar patients. Research, and learning would be precluded.

A further element of classification is its facility to communicate; thus, describing a person as tall or small implies a system of classification which is distinct from that describing them as male or female. In psychiatry, as in all branches of medicine, the capacity succinctly to describe a patient and to use terminology which conveys meaning is of fundamental importance. For this it is mandatory to have a basic understanding of how psychiatric disorders are grouped and to be aware of the difficulties inherent in this process as well as recent changes in the approach to the classification and description of the common psychiatric conditions. These issues will be discussed in the context of the DSM and the ICD systems.

DEVELOPMENTS AND CHANGES

Multi-axial classification

The argument that single labels are inappropriate to describe a patient's difficulties will be recalled. As outlined above, the psychiatric profession responded by devising a dimensional or multi-axial system of classification. This means that several aspects of the patient can be described. In ICD 10 the axes are poorly developed and there are three: 1, mental state and personality disorder; 2, psychosocial/environmental problems; 3, impact on functioning. DSM IV however has different and more comprehensive axes: axis 1 refers to mental state diagnosis; axis 2 to personality disorder; axis 3 describes physical illnesses contributing to the emotional problems; axis 4 refers to the level of social functioning at a designated point, e.g. at admission or discharge, and axis 5 refers to stressors in the previous 6 months. In this way a clear and succinct picture of the patient, his background and problems can be presented and communicated to those charged with his management.

The neuroses

The term neurosis was coined in 1772 in Edinburgh by Cullen, a physician. Freud used the term psychoneurosis to describe specific disorders (anxiety, phobic, hysterical and obsessional neurosis) as well as to indicate unconscious conflicts which he believed were aetiologically important. This dual usage has continued.

Some clinicians use 'neurosis' to describe those disorders which are associated with distressing symptoms but where reality testing is intact, i.e. it is used as a descriptive term. Others however use it aetiologically. Those of the psychodynamic school adopt the aetiological usage and believe that unconscious conflicts always underlie the traditional neurotic illnesses, but most clinicians now accept that there are other theories to explain the development of these disorders. These include cognitive, learning and biological models. Unfortunately, the word neurosis is also often used pejoratively as a way of describing difficult patients. This confusion paved the way for some clinicians to suggest that the term neurosis be abandoned, as obfuscation rather than clarification was its legacy. Inevitably this caused dismay to many but was welcomed by others.

When the American Psychiatric Association published DSM III in 1980 the term neurosis did not appear and the cluster of disorders subsumed by this rubric were classified under affective, anxiety and other disorders. In ICD 10 the traditional dichotomy between neurotic and psychotic has been abandoned although the former does find occasional use, as in the cluster headed 'Neurotic, stress-related and somatoform disorders'. However, categories such as 'neurotic depression' have been abandoned and the concept of neurosis can be said to be almost defunct in the current system of classification. This change in terminology may not directly affect family doctors in the immediate future, but in the longer term this will have an inevitable impact on the way psychiatric illnesses are conceptualised and on the terminology used when describing our patients.

Personality disorder

Many textbooks of psychiatry still contain a chapter entitled 'The Neuroses and Personality Disorder' suggesting that the two are linked. This has its foundation in the work of the 19th century psychiatrists who felt that personality predisposition was the real source of the malady and that psychiatric disturbances were reactions to stress. In the 1930s some questioned the interlinking of personality and mental state diagnosis and held that both were separate although of course in individual patients there may be an association. This separation has been the approach of the ICD and DSM classifications for many years. The clinical implication is that individual patients are no longer viewed in terms of either mental state diagnosis or personality disorder but may have one or other or both. Unfortunately many clinicians still retain a single dimension model in which the person is believed to either have a personality disorder or to have some other condition such as schizophrenia.

Psychoses

The distinction between manic depressive and schizophrenic psychosis was made by Kraepelin and this separation has rarely been subject to dispute. The only change has been the recognition that schizophrenia may have a good prognosis in some and successful attempts have been made to the identification of factors which make for this – a view not held by Kraepelin in his original description of 'dementia praecox' which he believed always had a poor outcome. Schizophrenia and manic depressive psychosis are thus retained as distinct entities in both the European and American systems of classification.

Other changes

Psychotic and neurotic illnesses following childbirth have been referred to as puerperal psychosis and postnatal depression, respectively. In other words they were classified by aetiology. There is now evidence that the treatment and outcome of disorders following childbirth are no different from those occurring at other times. The practice of classifying by aetiology has now been abandoned and has been replaced by symptomatic classification. If a patient has symptoms of schizophrenia or of depressive illness, they are described accordingly rather than by the precipitant.

For this reason the term 'reactive' depression is no longer used either. The latter had a number of meanings and for some it described a depressive illness which had a precipitant, for others an understandable reaction to stress and for still others was used interchangeably with neurotic depression. Thus a person who developed a depressive illness with psychotic features following a bereavement could have been described as having a psychotic depression or a reactive depression depending on local practice. Similar arguments have led to the abandonment of 'endogenous' depression, although the American system retains a similar concept in its recognition of depression with melancholic features. As with 'reactive' and 'neurotic' depression the term 'endogenous' was used variously to describe depression with a particular pattern of biological symptoms or to delineate an illness which had no precipitant.

A category of particular importance to general practice is the 'adjustment disorder' and 'acute stress reaction' cluster. Although included in the previous edition of ICD, this section has been expanded considerably in recognition of the multifaceted aspects of stress reactions. Unlike depressive illness, these do not have their own momentum but resolve when the precipitating stressor is removed or with the passage of time as a new level of adaptation is gradually achieved. These must be distinguished from depressive illnesses and from other disorders precipitated by stressors, such as generalised anxiety, whose resolution is not contemporaneous with removal of causation. In clinical practice the distinction can often be difficult (see Chapter 5, Case 1). Along with adjustment disorder, post traumatic stress disorder remains one of the few to be classified by aetiology.

CONCLUSION

It is clearly recognized that general practitioners see large numbers of patients with psychiatric disorders and that many are distinct in their mode of presentation from those seen in secondary care. For this and other reasons, the classifications used by psychiatrists, ICD 10 and DSM IV, are not appropriate to general practice. The World Health Organisation and the American Psychiatric Association have modified their classifications specifically in recognition of this.

Adhering to internationally recognised systems of classification is important as a first step in overcoming the confusion about diagnostic labels that has existed heretofore. To some the debate about classification may seem ephemeral, but the true value of a valid and reliable system rests in the accuracy of communication about patients at the interface between psychiatrists and general practitioners.

SUMMARY

1. There has been debate about the usefulness of psychiatric diagnosis, but there are forceful arguments against abandoning it.
2. Psychiatric diagnosis has been unreliable but by specifying the criteria, known as operational definitions, this can be improved and can be a springboard from which to validate these syndromes.
3. Both the American and the European systems of classsification, known respectively as DSM IV and ICD 10, have adopted this approach.
4. The modern approach to diagnosis favours describing the patient along dimensions (known as a multi-axial system) and in this way captures the multifarious aspects of the patient's condition.
5. Modern classifications avoid commonly used terms such as 'neurosis', 'postnatal depression' and a number of others.
6. A classification for use in primary care has been developed but its value has yet to be convincingly demonstrated.

REFERENCES

American Psychiatric Association. (1994). *Diagnostic and Statistical Manual, 4th Edition (DSM IV)*. American Psychiatric Association, Washington, DC.

Croudace, T., Evans, J., Harrison, G. *et al.* (2003). Impact of the ICD-10 Primary Health Care (PHC) diagnostic and management guidelines for mental disorders on detection and outcome in primary care. *British Journal of Psychiatry*, **182**, 20–30.

Kendell, R.E. (1975). *The Role of Diagnosis in Psychiatry*. Blackwell Scientific Publications, Oxford.

Ustun, T.B., Goldberg, D., Cooper, J. *et al.* (1995). New classification for mental disorders with management guidelines for use in primary care: ICD-10 PHC chapter five. *British Journal of General Practice*, **45**, 211–215.

World Health Organisation (1992). *Mental Disorders: glossary and guide to their classification in accordance with the tenth revision of the International Classification of Diseases.* World Health Organisation, Geneva.

FURTHER READING

Ustun, T.B., Goldberg, D., Cooper, J. *et al.* (1995). New classification for mental disorders with management guidelines for use in primary care: ICD-10 PHC chapter five. *British Journal of General Practice,* **45**, 211–215.

5

Stress Reactions and Adjustment Disorders

Stress is the term used to describe the overall reaction of individuals as they adapt to or attempt to adapt to circumstances or events which threaten to disrupt their physical or psychological wellbeing. These circumstances or events are referred to as stressors. However the association between the event and the response is not a simple cause and effect relationship but is governed by intervening variables known as mediators (see Fig. 5.1). It is these mediators which determine the magnitude and duration of the response – in other words the mediators rather than the stressor determine whether the reaction will be pathological or normal.

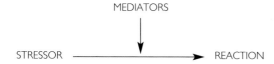

Figure 5.1. The stress model.

The effects of stress may be physical, behavioural or psychological but for the reaction to be considered abnormal, as distinct from proportionate to the circumstances, it is necessary that there be impairment in functioning. This is best encapsulated by the Yerkes–Dodson curve (Fig. 8.1, page 100) which shows that as the stress reaction (anxiety) increases performance improves and plateaus but thereafter diminishes. In other words it demonstrates that the presence of a stressor facilitates an optimum response. However beyond a certain point the reaction is pathological and behaviour is adversely affected. The point at which this is reached is a personal one and is determined by the mediators. This has important clinical ramifications.

MEDIATORS

Mediators are the factors which the link the stressor to the reaction. Without these, each stressor would have an entirely predictable effect on the recipient.

Table 5.1. Internal and external mediators.

Internal	External
Personality and defences, e.g. denial	Social supports
Cognitive interpretation	Religious beliefs
Biochemical predisposition, e.g. depressive illness	Cultural attitudes

Mediators may be classified into those which are internal and external and are listed in Table 5.1. The importance of mediators, particularly of those linked to personality, to cognitive interpretation and to social supports, lies in their relevance to treatment and prevention of recurrence.

DEALING WITH STRESSORS

The response to a stressor can be problem-focused, mediator-focused or response-focused. A problem oriented response implies avoiding or minimising the stressor *ab initio*. This may not always be possible since events occur without warning and are often not amenable to outside control. When events occur that are not predicted, early intervention to reduce their impact can offset the negative effect, e.g. if the loss of a workmate has caused a sudden increase in workload, rapid replacement would be essential.

Mediator-based responses to stress are not often applied since they may be ill defined. Essentially their purpose is to reduce the vulnerability of the person to the effects of stressors. Included in this group are the use of prophylactic medications such antidepressants for known psychiatric disorders which render the person vulnerable to abnormal stress responses. Bolstering support from others is also helpful, particularly when used to provide advice on practical solutions. Many assume that all support is helpful but when used only for emotional ventilation it is of much less benefit than when used in a practical way.

In addition, by using healthy coping skills the mediators may be modified and this should include a knowledge of the faulty strategies which are used as well as healthy defences. These are listed in Table 5.2.

Table 5.2. Defence mechanisms.

Positive	Negative
Planning	Denial
Suppression of competing activities	Substance misuse
Social supports for instrumental reasons	Social supports for emotional reasons
Active coping	Disengagement

A cognitive strategy for problem solving involves a staged process for resolving the problem. These are, (i) assessing the problem, (ii) setting realistic goals, (iii) planning a strategy, (iv) action to solve the problem, (v) evaluating the effects of this action, and (vi) re-adjusting the strategy on this basis.

The third approach to stress responses, and perhaps the best known to doctors, is the symptom-focused one in which either medication or relaxation is used to reduce the symptoms consequent upon the abnormal stress. These approaches can be very effective with rapid symptomatic control especially using anxiolytics. This is usually a short-term intervention but its benefit in reducing symptoms may enable the doctor to engage in other strategies as described above. Once a depressive illness has supervened, the approach to management is as outlined in Chapter 6 since there is no difference in response to pharmacotherapy or in outcome between those episodes which have a precipitant or those which occur spontaneously.

PATHOLOGICAL STRESS REACTIONS

The effects of stressors may be to produce reactions which stimulate performance and in these circumstances the stress is beneficial. However, when performance is impaired the result is an abnormal reaction and these are divided into three groups: physical, behavioural and psychological.

Abnormal physical reactions include peptic ulcers, hypertension, coronary artery disease and deterioration of established physical illness. However, abnormal stress may also lead to behavioural changes including lack of punctuality at work, absenteeism, alcohol misuse and occasionally overdosing and suicide. The psychological reactions are perhaps the most obvious and include adjustment reactions (this chapter), depressive illness (Chapter 6) and anxiety disorders (Chapter 8). Burnout although not included in the modern psychiatric classifications is frequently mentioned in self-help books dealing with stress. It is defined as an increasingly intense pattern of psychological, physical or behavioural dysfunction in response to a continuous flow of stressors. In practice it is best regarded diagnostically as a variant of either adjustment reactions or depressive illness, requiring treatment accordingly.

In the modern classifications ICD 10 and DSM IV, the only disorders listed under the 'stress reaction' heading are post traumatic stress disorder (PTSD), acute stress reactions and adjustment disorders. Even though disorders such as generalised anxiety or depressive episode can also be triggered by stressors they are categorised separately since the presence of a stressor is not essential to their genesis unlike adjustment disorders and PTSD where the diagnosis cannot be made in the absence of a stressor.

It is important to recognise that patients often describe themselves as suffering with 'stress' when in fact they have depressive illness. This is particularly true when anxiety, tension and insomnia are part of the symptom constellation of depressive illness. In these circumstances, pharmacotherapy may be strenuously resisted by the patient even when there is a clear indication for its use.

ADJUSTMENT DISORDERS

This category is seldom diagnosed in clinical practice although in the past the diagnosis of reactive depression, a concept similar to adjustment disorder, was frequently made. However, in response to concerns that depressive illnesses were under-diagnosed on the grounds of the symptoms being 'understandable' and 'reactive', this term was abandoned and its modern equivalent has never achieved the same status in terms of frequency of diagnosis or in research interest. Adjustment disorder was added to the DSM classification in 1968 and to the ICD system in 1976. Since then many biologically orientated psychiatrists have dismissed this group as a 'waste-basket'. However a few have attempted empirical studies and there is now convincing evidence that this category does warrant clinical description and that it is not only useful but also valid (Andreasen and Wasek, 1980).

There are three sub-categories of adjustment disorder: adjustment disorder with depressive features, with anxiety and with other disturbances of conduct.

Clinical features

Adjustment disorders are those disturbances which are closely related in time to a stressful event. They are described according to the content of the main symptom. Thus they may be depressive, anxious or behavioural in content and the latter are described mainly in teenagers. These reactions occur in the absence of any pre-existing psychiatric disturbance although personal vulnerability also plays a role. They occur generally within 3 months of the original stress and they continue until resolution, either when the stressor is removed or until a new level of adjustment is reached. When symptoms persist longer than 6 months they are then classified as either major depression or an anxiety disorder, although this may be an oversimplification since some very vulnerable people require much longer to adjust to stressors.

The symptoms themselves are often chronic, due to the chronicity of the stressors, and between 25% and 50% of those with this disorder have had symptoms for over a year at the time of presentation. The stressors are related mainly to school problems and parental problems in adolescents and in adults to marital, relationship and financial difficulties, but others are also described. Demographically, women outnumber men by a ratio of 2:1. The diagnosis is made largely in the under 30 age group and over 50% are single, separated or divorced.

Epidemiology

There is no information on the prevalence of adjustment disorders in the general population. Among the totality of general practice attenders this diagnosis was made in 17.9% of patients, making it the single largest diagnosis, followed by major and minor depression in 10% of consulters (Blacker and Clare, 1988). Among general practice attenders identified as having an emotional disorder, adjustment disorders were diagnosed in just under 25% of patients (Casey *et al.*, 1984). Recent figures from the United States showed that the diagnosis was made in 5% of in-patients in a unit with an interest in the disorder and for this reason is likely to be higher than in most other centres. No figures are available for psychiatric out-patients.

Differential diagnosis

The main problem is distinguishing adjustment reactions from depressive illness, since the latter also frequently has a precipitant. Appetite, sleep and concentration disturbance may be present in both. Anxiety is also common to each. If the classical biological symptoms of depressive illness such as diurnal mood swing, etc. are present the distinction may be more obvious. The recency of the stress may also be a guide since emotional upset is to be expected immediately following bereavements, other losses, failed exams and the common problems of life. If the stress is longstanding, arriving at a definitive diagnosis is more difficult. There is little guidance for the doctor in this regard although some rules of thumb may be of clinical assistance and these include the ability of the patient to respond to reassurance and to attempt to act upon advice given, the limited impact on functioning when compared with depressive illness and the reactivity of mood to pleasant stimuli and to changes in surroundings such as going on holiday. When accompanied by a recent identifiable stressor which antedates the symptoms, an adjustment reaction should be considered in the differential diagnosis along with a depressive episode or generalised anxiety. Conversely the absence of a stressor rules out adjustment disorder as a diagnosis. Biological investigations such as the dexamethasone suppression test and thyroid releasing hormone assessment are unhelpful since they are shown to be abnormal in only a proportion of depressives and their role in adjustment reactions has never been measured.

Generalised anxiety must also be distinguished from adjustment reactions with anxiety. The former is of longer duration and occurs after any stresses have been removed.

Treatment and prognosis

By definition the minimum of treatment is required since this condition is not conceptualised as an illness but rather as a reaction which is self-limiting. Pharmacotherapy has little role to play except in the acute phase if symptoms such as anxiety or insomnia are overwhelming. Antidepressants are not indicated. Relaxation techniques should be encouraged and an explanation of the basis for the symptoms along with reassurance that these are understandable in the circumstances should also be given. Frequently patients will ask if they are likely to 'break down' and again this fear must be dispelled since failure to do so may result in requests for and pressure to prescribe.

The importance of providing support for this group is obvious as is the necessity to effect environmental change where possible. Frequently the doctor will find himself unable to 'do' anything to effect change in the patient's circumstances or often there is nothing to be done. The value of 'just being there' should not be underestimated since many who consult with such reactions will be isolated socially or unsupported and have few personal resources. Acting as a confidant and a 'shoulder to cry on' is important for such people and may at times be life-saving. The general approach to counselling is discussed in Chapter 17. The value of talking and of social, family or cognitive therapy as required rather than pharmacological intervention is supported by findings that the prognosis is good with such non-biological approaches. However, most improve over time even without any formal therapy.

Up to 80% of adults given this diagnosis were well 5 years later and few had had problems in the interim (Andreasen and Hoenk, 1982). The outcome for adolescents was slightly less hopeful with 57% being well at follow-up. Those with poor outcome were given a subsequent diagnosis of depressive illness or alcoholism if adult, and adolescents were diagnosed as having antisocial personality disorder or drug abuse. The identification of those who may potentially become clinically depressed is a challenge which psychiatry has yet to meet.

On occasions if the diagnosis is still unclear, especially when depressive illness has not been ruled out, then a pragmatic course may have to be followed and treatment with antidepressants commenced. The hazards of not identifying and treating a depressive illness lie in the effect that a debilitating and life-threatening condition has upon the patient's life. Alternatively making the converse mistake and providing a prescription for a non-illness allows the patient to opt out of making personal changes which may be of benefit (see Case 1 below).

ACUTE STRESS REACTIONS

Acute stress reactions are those disturbances which develop in response to exceptional physical or mental stress. The symptoms are present in the early days following such a stressor, usually appearing within minutes of the impact of the stressful event and may resolve within hours or days

Initially there may be a dazed feeling and withdrawal from the surrounding situation. Associated panic and autonomic symptoms are also present. The symptoms are identical to those of PTSD but then resolve within weeks of onset. When they persist for longer than 1 month the diagnosis changes to PTSD although there may be a gap of months between the resolution of the acute reaction and the onset of PTSD. A diagnosis of acute stress reaction is a risk factor for the later development of PTSD although the latter is not inevitable.

POST TRAUMATIC STRESS DISORDER

Post traumatic stress disorder (PTSD) is distinct from most others in psychiatry in that a stressor is required, without which the condition would not have developed. The current classifications specify that the stressor be such that 'the event is of an exceptionally threatening or catastrophic nature, which is likely to cause distress in almost anyone'. The range of stressors has increased significantly in recent years and includes traumatic hospitalisations for cancer treatments such as for autologous bone marrow transplantation, asthma, etc., as well as events that traditionally were associated with this condition such as warfare, kidnappings, torture and rape. In clinical practice the stressors most frequently associated with PTSD are traffic accidents, some of which may not be physically serious.

The concept of post traumatic stress disorder (PTSD) is not without its critics, of whom Summerfield (2001) is the most vociferous. He points to the social utility of the diagnosis and argues that its emergence following the Vietnam war was driven by the antiwar movement and its desire to see attention moved from the soldier's background and personality towards an acceptance of the traumatogenic nature of war. Moreover, Summerfield and others draw attention to the expansion in the nature of the traumas that are now credited with causing PTSD, some of which although upsetting, such as a verbal sexual harassment, cannot compare with torture and rape. His view has been challenged by pointing to the neurobiological abnormalities that are associated with PTSD and that point to the poor outcome in many when followed longitudinally. However, there are studies also showing that some magnify or fabricate their symptoms either deliberately for financial gain (factitious disorder, see page 209) or as a result of positive reinforcement from the constant focus that is part of the legal process. In the latter this is not a conscious effort and when the legal case is resolved the symptoms diminish or resolve also. This pattern is often found in those with unexplained or magnified pain following road traffic accidents. Interestingly, the prevalence of PTSD is no different among accident victims making claims when compared with those who are not.

A further criticism of PTSD surrounds the classification of the syndrome. Some argue that the core symptoms such as intrusive thoughts are also found in other disorders such as depressive illness and that it would be better described according to the symptoms than by aetiology, analogous to 'puerperal psychosis' which is now diagnosed by generic symptoms, e.g. schizophrenia, mania, etc. Moreover, since the course of PTSD is variable, with depressive illness, drug misuse and panic disorder emerging over time, it is arguably a heterogeneous condition and not a specific disorder (Breslau and Davis, 1987). A final consideration is the reliance upon memory to describe the stressful events that preceded the onset of symptoms, an attribute that is often unreliable even for highly traumatic and specific events such as atrocities witnesssed by soldiers (Southwick *et al.*, 1997).

Risk factors

The risk of developing PTSD is greatest in those who are vulnerable either because of personality dysfunction or where there is a prior history of psychiatric disorder. In addition, a number of pre-traumatic risk factors have been identified including negative life events and emerging psychiatric symptoms. Specific coping mechanisms are associated with a higher risk and these include the identification of an external locus of control, i.e. feeling powerless over one's life, emotion rather than problem-focused coping, and disengagement from the stress. The occurrence of an acute reaction immediately following the event also increases the risk of subsequent PTSD (see p. 40).

Central to the diagnosis of PTSD is the fact that the event must be outside the realms of 'normal' experience. The nature of the stress itself plays an uncertain role since it is the perception of the stress which determines the likelihood of developing PTSD. For this reason even relatively 'minor' accidents may sometimes be followed by marked symptomatic change. Undoubtedly however, the greater the real threat to life, the greater the risk – thus victims of violent rapes, torture, kidnapping and serious physical injury are at special risk even though this may be delayed for months or even years after the event. PTSD can also develop by proxy, such as witnessing the maiming or killing of others. Certain occupations carry a special risk; these include body handlers and army personnel, fire-fighters and ambulance staff. However PTSD is not inevitable and some, even those exposed to severe trauma, seem to adjust well. Those exposed to man-made rather than natural disasters are at greater risk.

The biological basis of PTSD

The neurobiology of PTSD is complex and still evolving. Neuroendocrine studies have focused on endogenous opioid depletion, abnormal cortisol secretion and catecholamine excretion. Changes to the sleep/dream cycle have also been cited as has activation of the areas of the brain concerned with memory encoding and retrieval. Abnormalities to the amygdala, the hippocampus, the lateral septum and the prefrontal cortex in animal models have been shown by neuroimaging studies. Noradrenaline is believed to play a role in inducing intrusive memories while downregulation of the GABA system is believed to play a significant role in encoding memory during extreme stress and there is dysregulation of the hypothalamic–pituitary–adrenal axis. Kindling, the repetitive sub-threshold stimulation of neurones, has also been explored. However, few of these putative abnormalities have assisted in finding suitable treatments, with the exception of the selective serotonin reuptake inhibitors (SSRIs) (see below) which may act indirectly as they have a modulatory effect on the locus ceruleus/noradrenergic system.

Epidemiology

Studies in the US suggest a life-time prevalence of 1–9%, a not surprising figure in view of the high prevalence of traumatic events such as mugging, violence, and traffic accidents. When assessments are made shortly after the accident the figure for those with psychiatric symptoms is much higher, but these are frequently self-limiting.

Although men more commonly experience traumatic incidents, women are more at risk of developing PTSD, possibly accounted for by the greater exposure of women to particularly traumatic offences such as abuse or rape or due to greater personal vulnerability.

Clinical features

Psychological

Symptoms of PTSD are very common in the early days following a traumatic event but in this instance the diagnosis is not PTSD but 'acute stress reaction' (see p. 40). Most of these symptoms reduce markedly over the subsequent weeks and a diagnosis of PTSD is made only if symptoms persist for at least one month. Inappropriate labelling at this early stage may only prolong the illness behaviour and may stimulate medico-legal action.

In many there may be a delay between the events and the onset of symptoms of up to 6 months but in a small proportion (1–4%) it may be delayed for several years. This is most likely when physical injury has occurred and the focus is not directed to the emotional reaction. The prognosis is also poorer.

Three broad symptom clusters are described in those with PTSD:

(a) Intrusion
(b) Avoidance
(c) Hyper-arousal

The intrusive cluster is regarded as the most unique to PTSD since symptoms from this group must be present to make the diagnosis. These consist of nightmares, flashbacks and intrusive thoughts of the experience which are very distressing. Flashbacks are often confused with intrusive memories when they should only be used to describe the phenomenon of re-experiencing the event. Thus, the smell or action or emotional state at the time of the event may be recapitulated. Avoidance results in numbing, inability to recall details of the trauma, restricted range of affect, depersonalisation or derealisation and active avoidance of reminders or symbols of the event. Hyper-arousal is associated with anxiety, an increased startle response, insomnia, an increased sense of one's security or hypervigilance and irritability. In addition there may be survivor guilt and personal life may be seriously affected with an inability to return to work due to debilitating anxiety or phobia. Other symptoms include panic attacks, poor concentration, a sense of foreshortened future and mood disturbance.

Physical

As well as developing psychological symptoms, physical symptoms are also dominant and these include chronic pain, gastrointestinal disorders including irritable bowel syndrome, fibromyalgia and chronic pelvic pain, the latter especially in women who were victims of child sexual abuse. Other unexplained physical symptoms include nausea, shortness of breath and limb pain.

Treatment and prognosis

Forming a relationship with the patient is the first requirement for any successful intervention. Among those with PTSD anger may often be dominant and this will be directed at the third party who caused the event. Even when the events are naturally occurring rather than man-made, anger may be directed at the hospital receiving the victims or at those organising the rescue. Frustration may be felt at the change in income or living standards that have ensued and the patient will usually wish to articulate this. The lost opportunities and the change in personal life may be a source of mourning, as in any major loss and this must be acknowledged and worked through.

Pharmacological interventions consist mainly of antidepressants and the SSRI paroxetine is now licensed for treatment of this disorder. Its effect is not just on co-morbid depression but also on the core symptoms of PTSD, thus bringing about a global improvement in the patient's condition.

As well as the SSRIs, other agents such as the tricyclic antidepressants (TCAs) (amitriptyline, imipramine and lofepramine) and the monoamine oxidase inhibitor (MAOI) phenelzine are used without specific licence particularly when depression supervenes, although they also reduce the intrusive symptoms. There are numerous open trials and case reports of the efficacy of clonidine, alprazolam, moclobemide, buspirone and lithium but there is no evidence for their efficacy from double blind studies.

Psychological interventions consist largely of behavioural and cognitive models. Behavioural treatments involve real or imaginal exposure and relaxation techniques. These approaches may also be combined with cognitive approaches that aim to modify the dysfunctional thinking about the event.

Other therapies include hypnotherapy but it is believed that exposure in imagination is the key element in successful outcome with the approach. Eye movement desensitisation and reprocessing (EMDR), first described in 1989, is one of the newer treatments described in the literature. The theory is that the distressing images and thoughts can be diminished if they are paired simultaneously with a series of rapid eye movements induced by the therapist. This treatment was greeted with enthusiasm initially but this has lessened over time as the early positive studies had methodological flaws. Moreover, there is no conclusive theoretical model underpinning it and further controlled studies are necessary.

Prevention

The role of critical incident stress debriefing (CISD) is assuming increasing importance in the wake of large-scale terrorist attacks and traumatic incidents during warfare. Indeed most hospital emergency plans incorporate CISD as part of the official response and failure to provide it is frequently incorporated in negligence suits against official organisations such as the army, police force, etc. CISD consists of a single session in a group setting that involves reviewing the event and the emotions associated with it. Ventilation is encouraged and guidance concerning coping and preparing for the future is given. Studies in the early 90s suggested that this was helpful in preventing later PTSD and the recipients reported finding it helpful. More recent studies have shown that not only is CISD unhelpful but that it may cause more harm by interfering with the natural healing and processing that occurs for most people subjected to severe trauma. A recent Cochrane review concludes 'Compulsory debriefing of victims of trauma should cease' (Rose *et al.*, 2004).

Prognosis

The current literature on the prognosis of PTSD is variable and inconclusive. The prognosis depends on a number of factors such as the presence of abnormal personality and the duration of symptomatology before treatment is instituted. Some remain chronically incapacitated and between 9% and 33% still have a definite psychiatric disorder several years later (Tarsh and Royston, 1985). The prognosis is generally better after traffic accidents than after burns, head injuries or disasters.

Finally, it should be realised that families often become over protective and frequently reinforce the sick role thereby causing entrenchment and reducing the capacity for psychological rehabilitation. One of the influences on this is the lengthy litigation process and attempts at hastening settlement should be encouraged so as to facilitate early reintegration at work and in the community at large.

BEREAVEMENT

For most people the grieving process is uncomplicated albeit emotionally painful and will have resolved within 6–12 months, with a re-adaptation to life without the deceased. For some, grief is complicated by not occurring at all or by being excessively protracted. In addition some people develop physical problems or behavioural problems such as substance misuse, depressive illness and anxiety symptoms.

Normal grief

The earliest descriptions of grief continue to hold good to the present day with their focus on the four stages of the process although these do not imply any sequential phasing but are overlapping and intermixing. The first or numb phase describes the initial reaction of shock or disbelief, lasting for hours or even weeks. A second or yearning period is characterised by pangs of sadness and pining during which anger, and/or self-blame may occur as well as crying, sighing and disturbance of sleep and appetite. Disorganisation is prominent in the next period when the full realisation of the death occurs, resulting in despair, withdrawal and apathy. Finally with resolution the person adapts to life without their loved one and hopelessness declines. At this point there is a gradual return to social activity.

Other features described by those who are bereaved include seeing or hearing the deceased, especially when among crowds (illusions), deriving comfort from talking to the deceased and feeling the he/she is looking after family members left behind.

Abnormal grief

A small proportion of those bereaved describe either protracted grief or no grief at all and in this group professional help is required with the aim of preventing the later development of major emotional problems. Failure to experience any grief is uncommon and may stem from actively avoiding reminders of the deceased or striving to conceal emotion through fear of losing control.

Those who continue to describe acute symptoms of grief such as yearning and despair often require antidepressants and diagnostically they are regarded as then having a depressive episode. As well as depression, some describe symptoms of anxiety but these almost always co-exist with depressive symptoms and should be treated as such. The misuse of alcohol is a further complication of bereavement although it is not as common as previously thought and for most the increased use of alcohol post-bereavement is a temporary aid to sleeping and to reducing the 'edge' of the grief. Most studies report an increase in suicide and parasuicide following the death of a spouse or parent.

Grief in other situations

The circumstances of the death can also affect the outcome and pathological reactions are particularly associated with a number of these including:

- Death of a child, baby or sibling
- Prenatal loss of a baby through stillbirth, abortion or miscarriage
- Violent death
- Unexpected death
- Where the bereaved is responsible for the death

- Death by suicide or murder
- Where post-mortem or inquest is involved
- When the body is not recovered
- When there is uncertainty as to whether death has occurred, e.g. disappearance

Risk factors for abnormal reactions

A number of factors, apart from the circumstances of the death, are associated with abnormal reactions and foremost among these is whether the funeral was attended or not. Those who have many previous bereavements and a history of psychiatric disorder are also at increased risk as are those who were excessively dependent or ambivalent in their relationship with the deceased. Being male, under the age of 65 and lacking social supports also increases the risk and where the relationship does not allow for full participation in the mourning process, e.g. extramarital or same sex relationships, 'disenfranchised' grief can occur.

Management

For most the grieving process takes place spontaneously and without any recourse to counsellors. Unless there are very grave reasons, the bereaved should attend all parts of the funeral and should be encouraged to touch the deceased and say goodbye and some may even wish to take photographs prior to the closing of the coffin. The short-term use of hypnotics in the early stages of bereavement can help greatly but no other medication is usually required.

Where grieving has failed to occur or where it has remained unresolved, so that the person is still tearful, unable to visit the grave or look at a photograph, professional intervention may be necessary. Using the facilitating techniques described in Chapter 17 (page 264), the emotions should be encouraged and support given while the stages of numbness, anger, etc. are worked through. During therapy it may also be appropriate to give permission to reduce the frequency of visits to the cemetery or to remove the clothes and other possessions of the deceased.

However, it must be remembered that continuing grief may indicate a need for antidepressants.

Bereavement counselling may be necessary in situations of loss other than those of a loved one, including physical losses such as amputations, mastectomy, etc.

SUMMARY

1. Adjustment disorder is defined by the presence of a stressor and by a symptom cluster which improves with time as a new level of adjustment is reached, or when the precipitating stress is removed.

2. It can sometimes be difficult to distinguish from depressive illness.
3. Medication, such as antidepressants, has little part to play in treatment.
4. Research is needed to identify those at risk of progressing to a depressive illness subsequent to an adjustment reaction.
5. Post traumatic stress disorder occurs in the face of extraordinary stress.
6. Support and treatment of the primary symptom cluster is the mainstay of management.
7. Psychological debriefing may be harmful.
8. The prognosis is variable and some remain permanently incapacitated even after litigation has been completed.
9. Bereavement may be complicated by being absent or by being protracted.

CASE HISTORIES

Case 1

Mrs X was referred with a 5-year history of depression which had failed to respond to therapeutic doses of antidepressants or to in-patient group psychotherapy received in a private institution. Her symptoms consisted of feeling low in spirits, crying and feeling irritable with her husband. These began after she married against the advice of her parents. She was pregnant at the time and felt obliged to do so. Her relationship with her family had always been poor, the patient having trouble accepting discipline from them as a teenager and later their advice in many important matters. She had two children and had no problems relating to them or caring for them although she had help with this since she worked every day. She coped with her job, which was professional in nature, and felt that but for this she would have been much more gloomy. She had no concentration difficulties and socialised with her colleagues on a regular basis. She felt well when out socially and was then able to forget her worries. Her relationship with her husband had steadily deteriorated since she married such that they now did not go on holiday or socialise together. She knew that he had had at least one extramarital affair but did not discuss this with him at the time and had never sought help for her marital problems believing the relationship not to be worth working at. Her parents had suggested she separate but she refused because she did not wish to forfeit her comfortable lifestyle. Since this woman did not have any sleep, appetite or concentration disturbance and as her mood was reactive to her environment a diagnosis of adjustment reaction was made and marital therapy offered. She declined this and was offered psychotherapy which would focus on her reasons for remaining in the marriage and on ways of dealing with the difficulties which presented themselves. She also refused this, saying she wanted relief from her depression with medication and nothing else. This was refused and the patient returned to her general practitioner's care.

Comment

This woman had no symptom suggestive of a depressive illness, lacking both the commonly described biological symptoms and the more recently delineated atypical symptoms (see Chapter 6). The onset of symptoms coinciding with the realisation of an unsatisfactory marriage, the focus of symptoms upon her husband and the reactivity of mood all lend weight to the proffered diagnosis. It was noted that this lady always had problems accepting her parent's advice and, although not articulated, it is possible that this was an element in preventing her from separating from her husband. Her insistence that she was ill and in need of medication served to prevent her making decisions about her life which she might otherwise find painful or humiliating. The offer to explore this woman's need for status was, not surprisingly, refused. Prescribing would not only have been bad medically since antidepressants do not relieve depression when it is a symptom in such disorders but also would have reinforced her belief that she was ill and that her feelings were due to pathology rather than the psychic pain of unhappiness.

Case 2

Mr X, a 32 year-old chemical engineer, was involved in an explosion at work and severely burnt on his right shoulder, arm and chest. This necessitated a skin graft and a 2-month hospitalisation. After discharge he had frequent nightmares in which he and his child were burnt alive. At this time he was waking early mainly from the discomfort of his graft and feeling tearful. His concentration and appetite remained intact throughout. At the time of referral he described flashbacks and nightmares as well as anxiety about returning to work. He had on one occasion cancelled a meeting in his laboratory to discuss this because of overwhelming anxiety which prevented him from sleeping the previous night. He showed no panic in other situations although he was unable to read about fires or explosions in the press. He functioned normally in his home but his interest in sport had somewhat diminished. He felt angry at what had happened especially as he had warned his superiors of some shortcomings in safety procedures. He was happily married and had no previous psychological problems. This man would fit the criteria for post traumatic stress disorder. Since he also had typical phobic symptoms this diagnosis was also made and treatment commenced as for this. Initially he was shown relaxation techniques and encouraged to carry these out twice daily. In addition, a hierarchy of anxiety provoking situations relating to work was constructed. The lowest on the hierarchy was seeing photographs of the plant, then driving into his office, etc., and finally going into the laboratory next to the reactor which exploded. He was desensitised in imagination over a 4 week period and subsequently given instruction in graded exposure to these situations in vivo. His wife acted as therapist for those lowest in the hierarchy but discontinued this when he was on the point of entering the factory. By combining relaxation with graded exposure he successfully returned to work and has remained symptom free.

Comment

Mr X was highly motivated to return to work and had a helpful wife who reinforced this wish. This was one of the main factors contributing to his success in treatment. Imaginal treatment was tried initially because he was so motivated and also psychologically minded. Using his wife as co-therapist reinforced his motivation. He was encouraged to talk about his experience and his feelings subsequent to the accident. More formal cognitive therapy was not required. At the time of writing he had returned to his pre-accident level of functioning.

Case 3

Mr X was a 40 year-old printer who was involved in an accident at work in which he cut his hand very badly and almost severed it. He was hospitalised for 2 weeks following the injury. For the first 2–3 weeks he had no psychological symptoms and was thankful that he had not lost a limb. However, following discharge from hospital he began to feel anxious and panicky. He had difficulty sleeping and he was drinking 6–7 cans of beer every evening. He began to feel extremely angry at his employers, complaining that they had no concern for him. He was unable to go back to work because of his poor concentration and he spent his day sitting in his house. His personal hygiene was poor and he looked dishevelled. He lived alone but had a young son from a previous relationship whom he saw regularly although his irritability recently had alienated him from his former girlfriend. He was offered cognitive therapy but defaulted after a few sessions saying his problem wasn't being dealt with appropriately. He was then referred for psychodynamic psychotherapy and he engaged well with this. He was not offered antidepressants as he was drinking to excess and it was felt this was contributing to his low mood. In spite of his anger at his employers and at his psychiatrist who refused medication he continued to attend. His symptoms were largely unchanged for the 3 years that he was attending. The medico-legal case was settled in his favour although the financial award was very small as he was held to have contributed to the accident. At the subsequent out-patient visits his mood had improved significantly even though he was in debt to his legal team due to the small settlement. He was neatly dressed and had cut down his alcohol intake. He was again on speaking terms with his former girlfriend. He explained the dramatic change by the fact that the case was now over and he could get on with life again.

Comment

This history illustrates two points. First, there is often a delay in the onset of psychological symptoms when there is a serious physical injury and the focus of the patient and medical staff is on that. Secondly, the dramatic improvement in symptoms following the settlement of his medico-legal case, albeit financially unsatisfactory, is a common finding. The frequent visists to doctors and solicitors with the constant recounting and recalling of the traumatic event serves to reinforce the symptoms. For this reason early settlement is the ideal.

REFERENCES

Andreasen, N.C. and Hoenk, P.R. (1982). The predictive value of adjustment disorders: A follow-up study. *American Journal of Psychiatry*, **139**, 584–590.

Andreasen, N.C. and Wasek, P. (1980). Adjustment disorders in adolescents and adults. *Archives of General Psychiatry*, **37**, 1166–1171.

Birtwistle, J. and Kendrick, T. (2001). The psychological aspects of bereavement. *Primary Care Psychiatry*. **7**, 91–95.

Blacker, C.V.R. and Clare, A.W. (1988). The prevalence and treatment of depression in general practice. *Psychopharmacology*, **95**, 514–517.

Breslau, N. and Davis, G.C. (1987). Post-traumatic stress disorder. The stressor criterion. *Journal of Nervous and Mental Disease*, **175**, 255–275.

Casey, P.R., Dillon, S. and Tyrer, P.J. (1984). The diagnostic status of patients with conspicuous psychiatric morbidity in primary care. *Psychological Medicine*, **14**, 673–681.

Rose, S., Bisson, J. and Wessely, S. (2004). Psychological debriefing for preventing post traumatic stress disorder (PTSD) (Cochrane Review). In: *The Cochrane Library*, Issue 1. Wiley, Chichester.

Tarsh, M.J. and Royston, C. (1985). A follow-up study of accident neurosis. *British Journal of Psychiatry*, **146**, 18–25.

Southwick, S., Morgan, C., Nicolaou, A. *et al.* (1997). Consistency of memory for combat-related traumatic events in veterans of Operation Desert Storm. *American Journal of Psychiatry*, **154**, 173–177.

Summerfield, D. (2001). The invention of post-traumatic stress disorder and the social usefulness of a psychiatric category. *British Medical Journal*, **322** 95–98.

FURTHER READING

Burnard, P. (1989). *Counselling Skills for Health Professionals*. Chapman and Hall, London.

Casey, P., Dowrick, C. and Wilkinson, G. (2001). Adjustment disorders: fault line in the psychiatric glossary. *British Journal of Psychiatry*, **179**, 479–481.

Hageman, I., Andersen, H.S. and Jorgensen, M.B. (2001). Post-traumatic stress disorder: a review of psychobiology and pharmacotherapy. *Acta Psychiatrica Scandinavica*, **104**, 411–422.

Lally, S.S. and Sims, A.C.P. (1999). The treatment of post-traumatic stress disorder: a UK perspective. *Primary Care Psychiatry*, **5**, 89–100.

Rose, S., Bisson, J. and Wessely, S. (2004). Psychological debriefing for preventing post traumatic stress disorder (PTSD) (Cochrane Review). In: *The Cochrane Library*, Issue 1. Wiley, Chichester.

SUGGESTED READING FOR PATIENTS

Kinchin, D. (1994). *Post-Traumatic Stress Disorder. A Practical Guide to Recovery*. Thorsons, London.

Mason, L.J. (1988). *Stress Passages: Surviving Life's Transitions Gracefully*. Celestial Arts, Berkeley, California.

Collick, E. (1988). *Through Grief: The Bereavement Journey*. Darton, Longman and Todd, London.

Lewis, C.S. (1966). *A Grief Observed*. Faber and Faber, London.

Wallbank, S. (1991). *Facing Grief: Bereavement and the Young Adult*. Lutterworth Press, London.

USEFUL WEBSITES FOR PATIENTS

Stress management: www.ivf.com/stress.html

National Centre for PTSD: www.ncptsd.org

Royal College of Psychiatrists' information on bereavement:
www.rcpsych.ac.uk/info/bereav.htm

USEFUL CONTACTS

Victim Support (UK)
Cranmer House
39 Brixton Road
London SW9 6DZ
Tel: 020 7735 9166
Email: contact@victimsupport.org.uk
Website: www.victimsupport.org.uk

Victim Support
Haliday House
32 Arran Quay
Dublin 7
Tel: 01 8780 870
Email: info@victimsupport.ie
Website: www.victimsupport.ie

Cruse Bereavement Care
126 Sheen Road,
Richmond
Surrey TW9 1UR
Tel: 020 8939 9530
Email: info@crusebereavementcare.org.uk
Website:
www.crusebereavementcare.org.uk

The Compassionate Friends
(provides support for bereaved parents)
53 North Street
Bristol BS3 1EN
Tel: 0845 123 2304
Email: info@tcf.org.uk
Website: www.tcf.org.uk

6

Affective Disorders

Next to adjustment reactions, depressive illness is the most frequent psychiatric disorder seen in general practice. In this setting it has many faces, making it difficult to diagnose. Unipolar depression (also termed depressive episode) is the term used to describe a single episode of depression and when it recurs it is termed recurrent depressive disorder. Bipolar illness or manic depression refer to depressive illness intermixed with mania or hypomania, called bipolar I and II, respectively. Dysthymia is a chronic, low grade depressive illness which usually begins in early adulthood and is generally refractory to treatment. It is associated with long-standing personality difficulties which may amount to personality disorder and the distinction between them is very difficult. Some believe that dysthymia is another category of personality disorder. When an acute episode of depressive illness is superimposed on dysthymia the term 'double depression' is invoked. The term reactive depression is no longer used since in its meaning it could represent either an adjustment reaction or a depressive episode triggered by a stressful event, thereby causing therapeutic confusion. Similarly, endogenous depression has fallen into disuse since it is recognised that even a depressive episode that is triggered causes biological sensitisation and increases the risk of subsequent non-precipitated episodes.

PREVALENCE

Using various approaches to case identification among general practice consulters a one year prevalence of between 3 and 17% has been found although there are very wide cross-national differences. For example, a recent study using the same methodology in all 15 centres worldwide found the rate for current major depression lay between 1.6% in Nagasaki and 26.3% in Santiago. Manchester had a prevalence of 17.1% (Simon *et al.*, 2002). Although it is tempting to ascribe these cross-national differences to differing risk factors and therefore to be a true finding, this study found that in the centres of high prevalence, which included

Manchester, milder cases were being identified while in the other centres only illnesses of greater severity were diagnosed. However, variability in single country studies are more likely to be accounted for by demographic, urban/rural and methodological differences. More recent studies have suggested a one year prevalence of around 10%. The life-time risk is about 10% for men and 20% for women although a recent Swedish study spanning 17 years found a much higher probability risk of 25% for men and 45% for women up to the age of 70. It has been convincingly shown that there is failure to identify between a third and a half of those patients with emotional disorders and figures as low as 3.5% for the total morbidity have been described. The reasons for non-identification are outlined below.

Bipolar I disorder is much less common and has a lifetime risk of around 1%. The sex ratio is also slightly different with a female:male ratio of 3:1 for unipolar depression and of 1.5:1 for bipolar disorder. The mean age of onset at 30 is slightly earlier also. There is no established link with social class and depressive illness in general predominates in women under the age of 45 and in men over the age of 55. The more severe episodes peak in the elderly.

Bipolar II disorder, being a relatively recent addition to the current diagnostic categories, has been the subject of much less research. A recent study found a prevalence for this disorder of around 10% in the general population (Angst *et al.*, 2003) and suggested that it is under-diagnosed, being mistaken for recurrent depression in around 30% of those so diagnosed (Piver *et al.*, 2002). This group of conditions, ranging from classic manic–depression (bipolar I) through to depression with mild forms of hypomania, are referred to as bipolar spectrum in a manner analogous to the broad group of depressive disorders that spans psychotic depression through to dysthymia.

UNDETECTED DEPRESSION

There are several explanations for the non-detection of psychiatric illness in general, and depressive illness in particular. One is that some patients do not consult despite obvious distress. In particular, men find difficulty in describing their emotional difficulties and are therefore reluctant to consult. It has been suggested that the predominance of alcohol abuse among men results from their tendency to use it for symptomatic relief. More surprisingly however the majority of people with significant symptoms do consult their doctors.

Amongst consulters the reasons for non-detection are four-fold. First, the *accuracy* and *interest* of the doctor have inevitable implications for detecting depressive illness (see Chapter 2). *Sociodemographic factors* may be a source of bias and males, those from high socio-economic groups, the young, the elderly and the unmarried are less likely to be labelled as psychologically unwell than their female, separated and poor counterparts. In addition, the *manner in which patients present their symptoms* is of crucial importance and complaints of physical symptoms, such as insomnia, tiredness, palpitations, etc., may reduce the probability of being correctly diagnosed. Moreover, those who normalise their symptoms are also less likely to be diagnosed with an emotional disorder (Kessler *et al.*, 1999). Undetected patients are often less obviously depressed and may have an associated physical illness which distracts from the emotional difficulties. Finally, there is the obvious difficulty of *confusing depressive illness with anxiety disorders or adjustment disorder* because of the symptom overlap.

CLASSIFICATION

The traditional subdivisions of depressive illness into categories, i.e. neurotic/ psychotic and reactive/endogenous, although still used by some have been abandoned by most clinicians and also by the official documents on classification, i.e. ICD 10 and DSM IV (see Chapter 4). The neurotic/psychotic dichotomy was based on the type of symptoms described. An alternative, and separate classification was derived from the presence or absence of precipitants, i.e. reactive/ endogenous. Provided both were used independently these differing systems would be acceptable. However, since both were used interchangeably so that neurotic and reactive became synonymous, as did psychotic and endogenous, confusion reigned. In addition those who developed depressive symptoms resulting from stressful events were diagnosed as having 'reactive' depression. This caused confusion in labelling and therapeutic inertia in relation to those designated neurotic/reactive even though it is now recognised that stressful events can precipitate a full-blown and sometimes severe depressive illness (see also adjustment disorder, Chapter 5). Studies examining precipitants to depressive illness, symptom patterns and response to treatment suggested that there was no clinical justification for retaining the distinction. The decision to have a separate category for adjustment disorders and to classify depressive illness by severity of symptoms alone was hailed by many as an advance from the doldrums enveloping this disorder. In simple terms the distinction is now between stress/unhappiness, termed adjustment disorder, and illness.

Bipolar disorder is also going through a process of reclassification although the European system (ICD 10) recognises it as a single entity while DSM IV has subdivided it into bipolar I and II. There are now moves to increase the number of subcategories further to incorporate milder forms of hypomania as well as those that are triggered by antidepressant treatment. The latter causes division within the profession, some of whom regard it as a form of bipolar disorder with the attendant implications for treatment while others simply believe this as an unwanted side effect of antidepressant treatment with no implications for bipolarity.

AETIOLOGY

Genetic

The genetic basis for unipolar depression, although present, is weaker than in bipolar depression, with a concordance among monozygotic twins of about 50% and among dizygotic twins of 10-25%. For bipolar I disorder there is an increased risk among the relatives of affected patients and a higher concordance for the condition among monozygotic twins (up to 90%) than dizygotic twins (up to 25%). Moreover, 50% of bipolar I patients have at least one parent with a mood disorder, usually depressive illness and if one parent has bipolar I disorder there is a 25% chance that a child will be similarly affected while if both parents have this disorder the risk is 50-75%. Molecular biology has enabled greater study of the exact mode of inheritance for these disorders and although no certainty as yet exists, associations for mood disorders, especially bipolar I, with chromosomes 5, 11 and the X chromosome have been reported.

Neurochemical

The most acceptable hypothesis derives from the observation that antidepressants exert their central neurochemical effect on the 5-hydroxytryptamine (5HT) and noradrenergic receptors. Suggestions that the reduced availability of 5HT at synapses is responsible for depressive illness have been countered by theories that it is increased due to the reduced sensitivity of the postsynaptic receptors. The possible role of noradrenaline (NA) has also been investigated and findings of depletion of NA and of an increase in the number of presynaptic receptors have been reported. Newer antidepressants act by raising central catecholamine levels, particularly 5HT and noradrenaline. The roles of sodium, calcium and magnesium have also been subject to testing and their involvement remains to be clarified.

The 'time-keeper' hormone, melatonin, has been the focus of attention, mainly due to the seasonal variation in depression in some patients and the diurnal changes in symptoms. So far, the results are unconvincing. Since a variety of neuroendocrine dysregulations have been found in those with mood disorders this has been the subject of considerable interest. However, as the hypothalamo–pituitary axis receives many inputs that involve noradrenaline, serotonin, etc., it is possible that this dysregulation is the result of more fundamental abnormalities elsewhere. The predominance of depression among women and the special risk following childbirth suggest a hormonal cause, but there is yet no convincing evidence for this.

Life stresses

It is accepted from a wide body of research that major events have an impact on mood and can trigger both depressive illness and bipolar disorders. Events such as bereavement and childbirth have long been known to provoke depressive or hypomanic episodes and terms such as postnatal depression and prolonged grief reaction were used descriptively in recognition of this. Naturalistic studies have shown that those illnesses which were so precipitated are no different from those which were unprovoked. Moreover, all life events, but especially unpleasant ones, have been implicated. Included amongst the most stressful are those already mentioned, but also moving house and loss of a job. Subsequent episodes of illness can occur without any precipitant.

Vulnerability and personality

Recent work suggests that certain factors increase the likelihood of becoming depressed in the face of a life stress. These include the absence of a confiding relationship, unemployment, caring for young children and the loss of a mother in childhood. The importance of outlets and of support from family and friends is obvious from this work and should be borne in mind by the GP who is involved in the work of prevention. For many years it was believed that obsessional person-alities had a tendency to exhibit 'endogenous' type symptoms and that neurotic symptoms were linked to those with 'neurotic' traits. There is no doubt that in some vulnerable individuals personality attributes increase the likelihood of becoming depressed. For example those of obsessional disposition may be at risk of developing depression in response to 'change' events although no one person-ality type is consistently associated with depression. In particular, the difficulty of assessing personality in the presence of depression must be remembered (see Chapter 11); this was a problem in many of the early studies. The supposed associ-ation between depression and pyknic body build has also been disproven.

Psychological causes

Freud proposed that depression was analogous to mourning and even where there was no obvious loss the depression was a response to a symbolised loss. However, investigators have found that fewer than 10% of those experiencing recent losses develop a depressive illness. This suggests that the contribution from this type of event to the totality of depressions is small. Other theorists have emphasised the importance of emotional deprivation or maternal loss in causing depression but these have been associated with many psychiatric conditions such as alcoholism, antisocial personality, etc., and seem to be non-specific. The theory of 'learned helplessness' has attracted much attention but is equally unsatisfactory as an expla-nation. This theory states that depression develops when rewards and punishment are no longer dependent on the actions of the individual and the lack of control over whether these are received is at the core of this hypothesis. More plausible than these theories is the theory of Beck (1967) that depressive cognitions may be the cause of the disorder or, at least, are important factors in maintaining the disorder once established. These negative cognitions refer to oneself, one's experiences, and the future and are termed the 'cognitive triad'. This theory has led to an approach to treatment which is described below.

PRESENTATION OF DEPRESSION IN GENERAL PRACTICE

Three forms of presentation can be identified.

Physical symptoms

Patients sometimes describe physical symptoms such as anorexia, loss of energy, aches and pains and stomach problems rather than depression itself. If they do complain of disturbed mood it is attributed to the physical symptoms. These people are known as somatisers and are often resistant to the idea of their symptoms having a psychological origin. Symptoms of anxiety are almost universal in depression and it is hardly surprising that these will often be the prime focus of the patient's attention rather than the accompanying emotional changes.

There are a number of reasons why the patient may present with somatic symptoms, including low IQ, a (mistaken) belief that the doctor only wants to hear about physical symptoms and absence of psychological mindedness. Cultural factors also have a bearing and Eastern races frequently present in this way. Included in this group of somatisers are those who present with pain only, especially in the mouth and face. Atypical pain is an uncommon but clearly documented symptom of depressive illness and should be considered whenever there is no organic cause.

Emotional symptoms

Those who articulate emotional difficulties make the doctor's work easy although this mode of presentation is relatively uncommon. The patient will describe depression, anxiety and tearfulness but may also feel that there is an obvious cause for these. The doctor should beware of too easily ascribing causation, especially if the stresses seem relatively small or if their occurrence is remote in time. Anxiety is universal in depressive illness and, when this is the presenting symptom, may suggest anxiety neurosis as the primary diagnosis. The age of the patient together with assessment of sleep, mood and other symptoms should clarify the diagnosis. Among general practice patients diurnal changes in mood may not be obvious but changes in the level of anxiety should alert the doctor to the possibility of depression.

Other emotional problems

Presenting with some other emotional problem, e.g. loss of libido, excessive drinking, forgetfulness or an increased dependence on the spouse, may lead the doctor to suspect a sexual difficulty, primary alcohol abuse, dementia or personality disorder unless a careful history is obtained from the patient and from a collateral source also. A history of change from usual will help confirm the diagnosis. Confusion is a well documented symptom of depression and is referred to as depressive pseudodementia.

SYMPTOMS

Depression

The symptoms of depressive illness are listed in Table 6.1. The prominence of anxiety and panic attacks has already been emphasised. Psychotic symptoms are rare among general practice depressives and for this reason it is easy to forget that they can occur in severe forms of this illness and may lead the GP to suspect schizophrenia. The content of the psychotic symptoms is negative, gloomy and centres around the devil, evil, serious illness and the parlous state of the world. Hallucinations are heard in the second rather than the third person.

Hypomania

Hypomania represents a milder form of mania in that psychotic symptoms are absent. Hypomania and mania are uncommon and may be confused with schizophrenia. When hypomania/mania occur simultaneously with depression the clincial picture is of tearfulness, overactivity and irritabiliity alternating with elation and is termed dysphoric hypomania/mania or a mixed affective state. Management of mixed states is with major tranquillizers in the first instance, until a clear picture of either depression or more commonly of hypomania (mania) emerges.

ATYPICAL DEPRESSION

This disorder has achieved prominence recently and the term is used to describe those who exhibit hypersomnia, overeating, evening worsening of symptoms, anxiety and irritability. They are often of longstanding. Monoamine oxidase inhibitors (MAOIs) have been shown to be beneficial in treatment and are probably superior to the tricyclic antidepressants. For the general practitioner the importance of this condition lies in the unusual symptom pattern and the consequent

Table 6.1. Common symptoms of depression, hypomania and mania.

Mild/moderate depression	Hypomania	Severe depression	Mania
Gloom/tearfulness	Elation or lability	Inability to cry	
Irritability	Irritability and hostility	Inability to feel (loss of emotional	
Anxiety: free-floating and phobic	Disinhibition	resonance)	Delusions of grandiose identity or ability
Depersonalization		Delusions of guilt	Delusions of persecution
Agitation or retardation	Overactivity	Delusions of persecution	Delusions of reference
Insomnia: early, middle or late	Insomnia	Delusions of reference	
Hypersomnia			
Aches and pains		Hypochondriacal delusions	
Anorexia or overeating			
Impaired concentration	Impaired concentration		
Lack of confidence	Grandiosity	Nihilistic delusions	
Inability to cope		Auditory hallucinations, 2nd person critical	
Overvalued ideas of guilt, reference,	Overvalued ideas of reference		
hypochondriasis			
Obsessional rituals or ruminations			

likelihood of misdiagnosis. Patients exhibiting some or all of these symptoms should be referred for specialist assessment rather than being regarded, as hitherto, as among the 'worried well' or the personality disordered.

EFFECTS OF UNTREATED DEPRESSION

The effects of untreated depression are multiple and potentially serious: a mortality from suicide of 15% has been reported in older studies of those with severe depression. Much lower rates of suicide have been reported in a recent study with follow-up for up to 6 years, being lowest in those with mild depression (0.5%), followed by moderate depression (1%) and highest in severe depression (2%) and with men having over twice the risk of suicide compared to women (Kessing, 2004). Other studies place the suicide risk somewhat higher at about 7%. Marital disharmony consequent upon irritability, loss of libido or excessive emotional dependence may lead to eventual marital breakdown. The effects upon the bonding process with the newborn of depressed mothers are potentially lifelong and may increase the propensity to depressive illness among these children in adult life. Many sufferers also have handicapping phobias secondary to their illness, leading to isolation and restriction of outlets and some may abuse alcohol in order to obtain symptomatic relief. The aggressive treatment of this common condition is therefore essential if much suffering is to be avoided.

ARE THOSE WITH DEPRESSION SEEN IN GENERAL PRACTICE LESS SEVERELY ILL THAN THOSE SEEN IN THE OUT-PATIENT CLINIC?

When psychotic depression is included the obvious answer to this question is 'Yes'. Excluding this small group however makes a definite answer more difficult. Many patients are referred to the specialist services for reasons other than the severity of symptoms. These include suicidal ideation or behaviour, social dysfunction or alcohol abuse. When these factors are controlled there is some overlap between referred and non-referred patients although in general those who are referred are more severely depressed and incapacitated.

The decision to refer to the specialist services is taken in part because of the social consequences of depressive illness. For this reason men whose livelihood is affected, the young, and those who are psychotic, suicidal or a danger to others are most likely to be referred. Older doctors and those in urban practices make greater use of the psychiatric services. Overall between 5 and 10% of those seen in general practice are referred although this seems to be unaffected by the doctor having a declared interest in psychiatry. About one-third of those referred are thought to be beyond the scope of the general practitioner and a similar proportion are described as non-responders to pharmacological treatments, although the latter is often a consequence of inadequate treatment rather than an inherent part of the illness.

DEPRESSION AT SPECIAL TIMES

Postnatal depression

This refers to the occurrence of depressive illness in the 12 months following child-birth although the symptoms may sometimes have preceded childbirth. Symptoms are similar to those at other times of life but the feelings of uselessness and inability to cope centre round the patient's role as a mother. In its severe form, known as puerperal psychosis, the presence of delusions may place the baby and also the mother at risk of physical harm and admission to hospital is invariably necessary in these circumstances. The provision of a mother and baby unit provides the optimum setting for the management of depression following childbirth. While these disorders are no longer believed to be specific to childbirth this does not exclude the impor-tance of helping the depressed mother adjust to her new role as mother or to the stresses inherent in tending a new baby. The pharmacological treatment of the symptoms is however similar to that used in all patients with depressive illness and the long-term prognosis is similar to that of depressive illness in general.

The menopause

The menopause has traditionally been believed to be associated with an increase in emotional problems especially depressive illness. A number of studies are now available which refute this belief and in fact depressive illness is a condition which predominates in younger women. There is no doubt that women do suffer emotional difficulties at this time but these may be due to the change in status as children leave home, to the loss of family and friends through bereavements which often gather momentum in the middle years and perhaps to previously untreated depression which is augmented at times of personal stress. Although some studies suggest that the pre-menopausal period may be associated with a higher incidence of depression than other times, attempts to relate symptoms to hormone levels or to treat them with replacement therapy have been inconclusive.

Involutional depression

Involutional depression, once believed to be a specific disorder but now relegated to the same fate as postnatal depression, was characterised by delusions about bodily functions, psychomotor retardation or agitation and hallucinations. Its nearest equivalent is severe depression and the period of greatest risk for first episodes of severe depression is between 55 and 65. The reason for this is unknown since investigation of the possible aetiological factors such as genetic or personality predisposition, organic brain damage, life events, loss of physical independence have not been proven to be the exclusive reason. The suggestion that the ageing process itself, through an effect on monoamine metabolism, places the elderly at risk is worthy of consideration. Whatever the reason for this excess of severe depressive illness, the social conditions of individual patients need careful consideration and manipulation if relapses are to be prevented and the risk of suicide reduced. In addition to antidepressants, ECT is more frequently used in this age group than in any other – a reflection of the severity of the illness which they suffer. The short-term prognosis is good and a marked improvement occurs in over 85% but subsequently about one-third lapse into invalidism with intermittent depressive episodes, a further third have episodes from which they recover and the remaining third remain completely well. In this age group the onset of depression may herald Alzheimer's disease well before the typical symptoms of memory impairment become obvious.

Physical illness

Physical illness is known to be connected to depressive illness and this is detailed further in Chapter 15. Painful bone disorders and neurological disorders especially cerebrovascular accidents and multiple sclerosis result in a striking excess of depressive illness. These do respond to antidepressants and to withhold such treatment is to court disaster since the final result may be death by suicide.

INVESTIGATIONS

Dexamethasone suppression and thyroid releasing hormone levels are disturbed in some patients with depressive illness and measurement of these has been advocated by some. These are unlikely to be helpful to the general practitioner since they are normal in most of those with depressive illness. Moreover they have not been investigated in patients with adjustment reactions. When depressive illness fails to respond to adequate treatment it is important to rule out the common physical causes of depressive illness especially thyroid disease and malignancy.

TREATMENT OF DEPRESSIVE ILLNESS

Before considering the treatment of depression the patient must be given information about the illness. It is important not only to be honest but also to correct some of the myths which exist:

1. Emphasise that it is an illness and not indicative of any inherent weakness in character. A simple description of the neurochemical abnormalities may be required. The patient may also enquire about the risk of transmitting the disorder to offspring.
2. The likely success of treatment should be explained along with the discussion of the necessity for treatment. Many patients may believe it is up to themselves to change but an explanation of the rationale and importance of treatment should correct this view.
3. When discussing medication distinguish between tranquillisers and antidepressants since only the best informed patients will be aware of the distinction. In particular, patients are likely to enquire about the risk of dependence.
4. Draw attention to the likely side effects of the chosen antidepressant and explain the delay in onset of antidepressant effect especially with TCAs and SSRIs as this will improve compliance.
5. Women of childbearing age will want to know of the risks to a pregnancy, if taking antidepressants, and also the possibility that the disorder will be passed to their children. Problems with breastfeeding while taking antidepressants will also need to be explored and the general practitioner should provide as much information as possible by contacting the pharmaceutical company directly or by seeking advice from specialist services.

Drug treatments

The importance of antidepressants for treating depressive illness in general practice has been bolstered by placebo-controlled trials in this setting (Paykel *et al.*, 1988). The belief of many patients that it is their responsibility to make the necessary adjustments to life to improve mood bears a strong resemblance to the 'pull yourself together' attitude common in the past. Placing the responsibility for this upon the already apathetic and incapacitated patient will lead to an increased sense of guilt and uselessness. Moreover, the depressed patient is unable to respond to such advice since the ability to step outside the symptoms and be objective is diminished. While changes may be desirable in the patient's life, counselling should be deferred until after symptoms have improved. It is for this reason that antidepressants are essential and the choice in treating depressive illness is not between drugs or psychotherapy but for many patients a combination of both. In the early stages psychotherapy will be of a supportive type but as symptoms improve it will be more problem-oriented, psychodynamic or cognitive as deemed necessary.

Many patients believed to be chronically depressed may not be receiving the minimum therapeutic dose of antidepressant, although this problem should be significantly reduced with the increased use of the SSRIs where the therapeutic dose is identical to the initiation dose. It is essential to prescribe antidepressants in adequate doses and for up to one month before changing to another (Table 6.2). The elderly

Table 6.2. Antidepressants in common use.

	Sedative/ alerting	Starting dose (mg)	Minimum therapeutic dose (mg)	Maximum therapeutic dose (mg)
Tricyclics				
Amitriptyline	Sedative	50–75	100	200
Dothiepin	Sedative	50–75	100	200
Doxepin	Sedative	50–75	100	200
Trimipramine	Sedative	50–75	100	200
Imipramine	Mildly sedative	50–75	100	200
Clomipramine	Mildly sedative	50–75	100	200
Lofepramine	Mildly sedative	70 b.d.	210	280
Tetracyclics				
Mianserin	Sedative	30	60	120?
Maprotiline	Mildly sedative	75	75	150
MAOIs				
Irreversible				
Tranylcypromine	Alerting	10 b.d.	30	60
Phenelzine	Alerting	15 b.d.	45	60
Reversible				
Moclobemide	Neither	300	150 b.d.	600
SSRIs				
Fluoxetine	Neither	20	20	80
Fluvoxamine	Neither	100	100 t.i.d.	300
Paroxetine	Neither	20	20	50
Sertraline	Neither	50	50	200
Citalopram	Neither	20	20	60
Escitalopram	Neither	10	10	20
Phenylpiperazines				
Trazodone	Sedative	100	200	600
SNRIs				
Venlafaxine	Neither	75	75	375 (taken in divided doses)
Venlafaxine XL	Neither	75	75	225 (XL is taken once per day)
NaSSAs				
Mirtazepine	Sedative	15	30	45
NaRIs				
Reboxetine	Slightly alerting	4 b.d.	8	12

and those with idiosyncratic reactions should be prescribed lower doses but these are the exception and do not invalidate the general principles. The usual practice is to begin with the recognised starting dose and to increase this to the therapeutic dose after 5–7 days. Despite claims that patients do not tolerate these doses, warning of the possible side effects and of the delay in onset enhances compliance dramatically although this may be less relevant now that the speed of onset of action is much enhanced with the newer antidepressants such as escitalopram and venlafaxine.

Tricyclic antidepressants

Tricyclic antidepressants are widely used in the treatment of depressive illness. They should not be used where serious contraindications exist such as glaucoma or cardiac arrhythmias. Neither should they be prescribed where there is a risk of overdose in view of their toxicity. Postural hypotension is sometimes also problematic, leading to dizziness. Some of their side effects can be used to advantage such as their hypnotic and sedative effects in bringing about rapid relief from the insomnia and anxiety associated with depressive illness. Indeed the hypnotic effect is immediate, the anxiolytic effect becomes apparent in three to four days and the antidepressant effect after 14 or more days. Lofepramine is the exception among tricyclic antidepressants having fewer sedative or anticholinergic effects than its older counterparts.

The rule that if one tricyclic fails there is little point in prescribing another is an over-simplification. If the reason for failure has been non-compliance due to side effects, then there is a good reason for prescribing another with a different profile. For example a patient may be unable to tolerate a drug because of accompanying insomnia and replacing it with a more sedative tricyclic may overcome this. If however the failure to respond is a true therapeutic failure then a change to a different group is indicated.

Most tricyclics (except lofepramine) can be prescribed in a once daily dose. Common sense dictates that the alerting antidepressants should not be prescribed at night and are best avoided after mid-afternoon. There may of course be individual differences but the principles outlined here apply to the generality of patients.

Selective Serotonin Reuptake Inhibitors (SSRIs)

The launch of the SSRIs in the mid-1980s heralded a major advance in the treatment of depressive illness, but also in the treatment of other disorders such as obsessive–compulsive disorder (see Chapter 14), panic disorder (see Chapter 8), PTSD (see Chapter 5) and bulimia nervosa (see Chapter 14). These advances stem from the side effects profile rather than from their speed of onset or their efficacy which are similar to the tricyclics. The absence of anticholinergic effects makes them suitable for use in those with cardiac arrhythmias or glaucoma. Some elderly patients with limited intellectual reserves may develop confusion in association with the anticholinergic properties of the tricyclic antidepressants and the SSRIs are especially useful in this group. In addition they are not toxic in overdose but care must be exercised in this regard lest a false sense of security is instilled in the prescribing doctor. They should not be prescribed when a patient is suicidal since the sufferer may die by some other means; rather an urgent psychiatric referral should be requested and hospitalisation may be necessary while the antidepressant takes effect.

A disadvantage of the SSRIs is the absence of sedative properties and the reported increase in anxiety in the early stages of treatment, sometimes necessitating hypnotics initially. Sedative and anxiolytic effects become apparent once the antidepressant effect is established. Common side effects are nausea, headaches, anxiety, restlessness and sexual dysfunction. Extrapyramidal side effects and discontinuation symptoms have been reported with both tricyclics and SSRIs although this does not imply dependence due to the absence of craving or tolerance, as patients often believe. Caution should be exercised in combining them with tricyclic antidepressants as the combination may cause a serotonin syndrome, characterised by restlessness, tremor, shivering, myoclonus, convulsions and possibly death. As with the tricyclic antidepressants it is advisable to become familiar with a few of the current products available. There are concerns however that the older SSRIs are not as potent in treating severe depression as the tricyclics and there may be wear-off in the effects over time, although neither of these have been definitively confirmed. A new SSRI, escitalopram, is unique among the SSRIs in having a more rapid onset of action, showing an effect within one week. It is also possibly more potent than the older SSRIs, bringing about total remission in both symptoms and social dysfunction.

Tetracyclic and phenylpiperazine antidepressants

The tetracyclics do not have any anticholinergic side effects but are sedating. Unlike the tricyclic antidepressants and the SSRIs they do not block the reuptake of 5HT but block postsynaptic noradrenaline and 5HT receptors. Mianserin is the best known tetracyclic but because of occasional leucopenia it is recommended that white cell counts be monitored monthly for the first 3 months of treatment. Trazodone and nefazadone belong to the phenylpiperazine groups and although sedating do not have any anticholinergic properties, making them useful in those with cardiac arrhythmias and with glaucoma. These act by blocking $5HT_2$ receptors and inhibiting the reuptake of 5HT and the most common side effects are dry mouth, nausea, drowsiness and dizziness.

Monoamine Oxidase Inhibitors (MAOIs)

These are divided into two groups: the irreversible and reversible MAOIs on the basis of their capacity to deactivate monoamine oxidase, an enzyme involved in the metabolism of 5HT, dopamine and noradrenaline. The irreversible MAOIs are not used as frequently as the other antidepressants because of their potential for serious interaction with foods and with other drugs. However they are very useful in specific situations especially in treating refractory depression, when anxiety predominates (see Table 6.3), in atypical depression and possibly in dysthymia. The newer reversible MAOIs, of which moclobemide is the best known, do not have any specific indications but are effective in depressive illness generally. Their advantage is that they do not have the food or drug interactions of their predecessors.

Table 6.3. Drug combinations useful in treating resistant depression.

- Lithium plus a tricyclic antidepressant (lithium level 0.4-0.6 mmol/l)
- An MAOI plus a tricyclic (tranylcypromine, imipramine or clomipramine should not be included in the combination)
- Add tri-iodothyronine (20-50 µg/day)
- Fluoxetine and olanzapine
- Add L-tryptophan (named patient basis)
- Add mirtazepine
- Reboxetine plus an SSRI
- Add lamotrigine

In the past 5 years there has been a surge in the number of new antidepressants on the market. These act variously on the serotonergic and/or the noradrenergic systems.

Serotonergic Noradrenergic Reuptake Inhibitors (SNRIs)

Venlafaxine is the only available antidepressant belonging to this group, so-called because it acts on both the serotonergic and noradrenergic systems blocking the re-uptake of these respective neurotransmitters. Unlike the tricyclics they have no effect on the histaminergic, the α_1-adrenergic or the muscarininc receptors. Serotonergic blockade occurs at low doses; at medium doses both serotonergic and noradrenergic blockades are inhibited, and at high doses dopamine re-uptake is also inhibited. The common side effects include nausea (must be taken with food), headache, sexual dysfunction, agitation and insomnia. On the positive side venlafaxine has a rapid onset of action, usually within one week and may bring about total remission quickly. It is very useful in all types of depression including refractory depression. Unlike other antidepressants, there is a dose response curve so the dose is chosen according to clinical need. A disadvantage is the discontinuation syndrome that may occur and the fact that it is sleep neutral may necessitate a hypnotic in the early stages of treatment.

Noradrenergic Specific Serotonergic Antidepressants (NaSSAs)

Mirtazepine is the only NaSSA available at present. It acts by antagonising the α_2-receptors (themselves autoreceptors) resulting in an increase in noradrenergic and the $5HT_{1A}$-mediated neurotransmission, both desirable properties in antidepressants. In addition it antagonises $5HT_2$ and $5HT_3$ improving its tolerability compared with SSRIs. It also has antihistaminergic properties, which counteract the anxiogenic effects of noradrenaline and contribute to sedation. However this property can also cause weight gain. Unlike other antidepressants which increase the uptake of neurotransmitters, mirtazepine achieves its antidepressant effect by blocking the α_2-receptors. It is useful especially in depressive illness with insomnia or with anxiety and panic attacks, due to the sedation that occurs at the starting dose. This decreases as the dose increases. As well as being associated with weight gain and requiring caution in those with diabetes, it should be prescribed with caution in immuno-compromised patients due to the rare complication of agranulocytosis.

Noradrenergic Reuptake Inhibitors (NaRIs)

Reboxetine is the only antidepressant in this group so far. Its benefits in treating depression are believed to extend to social functioning due to its impact on motivation mediated through its noradrenergic uptake inhibition. It has the advantage of having no interaction with alcohol.

Combination drug therapy and refractory depression

Resistant depression is defined as any depressive episode which fails to respond to a trial of two antidepressants from different classes given for an adequate period of time and in adequate dosage. The management of this condition rarely falls entirely to the general practitioner since failure to respond to treatment is one of the common reasons for referral to the psychiatric services. A number of drug combinations have been found to be helpful and are listed in Table 6.3. These include augmentation with tri-iodothyronine (T3) since the addition of 20–50 µg can convert a non-responder to a responder. Until recently L-tryptophan was used to augment the tricyclics but this has now been taken off the market and is only available on a 'named patient' basis. In all of those combinations involving lithium the serum level can be lower than that required for prophylaxis. Studies have also confirmed the potential usefulness of mirtazepine as an augmentation strategy in those with refractory depression and others suggest that a combination of reboxetine and an SSRI are possible combinations also.

Cognitive therapy

This is the currently sought after treatment for depression, partly because it does not involve drug taking, but also because of its claims to reduce the risk of relapse. Aaron Beck first described the technique and immediately it was the subject of controlled trials in combination with antidepressants and on its own. It is based on the hypothesis that the way we think affects our feelings. It is thus the opposite to the usual approach to depression where our moods are believed to affect how we perceive ourselves and the world. Some cognitive therapists suggest that the two views are not incompatible and that once in train the negative cognitions and the low mood reinforce each other. Therapy aims to examine these cognitions and the assumptions about confidence, self-worth, etc., that accrue from them. The difficulty is that therapy is very labour-intensive and up to 30 hours of treatment may be necessary before symptoms resolve. The other stumbling block is that only mild or moderate depression seems to respond. Cognitive therapy has also been used to prevent relapse in those with bipolar disorder while also receiving lithium. The general practitioner inevitably is not in a position to undertake this specialist treatment and referral to the secondary services is required.

A recent study (Dowrick *et al.*, 2001) examined the role of problem solving, a type of cognitive therapy that focuses on the problems causing and resulting from depression and on strategies for dealing with these. The therapists require special training and the one-to-one sessions took place over several weeks. The results were positive in the short term, but at one year follow-up there was no difference between treatment as usual (from the general practitioner) and problem solving. Clearly this approach is worthy of further investigation.

Physical

Electroconvulsive treatment (ECT) has unfortunately received an adverse press in recent years. It is not routinely used in treating depression but is very successful as an emergency method where life is at risk either from suicide, starvation or dehydration or where psychotic features are present. It should not be used unless depression is considered severe and a positive outcome is most likely when the typical biological symptoms are present. It does not prevent relapse and for this reason antidepressants are prescribed in conjunction and must be continued for at least 9 months. There is no definite evidence that brain damage occurs even with repeated usage of ECT.

A recent development has been the use of repetitive transcranial magnetic stimulation (rTMS) in which a controlled, rapidly fluctuating magnetic field is generated using a hand held coil. The left prefrontal cortex is targeted and preliminary studies suggest that it may be a safer and more acceptable alternative to ECT. It is not yet available at centres in Britain or Ireland and it remains to be seen if larger studies will confirm the promise that is presently held out.

NATURAL HISTORY

The mortality from untreated severe depressive illness is about 7% depending on the study and this emphasises the importance of adequate treatment as mood disorders have a close relationship to suicide. Among those with bipolar illness the periods between episodes tend to shorten in the early years of the illness but subsequently increase. Some patients, known as rapid cyclers, have individual episodes in quick succession and have a poorer prognosis than slow cyclers. The definition of rapid cycling is four alternating episodes in 12 months. Before the introduction of modern treatments the episodes of depression or elation remitted spontaneously in many cases.

PROPHYLAXIS

Prophylaxis in unipolar disorder

Those with recurrent severe unipolar depression may derive benefit from long-term antidepressants or, if these fail, from lithium although it may be less successful than in those with bipolar illness. The rule of thumb for prescribing long-term antidepressants is the occurrence of three or more episodes of depression in 5 years although even less frequent episodes may require prophylaxis if the symptoms during episodes are very severe and there are other risk factors for recurrence such as a family history of mood disorders.

Prophylaxis in bipolar disorder

Lithium is the longest established and most widely used prophylactic although there are problems associated with its use including its partial benefit or ineffectiveness in about one-third of patients, especially in those with rapid cycling disorder. In addition sudden discontinuation can provoke rebound mania although this can be lessened if withdrawal is gradual over a period of 2-4 weeks. Earlier concerns about treatment resistance to its prophylactic effect following discontinuation have receded. Recent studies suggest that lithium may be less teratogenic than was previously thought provided levels are carefully monitored and kept within the therapeutic range, nevertheless great care must be exercised when the possibility of pregnancy arises. It can be reinstated in the second trimester and should be discontinued again before delivery. Careful monitoring is required as renal function changes during pregnancy and toxicity may occur. Lithium salts are excreted in breast milk and bottle feeding of the newborn is to be preferred. Abnormalities of thyroid function are not absolute contraindications to lithium prophylaxis but do necessitate closer monitoring. Although there have been claims of renal damage occurring even with doses in the therapeutic range, it is now believed that these have been exaggerated and that they are unlikely unless function was already compromised at the outset of treatment or if toxicity occurred. Table 6.4 outlines the possible adverse effects of lithium.

Generally speaking, lifelong treatment with lithium is required and there are now numerous studies showing that, despite many years of treatment, discontinuation of lithium results in relapse. Its narrow therapeutic window and associated toxicity make it a less than ideal drug for prophylaxis. In addition, compliance has been shown to be poor and patients often complain of feeling slowed up.

For optimal prophylaxis blood levels between 0.8–1 mmol/l are required. Some may achieve control in the lower range of 0.4–0.6 mmol/l although the likelihood of relapse is generally higher in the low dose range. There is little to choose between once daily and multiple dosing in relation to prophylaxis but polyuria is less with single dosing. Blood levels should be checked as close to 12 hours following the last dose as possible, roughly every 3 months. Thyroid, cardiac and renal function should be checked annually as well as before treatment initiation.

Table 6.4. Adverse effects of lithium.

Side effects	Toxic effects[a]
Fine tremor[b]	Nausea and vomiting
Thirst and polyuria	Ataxia and impaired coordination
Hypothyroidism	Dysarthria
Teratogenesis	Coarse tremor
Weight gain	Muscle twitching
Emotional dulling	Fits
Leucocytosis	Nephropathy
Nephrogenic diabetes insipidus	Confusion
Rashes, especially psoriasis	Hyperreflexia and nystagmus
Cardiac arrhythmias	Coma

[a]These occur when the serum levels exceed 1.3 mmol/l but may occur with levels in the therapeutic range in some patients.
[b]This may be treated with propranolol.

Lithium is also used in partially responsive or non-responsive depressive illness (termed augmentation). Up to 50% of those treated in this way are responsive and all types of depression, with or without psychotic features, single or recurrent, severe or moderate, benefit. The blood level seems to be less important than in prophylaxis although a level above 0.4 mmols/l is suggested with the ultimate dose based on clinical response. Often the effect is noticed within a few days and 4–6 weeks is considered an adequate trial.

Other agents have been increasingly used, of which carbamazepine is the best known. It is now licensed for prophylaxis in bipolar disorder and is said to be more effective than lithium in those with rapid cycling disorder. However some authors have suggested that its efficacy may fade over time. Side effects include dizziness, blurred vision, ataxia, rashes and gastrointestinal disturbances and these are dose related. It can also precipitate Stevens–Johnson syndrome, blood dyscrasias and toxic epidermal necrolysis. In addition to being metabolised by the cytochrome P-450 it may reduce the effectiveness of other drugs metabolised in the same pathway by enzyme induction. These include other anticonvulsants and the oral contraceptives. It can also be teratogenic and folate is recommended in women contemplating pregnancy.

Sodium valproate is now the leading mood stabiliser in the USA although the bulk of evidence for its efficacy in prophylaxis comes from open trials. It is well tolerated and the commonest side effects are nausea, ataxia, gastrointestinal disturbance and tremor. Weight gain may also occur due to increased appetite. Less common side effects include thrombocytopenia, impaired platelet function, hair loss and the development of curly hair. Due to its impact on liver function it cannot be used in those with liver disease or a family history of same. It may elevate the plasma levels of other anticonvulsants and increase the anticoagulant effects of warfarin. It too is teratogenic and folate supplementation is required.

Lamotrigine has been found to be effective in bipolar disorder and has recently received a licence for prophylaxis, especially where depressive episodes have predominated. The most common side effects are headache, nausea, diplopia, dizziness and ataxia. Tiredness may also occur as may skin rashes, the latter in the early phase of treatment. It may also rarely lead to generalised illnesses such as angio-oedema and Stevens–Johnson syndrome and first trimester exposure may lead to teratogenesis making folate supplements essential in those planning pregnancy. It does not induce cytochrome P-450 enzymes although its metabolism is induced by carbamazepine and valproate.

In general, blood levels for the anticonvulsants are less important in the prophylaxis of bipolar disorder than they are for lithium, and therapeutic levels have not been established. A full blood count, renal and liver function and cardiac evaluation are required prior to commencing therapy with carbamazepine. Since leucopenia is a rare but dangerous side effect 'a white cell' count is advisable at regular intervals. Before commencing valproate and during the first 6 months of treatment, liver function should be monitored. Full blood count, liver function and renal function should be assessed at baseline before lamotrigine is introduced but there is no requirement for further evaluations thereafter.

In general, combination treatments that include lithium and another mood stabiliser are more effective than monotherapy although the down-side is that side effects and toxicity increase. Unlike lithium discontinuation, there is little evidence of rebound mania when anticonvulsants are withdrawn. The biggest evidence base for effectiveness lies with lamotrigine although large trials of the other mood stabilisers continue. Lithium remains the first choice for long-term prophylaxis in bipolar disorder but for rapid cycling or for treatment resistant bipolar disorder, then anticonvulsants, alone or in combination with lithium, are playing an increasing role.

RECOVERY AND PROGNOSIS (DEPRESSIVE EPISODE)

Full recovery takes several months although symptomatic improvement occurs relatively quickly and is usually noticed within two to three weeks of beginning treatment. The delay is due to the lag in social recovery and close questioning of the patient will reveal that although sleep, appetite and mood disturbance have gone, the patient still feels unable to cope totally with housework, employment or many of the other aspects of life which involve social functioning. The patient who expresses concern at returning to work, for example, is not being lazy but showing residual depressive illness. Failure to appreciate that symptoms and functioning do not show a synchronised improvement may cause harsh judgements and bad advice to be foisted upon the patient. This has important implications for practicalities about such matters as returning to work, or resuming social engagements, etc.

The outcome of individual episodes of depressive illness is good and full remission can be achieved in about two-thirds of patients (Limosin *et al.*, 2004). However, follow-up studies confirm a high relapse rate (Wilson *et al.*, 2003) with almost 25% having a recurrence over the subsequent 5 years demonstrating that even in a primary care setting depressive illness is a chronic and relapsing disorder pointing to the need for adequate prophylaxis. Interestingly those who are recognised as having depression fare no better than those not recognised (Dowrick and Buchan, 1995), pointing to the possibility that failure to make this diagnosis may be related to the wider context in which symptoms of depression are seen in primary care, often as short lived responses to stressful events (adjustment disorders) not warranting any formal intervention. A small but important group, less than 15% of those with severe depression, become chronically ill despite aggressive treatment. Outcome is governed by a number of factors including the inherent biological process of the illness, the presence or absence of personality disorder and the adequacy of the support the patient receives from family, friends and social environment.

DIFFERENTIAL DIAGNOSIS

Adjustment reactions

Adjustment reactions are the most difficult to distinguish from depressive illness since most of the aetiological factors are common to both disorders. In particular the presence of a stressor, which may be chronic, confounds the issue. The reactivity of the mood is probably the most helpful symptom in distinguishing one from the other although there is no symptom which is pathognomonic of either. Many textbooks point to the significance of a mood change which is disproportionate to the precipitant and which, it is claimed, is the hallmark of depressive illness. In the author's view this is an over-simplification and relies upon a personal judgement which may be value laden or naïve (see Chapter 5).

Anxiety

The pre-eminence of anxiety in depressive illness is another source of diagnostic confusion. Questions about accompanying symptoms such as sleep, appetite and mood changes will clarify the diagnosis as will the presence of morning intensification of anxiety or depression. The age of the patient may also be of assistance since anxiety disorders do not begin after the age of 40 (see Chapter 8).

Personality disorder

Personality disorder may be offered as a diagnosis in those who are chronically depressed since it is recognised that depression, whether short lived or chronic, can alter personality until treatment has resolved the symptoms. In the absence of any history that the symptoms and behaviour have been present since adolescence a diagnosis of personality disorder is incorrect and serves only to 'justify' the failure of treatment rather than help the patient. There may of course be a co-existing personality disorder but evidence of a change in functioning is indicative of illness.

SUMMARY

1. Depressive illness is present in 3–17% of consulters depending on the methods and the country of study.
2. A significant proportion of depressed patients are unrecognised due to the mode of presentation, which is most commonly with physical complaints.
3. The aetiology of depressive illness is multifactorial and includes a combination of risk factors and triggers such as life events, absence of supports, physical illnesses and genetic predisposition, the latter especially in manic depression. Many patients do not have any obvious precipitant to their episodes of illness.
4. There is no evidence that illnesses precipitated by childbirth or any other event have a different prognosis from those without these provoking stressors. For this reason labels such as postnatal depression or reactive depression are best avoided.
5. There is convincing evidence for the effectiveness of antidepressants. Before medication is prescribed, time should be taken to explain the nature of the illness, the treatment and its side effects to the patient. This will improve compliance.
6. There has been an expansion in the available antidepressants in recent years and the GP should familiarise himself with their uses and risks.
7. Cognitive therapy is a non-drug form of therapy that is effective, but it is time-consuming and requires training.
8. Lithium is the drug most commonly used in the prophylaxis of bipolar disorder although anti- epileptic medications are now also used.

CASE HISTORIES

Case I

Mrs X was a 62 year-old lady who presented to her family doctor with a 2 year history of 3 stone weight loss and tiredness. She felt depressed and had both anorexia and insomnia (initial and late). She had married a few years earlier and had a good relationship with her husband. She did domestic work for a neighbour and was free from any worries, financial, family or otherwise. She had no previous contact with the medical or psychiatric services and seemed to have been well adjusted all her life. Extensive investigations by the local physician included blood picture, barium studies and endoscopies which were all normal. Failure to improve resulted in a second round of investigations similar to those already done. Again the results were negative. She was referred by her general practitioner to the psychiatric services at this point, not because he suspected any psychological problem but in view of the negative findings on physical investigation. An immediate diagnosis of depressive illness was made and she responded to a tetracyclic antidepressant. At the time of writing she had been returned to the care of her general practitioner and was symptom free. Attempts to discontinue her medication after 1 year resulted in a recurrence of the symptoms but increasing it again led to an improvement. It is recommended that she remain on this medication indefinitely.

Comments

This lady illustrates the severity of physical symptoms which may accompany depressive illness. The likely reason for the diagnosis being missed initially was the absence of any stresses and the good premorbid adjustment shown by this lady. It is important to remember that many patients have depressive illnesses without any precipitants and who in all other respects are stable. The dictum that 'she is not the type' is a dangerous myth!

Case 2

Mrs X was a 72 year-old woman who had become a widow 1 year earlier after a happy marriage of 42 years. Her husband had died of renal failure and she had been prepared for his death for several weeks. She had no prior contact with the psychiatric services and had a supportive family of four daughters. She and her husband had lived with her older daughter and family and relationships were excellent. At the time of his death she grieved normally – she went to his funeral, cried, visited his grave regularly and prayed for him. After 18 months she still cried for many hours each day, had trouble getting to sleep and had little interest in meeting her friends. She had lost about 1 stone in weight and was unable to concentrate. Her family had taken her on holiday but she got little pleasure from this. She was referred to the psychiatric services by a locum whom she had visited for a tonic . Her usual GP felt that she would improve with time and advised her to join a local widows' group. This she did but took little interest in the meetings. She cried throughout the first interview. She described a close relationship with her late husband although she viewed herself as being independent also. A diagnosis of depressive illness precipitated by bereavement was made and she responded to tricyclic antidepressants. Over 3 months she returned to her usual activities and at the time of writing was off all medication (she was treated for 12 months) and was symptom free. She still spoke of her loneliness for her husband but got comfort from praying for him each morning, from visiting his grave every month and from her dreams about him.

Comment

This lady illustrates the rule that a cause for depression is no reason for therapeutic inertia. Bereavement is a common cause of depressive illness although this complication occurs more commonly where there has been an ambivalent relationship. Her recovery was uneventful and the loneliness of which she spoke as well as her sources of comfort indicated a normal adjustment to the loss of this longstanding and happy marriage.

Case 3

Mr X was a 45 year-old married man with a 5 year history of not coping with work, low self esteem and anxiety. The difficulties at work resulted in occasional days off but there was no other noticeable effect. He felt his education at an expensive boarding school had been wasted and that he had learned little while there. He felt that his wife had made all the major decisions and he regarded himself as weak despite having risen to senior management in his firm of employers and being materially affluent. His anxiety was the most crippling aspect of his problems and prevented him going on holiday or even planning the following weekend. Anxiety was especially bad in the mornings and he believed it caused him to wake early each morning and to be excessively irritable at work. He felt depressed about his state but did not describe any diurnal swing to his mood state. He tended to overeat and was most contented when he went to bed, sleeping for up to 9 hours each night (2 hours more than usual). He had been well until 5 years earlier. His mother was not supportive and his only sister lived a bohemian existence in another country and he had little contact with her. His wife was supportive but she was disorganised about the house and he found this difficult being a tidy and well organised man. He failed to respond to tricyclic antidepressants in therapeutic doses prescribed by his general practitioner. A diagnosis of atypical depression was made and MAOIs were prescribed (phenelzine 45 mg b.d.). He made a dramatic recovery and his view of himself, his education and his future altered completely. At the time of writing his MAOI had been reduced to 15 mg b.d. and he was in the process of further reducing it. He remains symptom free.

Comment

The symptoms were by and large those of atypical depression and the author had the advantage of hindsight in deciding to prescribe MAOIs. This patient illustrates the longstanding nature of depressive illness and the effect it can have on the patient's view of himself. Because of the predominance of anxiety and unusual symptoms such as overeating these patients are often regarded as having personality disorders and remain untreated. A guide is the age of the patient and a clear cut history of a change in behaviour from normal.

See also Chapter 5, Case 1 and Chapter 8, Case 2.

REFERENCES

Angst, J., Gamma, A., Benazzi, F. *et al.* (2003). Towards a redefinition of sub-threshold bipolarity: epidemiology and proposed criteria for bipolar-11, minor bipolar disorders and hypomania. *Journal of Affective Disorders*, **73**, 136-146.

Beck, A.P. (1967). *Depression: Clinical, Experimental and Theoretical Aspects.* Harper and Row, New York.

Dowrick, C. and Buchan, I. (1995). Twelve month outcome of depression in general practice: does detection or disclosure make a difference? *British Medical Journal*, **311**, 1274-1276.

Dowrick, C., Dunn, G., Ayuso-Mateos, JL. *et al.* (2001). Problem solving and group psycho-education for depression: multicentre randomised controlled trial. Outcomes of Depression International Network (ODIN). *British Medical Journal*, **321**, 1450-1454.

Kessing, L.V. (2004). Severity of depressive episodes according to ICD-10: prediction of risk of relapse and suicide. *British Journal of Psychiatry*, **184**, 153–156.

Kessler, D., Lloyd. K., Lewis, G. and Gray, D.P. (1999). Cross-sectional study of symptom attribution and recognition of depression and anxiety in primary care. *British Medical Journal*, **318**, 436-439.

Limosin, F., Loze, J.Y., Zylberman-Bouhassira, M. *et al.* (2004). The course of depressive illness in general practice. *Canadian Medical Journal*, **49**, 119-123.

Paykel. E.S., Hollyman. J.A., Freeling. P. and Sedwick, P. (1988). Predictors of therapeutic benefit from amitriptyline in mild depression: a general practice placebo-controlled trial. *Journal of Affective Disorders*, **14**, 83–95.

Piver, A., Yatham, L.N. and Lam, R.W. (2002). Bipolar spectrum disorders. New perspectives. *Canadian Family Physician*, **48**, 896-904.

Simon, G. , Goldberg, D.P., Von Korff, M. and Ustun, T.B. (2002). Understanding cross national differences in depression prevalence. *Psychological Medicine*, **32**, 585-594.

Wilson, I., Duszynski, K. and Mant, A. (2003). A 5-year follow-up of general practice patients experiencing depression. *Family Practitioner*, **26**, 685-689.

FURTHER READING

Anderson, I.M. and Edwards, J.G. (2001). Guidelines for choice of selective serotonin reuptake inhibitors in depressive illness. *Advances in Psychiatric Treatment*, **7**, 170-180.

Rorsman, B., Grasbeck, A., Hagnell, O. *et al.* (1990). A prospective study of first-incidence depression. The Lundby Study, 1957–72. *British Journal of Psychiatry*, **156**, 336–342.

Tylee, A. and Freeling, P. (1989). The recognition, diagnosis and acknowledgement of depressive illness by general practitioners. In: Herbst, K. and Paykel, F. (Eds), *Depression: An Integrative Approach.* Heinemann Medical Books, Oxford.

SUGGESTED READING FOR PATIENTS

Bates, T. (1999). *Depression: The Common Sense Approach*. New Leaf, Dublin.
Jamison, K.R. (1997). *An Unquiet Mind. A Memoir of Moods and Madness*. Picador, London.
Salmans, S. (1997). *Depression: Questions You Have ... Answers You Need*. Thorsons, London.
McKeon, P. (1997). *Bipolar Disorder: A Practical Guide*. AWARE Publications, Dublin.
Wolpert, L. (1999). *Malignant Sadness*. Faber and Faber, London.

USEFUL WEBSITES FOR PATIENTS

Royal College of Psychiatrists' information on depression: www.rcpsych.ac.uk/info/dep.htm

Online support for those affected by bipolar disorder: www.pendulum.org

Online psychological services and information about major depression: www.psychology-net.org/major.html

Up-to-date information about depression: www.allaboutdepression.com

USEFUL CONTACTS

The Association for Post Natal Illness
(Provides information and offers one-to-one support from mothers who have been through postnatal depression)
25 Jerdan Place
Fulham
London SW6 1BE
Tel: 020 7386 0868
Email: info@apni.orh
Website: www.apni.org

Aware
(Provides information and support to people affected by depression in Ireland and Northern Ireland)
72 Lower Leeson Street
Dublin 2
Ireland
Helpline: 00 353 1 67661666
Tel: 00 353 1 661 7211
Email: info@aware.ie
Website: www.aware.ie

Depression Alliance (UK)
(Information, support and understanding for people who suffer with depression and for relatives who want to help)
35 Westminster Bridge Road
London SE1 7JB
Tel: 020 7633 0557
Fax: 020 7633 0559
Website: www.depressionalliance.org.uk

Depression Alliance (Scotland)
3 Grosvenor Gardens
Edinburgh EH12 5JU
Tel: 0131 467 3050

Depression Alliance Cymru (Wales)
11 Plas Melin
Westbourne Road
Whitchurch
Cardiff CF4 2BT
Tel: 02920 692891

Fellowship of Depressives Anonymous
(A national mutual support group for people suffering from depression)
Box FDAI
c/o Self-Help Nottingham
Ormiston House
32-36 Pelham Street
Nottingham NG1 2EG
Tel: 0870 774 4320
Fax: 0870 774 4319
Email: fdainfo@aol.com
Website: www.depressionanon.co.uk

Manic Depression Fellowship
Castle Works
21 St George's Road
London SE1 6ES
Tel: 020 7793 2600
Fax: 020 7793 2693
Email: mdf&mdf.org.uk
Website: www.mdf.org.uk

Manic Depression Fellowship (Wales)
1 Palmyra Place
Newport
South Wales NP20 4EJ
Tel: 01633 244244
Fax: 01633 244 111
Email: info@mdfwales.org.uk
Website:
www.manicdepressionwales.org.uk

Manic Depression Fellowship (Scotland)
Studio 1019
Mile End Mill
Seedhill Road
Paisley PA1 1TJ
Tel: 0141 560 2050
Fax: 0118 670 3666
Email: info@bipolarscotland.org.uk
Website: www.bipolarscotland.org.uk

7

Parasuicide and Suicide

Until the 1960s the traditional view was that every act of self-harm was a failed suicide attempt. This attitude was challenged by the emerging clinical impression that many 'suicide attempters' were prompted not only by a desire to self-destruct but by other motivations such as the wish to manipulate another, the desire to escape from problems, the non-verbal communication of distress and many others. The term parasuicide was coined to describe this behaviour, the motivation for which is heterogeneous. The definition of parasuicide is that it is any non-fatal act in which an individual deliberately causes self-injury or ingests a substance in excess of any prescribed or generally therapeutic dose. This definition includes experimental drug use since the ingestion of these substances is either not prescribed or, if prescribed, is taken in excess. The inclusion of this latter category is however open to criticism as being over-inclusive since drug abusers clinically represent a different constellation of problems. However the concept of parasuicide, which makes no assumptions about motivation, has found almost universal approval both for its pragmatism and its usefulness in clinical practice and research.

EPIDEMIOLOGY

Parasuicide is a behaviour which predominates in women, in those under 35 and in the divorced, single or separated. The association with unemployment and low social classes is well recognised although the mechanism for this is not understood. The episode generally occurs in the context of a family or personal crisis and for many it represents a repetitive behaviour pattern.

Many parasuicides are treated either by the general practitioner or in the Accident Department and official figures based on hospital records underestimate the number of parasuicide episodes by up to 30%. A further source of attrition is the number who self-discharge before emergency assessment. This results in an underestimation of about 12% of episodes. A precise prevalence is thus difficult to obtain although careful recording of hospitalised parasuicides in Oxford estimate rates of about 250/100,000 for men and 450/100,000 for women in 2003 with some fluctuation over time (Hawton *et al.*, 2003). The female excess may be less apparent if descriptive data were based on the total parasuicide population rather than the hospitalised group. Parasuicide rates are highest in the under 35 age group and show an inverse relationship with social class. Rates vary with marital status with the divorced and single being most at risk. A past history of violence to others is increasingly a feature, especially in women who self-harm.

Parasuicide is estimated to account for over 100,000 hospital admissions each year in England and Wales. The seasonal variation in suicide has long been recognised but recently a similar variation has been described for parasuicide. A peak in late spring/early summer and a trough in late December/January have been shown for women and these are probably related to the sense of purpose which is associated with the traditional role of women at Christmas.

Repetition is frequent with 15–20% having a recurrence of parasuicide annually and this is especially associated with male gender, personality disorder and lower social class. The risk of repetition is highest in the immediate period following the index episode and a clustering of episodes is often observed. Over a year 1% will successfully commit suicide, especially in the period immediately following an earlier episode. Attempts at predicting repetition or suicide by devising and applying scales have so far proved unsuccessful although further efforts to do so continue.

METHODS

Overdosing still remains the most common method of parasuicide accounting for about 90% of episodes among women and slightly fewer among men. Antidepressants, especially the SSRIs, minor tranquillisers and paracetamol are most often used in both Britain and Ireland. Wrist-cutting is next in frequency accounting for 10% of the total and it is this latter group who often indulge in multiple attempts, presenting a difficult clinical challenge.

CLINICAL DIAGNOSIS

The most frequent diagnosis is that of adjustment disorder. Other axis 1 diagnoses are uncommon and if present are usually affective in nature. Axis 2 diagnoses, i.e. personality disorders, are present in up to 65% of patients. Between 3% and 10% are drug abusers and up to 22% are alcohol abusers. As well as being used to bring about relief from distressing symptoms, the simultaneous disinhibiting and depressing effects of alcohol result in its use at the time of the act in up to 30% of victims. It is crucial that those with treatable affective disorders are identified since this group would be at particular risk of suicide following the index episode.

Who is referred for specialist help?

General practitioners frequently undertake the treatment of the parasuicide patient themselves, especially in rural areas. However, self-poisoners rather than those using other methods are more likely to be referred for specialist medical/psychiatric attention, as are those parasuiciding for the first time, those without a family history of psychiatric disturbance and those from lower social classes. The relative lack of a family history or of a previous history of parasuicide suggest that general practitioners perceive hospitalisation with its attendant psychiatric assessment as having a potential preventive role for further episodes. Unfortunately this expectation is not fulfilled and there is no convincing evidence that admission *per se* reduces the risk of repetition. In view of the onus placed upon the practitioner, the competent assessment of parasuicide is imperative. In general hospitals these assessment are increasingly carried out by psychiatric nurse specialists (McDonough *et al.*, 2004) who have received training and have access to ongoing supervision. This is supplemented by psychiatrists, as required, and in cases of uncertainty.

AETIOLOGY OF PARASUIDICE

The aetiology of parasuicide is complex and ill-understood and can be divided in general risk factors and precipitants. The most common risk factors are social and include unemployment and social disintegration or anomie (normlessness), a term used by Durkheim (1951) in his work on suicide. Evidence for the importance of societal norms in controlling suicidal behaviour comes from the findings that it is highest in inner cities where the correlates of anomie (non-marital births, crime, unemployment and divorce) are prominent. The relationship to poverty independent of these factors remains unproven. A history of sexual abuse is often present in those who cut themselves, in particular.

Other possible theories focus on the personal meaning such an act may have, and the idea of the 'cry for help' has now become a cliché, although so far unsubstantiated. Messages other than a behavioural plea for assistance may also be conveyed by parasuicide and individuals who have poor verbal skills, who are devoid of close relationships and who have poor social skills may use this behaviour as a method of controlling or of bringing about change in their environment.

Psychological studies have examined the thought processes in those who parasuicide and found deficits in problem solving and, in particular, identified inflexible thinking leading to impairment in generating responses to stress. This cognitive approach is increasingly forming the basis for interventions aimed at reducing repetition and may also explain the association between parasuicide and personality disorder. Biological research has investigated the role of serotonin and of noradrenaline in impulsivity, leading to suicidal behaviour.

Most episodes of parasuicide are precipitated by some event, in particular those relating to interpersonal relationships. An episode which is apparently without an obvious trigger should be viewed with caution and may indicate a serious attempt at suicide stemming from an underlying depressive illness.

SUICIDE RISK ASSESSMENT

If the patient is admitted to hospital this will not ordinarily be a problem for the general practitioner since most are assessed while in the Accident Department. If the patient self-discharges or presents to the family doctor after the medical effects have worn off the practitioner will then have to make an assessment of the patient's suicide risk and of any possible treatment which may be necessary. The psychiatric assessment of parasuicide is considered under the four headings which follow.

Suicide ideation

The presence of suicide ideation should be assessed in every patient presenting to the general practitioner with an emotional problem. Many patients will describe unfocused, fleeting thoughts in the absence of any active wish or plan to kill oneself. The patient might say 'I wish I could go to sleep and not wake up' or 'I wish I were dead' but without any further elaboration. These are referred to as passive death wishes. Nevertheless inquiry must be made about more serious active death wishes which include detailed plans to execute the act, plans to avoid discovery, and even final plans about saying goodbye. In the event of an act of parasuicide a full assessment of the act itself must be made in order to identify those acts of high intent.

Suicide intent

This is the most pressing concern if completed suicide is to be avoided in the immediate post-parasuicide phase. The question 'Is the patient currently suicidal?' may be answered by considering the degree of intent at the time of the act and by assessment of the current suicidal ideation. Reticence surrounding direct questions relating to present suicidality is misguided and far from increasing the likelihood of a future attempt, failure to ask may lead to missing the seriously suicidal patient. The presence of a suicide note, indications of final plans, such as a will, and careful execution of the attempt alert one to a high intent to commit suicide. The medical seriousness may not be related to intent and an assessment of the patient's concept of medical lethality must be made. Violent methods are generally believed to be evidence of high intent along with the absence of another person in the vicinity and attempts to conceal the episode. Questions about the patient's current attitude to the episode, to living and dying and to their view of the future increase the precision of the evaluation. In particular the symptom of hopelessness has been consistently found to predict high intent and must be viewed with gravity. Sometimes when the patient has reached the decision to take his own life, in other words there is no longer any conflict between the wish to live or to die, the person appears calm and at peace when speaking of suicide. The significance of this may easily be missed by the inexperienced doctor as agitation is more common than tranquility in those who are actively suicidal. The person with high suicide intent must be hospitalised as a life-saving measure irrespective of whether a psychiatric illness is deemed to be present or not since even those who are enveloped in a temporary crisis may be actively suicidal and this may intensify if alcohol is consumed.

Psychiatric illness

Psychiatric illness, with the exception of adjustment disorder, is uncommon in parasuicide patients. Irrespective of the level of intent, an attempt must be made to assess any treatable underlying illness. Inevitably high intent is frequently associate with psychiatric illness, most commonly affective and this should be ruled out by the usual questions relating to appetite, sleep, etc. The importance of hopelessness has already been emphasised. Some patients at the time of assessment do not exhibit much by way of depressive affect or suicidal ideation but a recent history of such symptoms or brittleness of mood should alert the doctor to the suicide potential. In these circumstances the practitioner may not wish to commence treatment and may wish instead to refer the patient to the local psychiatrist. If the general practitioner decides to treat the patient himself, such as when intent has been found to be low, the parasuicide co-incidental to illness or occurring several weeks earlier, then the risk of further self-harm must be re-evaluated. If repeat overdose is a possibility the SSRIs, SNRIs, NaRIs or NaSSAs should be used. Psychotic illnesses, although uncommon, should always be referred for full assessment and treatment irrespective of the level of suicide intent.

Social problems

By far the largest component in the assessment will be an evaluation of the social difficulties the patient is experiencing. Social problems including poor housing, unemployment, alcohol abuse, and marital disharmony are frequent concomitants to parasuicide. Social isolation is of special significance since it suggests the absence of support at times of crisis. This does not mean geographical or physical isolation but refers to loneliness and is especially significant in the elderly and infirm. The practitioner may have to involve social services and local voluntary organisations in attempting to bring about change in the patient's social environment and in providing companionship to the lonely.

The general practitioner and prevention

Most of those who self-harm do not receive hospital follow-up and are returned to the care of their general practitioners. Of the approximately 30 % who are referred to the psychiatric services following emergency assessment, only about one-third keep the appointment. By contrast, however, those who are returned to their general practitioner for follow-up have a high rate of consultation with 33% attending within one week following discharge from casualty and over 50% within 4 weeks (Gunnell *et al.*, 2002). Most discuss the reason for the episode of self-harm and report the consultation as helpful (Houston *et al.*, 2003). This high consultation rate places general practitioners at the forefront in identifying those with major psychiatric disorders or those who might be at risk of subsequent suicidal behaviour. While parasuicide repetition cannot be predicted, the possibility of developing focused psychological interventions for those at risk of repetition should be considered. In particular the high rate of consultation suggests that primary care might be a more effective outlet through which to deliver such interventions.

Interventions

There have been many systematic studies of attempts to reduce the repetition of parasuicide. These have included task-oriented case work, behaviour therapy and insight therapy. Most successful have been problem solving or cognitive-behaviour therapy (Linehan *et al.*, 1993) although when controlled trials of adequate sample size are used cognitive therapy (in manualised form) was no more effective than treatment as usual but was more cost-effective (Tyrer *et al.*, 2003). These therapies require specialist training and packages are not yet available for use by general practitioners.

A further reason for assessing each parasuicide act is to reduce the risk of completed suicide in the immediate aftermath and there is evidence that this goal can be achieved in the short term (Suokas and Lonnqvist, 1991). The long-term prediction of suicide is impossible due to the problems inherent in predicting rare events and this group remains at high risk of suicide, in particular men with high initial suicide intent and a history of psychiatric illness (Suokas *et al.*, 2001). There is no evidence that the Samaritans prevent suicide although there are humanitarian reasons for welcoming the establishment of that organisation. For individual patients the best approach to secondary prevention is to prescribe with circumspection and to respond in a supportive way at times of crisis. The detection and treatment of illnesses, such as depressive illness, which may place the patient at risk, need to be reiterated as does the appropriate assessment of the episode. Advice to the effect that the patient should 'do it properly next time' is crass, insensitive and irresponsible.

SUICIDE

Despite public concern, suicide is still uncommon and the individual practitioner will rarely be confronted with it. The rates worldwide have been fluctuating over the past 40 years. In England and Wales the rates decreased during the 1960s and 70s, only to increase for men until 1990, while falling among women. Between 1990 and 1997 the rates decreased for both sexes in all age groups and in 1997 the male rate was 10.3/100,000 and for females was 2.9/100,000. These figures represent a reduction of 14% and 22%, respectively, since 1990, well within the targets set in *Health of the Nation* (McClure, 2000). Ireland has seen a dramatic increase in its suicide rate, due mainly to an increase in suicide in the 20–30 year age group among men and the standardised male suicide rate is now 23/100,000 while the female rate has been relatively stable over the past 15 years and stands at 4.5/100,000. This change has been attributed to changes in Irish life, both religious and social in recent years (Kelleher, 1996).

In all cultures those at particular risk are the divorced, widowed or single. Differences in social class rates have diminished and the highest rates are recorded in late spring and early summer, reflecting the peak for affective disorders. Some European studies have noted a biseasonal distribution for women, with a second peak in the autumn although this has not been replicated in Eastern countries. There is also evidence for the idea of 'copy-cat' suicide and the possibility that publicity about suicide might facilitate it in the suicidally ambivalent. This is known as the Werther effect.

Methods of suicide

Availability is the major determinant of methods of suicide and these have changed in the last 30 years. In Britain, domestic gas, which was detoxified in the 1960s, was replaced by car exhaust poisoning (carbon monoxide) until the mid 1990s. However, the introduction of catalytic convertors has led to a reduction in this method and hanging is now the method of choice among men while women continue to use more passive methods such as overdosing (McClure, 2000). In Ireland slightly different methods are used with men choosing hanging and drowning and women poisoning and hanging. In both Britain and Ireland antidepressants on their own are implicated in 4% of suicides and in 2.5% in combination with other substances. Concerns about the potential for at least some of the SSRIs to induce suicidal ideation and/or behaviour have not been substantiated following investigation of the data by the Food and Drugs Administration of the United States (Khan *et al.*, 2003). The increased risk of suicide in the early stage of treating depression stems not from any suicidogenic properties of the antidepressants themselves but from the disparity in response between motivation and suicidal thoughts, with the former improving before the latter.

Aetiology of suicide

Two aspects to the aetiology of suicide present themselves. The first explores the reasons for the general increase in suicide throughout Europe and the second explains why individuals die by their own hand, given that self-destruction is a rare event; in other words these theories address population versus individual trends in suicide.

Population studies and sociological theories

The doyen of the sociological theorists is Emil Durkheim (1951) whose work still underpins our understanding in this area. His theory of anomie, the loss of the force of normative values on society, is frequently used to explain the reduction in suicide at times of social cohesion, e.g. war, and the increase during periods of social disorganisation, e.g. economic recession. The current trends in suicide are believed to have resulted both from the present economic decline as well as the change in traditional mores and values – both reflecting aspects of anomie. The religious dimension has since been examined by other workers and the role of religious commitment in protecting against suicide confirmed scientifically. Current approaches to measuring anomie focus on social fragmentation and material deprivation although the former seems to have a greater impact than the latter (Whitley *et al.*, 1999).

A further theory – the egoistic theory – views social isolation as being of aetiological significance and may explain the high suicide rate in cities, in migrants and in the divorced and single. Current work on suicide has identified the role of isolation in individual suicides, and those who are bereft of close contacts must be considered at risk of suicide. The third component which Durkheim describes is the altruistic suicide. This is the use of self destruction to achieve an ideal, and classic examples of this are found in the suicide bombers of the Middle East. Such suicides are of little psychiatric importance since the victims are not psychiatrically ill in any recognisable sense and prevention does not rest with the medical profession.

The separatist view of suicide holds that sociological and psychiatric explorations of the aetiology of suicide are conflicting and mutually exclusive. The author does not subscribe to this analysis but believes the two to be complementary and that both enhance our understanding of this tragic behaviour. A sociological as well as a pharmacological basis for depressive illness is well recognised by most psychiatrists (see Chapter 6) and illustrates the interaction between both forces. The absence of confidants, the absence of religious beliefs, unemployment and loss of mother in childhood are aspects of anomie and egoism as described by Durkheim – such difficulties predispose to depression and also to suicide. It can be concluded that psychiatry provides clues to the cause of individual suicides, while sociology leads to an understanding of suicide trends in populations.

Individual trends

Recent research using the method of psychological autopsy has confirmed the earlier findings of the presence of psychiatric illness, especially alcohol abuse, depressive illness and schizophrenia in most victims of suicide. In addition, examination of personality status has figured in recent studies and axis 2 diagnoses co-occur in over 30% of victims although there is little information on which categories predominate (Henriksson *et al.*, 1993). Among those not in contact with psychiatric services about one-third have no current psychiatric illness, a figure much higher than was previously thought (Owens *et al.*, 2003)

Since depressive illness is the most common diagnosis among victims of suicide, government efforts have focused on the identification and aggressive treatment of this condition (see Chapter 6). At risk are those who describe hopelessness and guilt, and those in the early stages of recovery when lassitude has lifted and motivation has returned while other symptoms still persist. Among alcoholics it is the chronic middle aged alcoholic who is at particular risk and often the final action is precipitated by the conclusion of a relationship. In contrast to this group are the young schizophrenic patients who in a period of apparent well-being kill themselves using violent methods. It is believed that the presence of insight about the nature of the illness places this group at particular risk although post-schizophrenia depression is also likely to be a factor. The impulsiveness of the act in this group makes it difficult to predict.

The association between physical illness and suicide has been documented by many, particularly the presence of painful conditions or of cancer. However depression has been shown to co-occur in such patients and it is likely to be this that drives the suicidal behaviour. Some researchers have pointed to an increased risk of suicide among HIV-positive patients especially in the immediate aftermath of obtaining a positive result but others have failed to replicate this finding.

Although depressive illness has been overwhelmingly associated with suicide, recent studies point also to the role of co-occurring personality disorder, especially of borderline type, and alcohol abuse (Foster *et al.*, 1999). This has implications for prevention and this broader appreciation of the underpinnings of suicide may explain why national prescribing rates for antidepressants seem to have little impact on suicide rates (Van Praag, 2003).

Recently there has been a growth of interest in the biology of suicide and the role of serotonin in suicidal behaviour has been investigated as has that of noradrenaline and cholesterol but the results are as yet inconclusive especially in relation to the latter two variables.

RELATIONSHIP BETWEEN SUICIDE AND PARASUICIDE

For many years emphasis was placed on the separation between completed suicide and parasuicide and distinctions are evident from the epidemiological profile of each group, from the motivation and from the differing clinical status of each. However, this is an oversimplification and it is recognised that there is a small but important overlap between both populations. During a one year follow-up, roughly 1% of parasuicides will go on to kill themselves. Moreover, of those who do commit suicide, up to 50% have had prior parasuicides. Although many parasuicides do not wish to die, some are clearly ambivalent about life and have been saved from death only by the advances in resuscitation procedures. Further evidence of some overlap between suicide and parasuicide is the fact that almost 40% of those who subsequently kill themselves have been shown retrospectively to have attended a Casualty Department in the previous year for any reason, and some 15% for an episode of deliberate self-harm. In addition 5% of those who take their own lives have visited Casualty in the last month of life because of a deliberate self-harm episode (Gairin *et al.*, 2003). In general, the closer the resemblance sociodemographically and clinically between the parasuicide patient and completed suicide, the graver the risk. The prime risk factors include being male, elderly, socially isolated, physically or psychiatrically ill, hopeless and using violent means of parasuicide. The pitfalls of adhering to these naïvely will be discussed later (Case 2) although they are useful as general guidelines.

PREVENTION OF SUICIDE

The Department of Health in its White Paper *The Health of the Nation* published in 1992 set a target for a 15% reduction in suicide and current trends in England and Wales suggest that this target is being achieved. It is unclear if medical intervention is fully responsible for this given the rarity of the event, the low contact with the medical profession and the problems of prediction. Some have suggested that sociopolitical and moral considerations are likely to make a greater impact on prevention (Wilkinson, 1994) and point to the failure of antidepressants to dent national suicide rates internationally (Van Praag, 2003).

The *adequate assessment* of individual acts of parasuicide is of paramount importance if completed suicide is not to be the short-term outcome in such patients. This has been described already.

The necessity to *recognise* and *adequately treat depressive illness* is evident since such illnesses have a high mortality if untreated. Recognising this illness may be difficult at times especially when the presenting symptoms are physical rather than emotional. This is especially the case among general practice attenders. The neurotic/psychotic dichotomy, adhered to by so many, does not assist in diminishing suicide risk. The presence of even a single biological symptom, e.g. sleep disturbance, should alert the physician to make further enquiries about depressive symptomatology. Also the presence of unusual physical symptoms which do not constitute any of the commonly recognised medical syndromes along with a prior history of psychiatric disorder should arouse suspicion. Failure to ask the necessary questions about the common symptom constellation found in depression may result in a woeful disregard for the fatal potential in this illness.

The adequate treatment of depression necessitates the use of antidepressant drugs in therapeutic doses. There is some evidence that this medication is under-used in such patients and that anxiolytics are used in preference, especially when anxiety symptoms dominate the clinical picture. Anxiolytics have no part to play in the primary treatment of depressive illness and although safe in overdose, this is not a justification for the inappropriate treatment of this disorder. It is clear that at the commencement of treatment due care must be taken to assess the risk of suicide and if in doubt relatives must be given charge of medication and/or in-patient treatment sought. The importance of using therapeutic doses must also be highlighted since to underprescribe is to heighten the suicide risk especially among those with psychomotor retardation.

Much debate has centred around the possibility of *restricting the availability of potentially lethal substances* such as paracetamol. There is a convincing body of knowledge which holds that limiting the availability of these and similar drugs may prevent individual suicides and this is laudable. However, the likelihood that the overall rate would significantly diminish is in question since such attempts in relation to coal gas in Britain and Holland did not have any lasting impact. It is accepted that the methods of suicide reflect the current availability of lethal materials, e.g. firearms being the most common method in the USA, but when they are limited potential victims choose other available means. It would seem that the prevention of suicide and halting the increasing spiral must rely on methods other than legal restrictions.

COMMON PITFALLS

Failure to ask

There was an erroneous belief that enquiring about suicidal thoughts would increase the risk by suggesting this as an alternative strategy where otherwise it would not have been considered. Such fears have fortunately been widely repudiated. The most direct way of finding out about suicidal ideation is by such questioning. The patient may provide other clues but these are more likely to be demonstrated to those in close contact with the patient than to the physician. A common way of introducing such a line of questioning is to ask, 'Do you ever feel it is difficult to just go on?' or, 'Has life ever seemed hopeless?'. More direct questions about the exact thoughts, 'Did you ever feel that you would be better off dead?' or, 'Did you ever think you might harm yourself?' should then follow along with questions about the plans, if any, for executing this.

Understandability

The doctor who knows and understands his patient may feel that there are compelling reasons why he might choose to harm himself. He may feel that in the circumstances, taking into consideration the patient's personality and the stresses to which he is exposed, nothing can or should be done. He may feel that his distress is the direct result of these burdens. It should be remembered that treatable illness can be provoked by such stresses (see Case 1 below) and to ignore warnings of suicide in such people is tantamount to negligence. Moreover, many of these stresses are transitory and with support and counselling can be diminished. Thus, the understandability of the reasons for depression and suicidal thoughts/behaviour is not a justification for ignoring them.

Relying on predictors

Too frequently the doctor may feel that the patient does not exhibit the features commonly associated with completed suicide. Thus, confronted with a young married woman, he may feel that her gender, marital status and age are not among the commonly cited risk factors. However, since women are more likely to consult their doctors than men and as most will be married, it follows that relying on the common predictors will be seriously erroneous. In general, the well known risk factors are useful as general guidelines but may lull the unwary into complacency if relied upon too rigidly.

Ignoring warnings

The received wisdom that those who speak about suicide will not execute it is a myth which must be dispelled. It has been shown that those who successfully harm themselves give warnings which include direct threats and also indirect forewarnings such as refusing to buy new clothes, etc. These are ignored at the patient's peril. Since suicide victims have a high degree of contact with their doctors in the immediate period before the act, it behoves every doctor to be alert to these forebodings.

THE FAMILY OF THE VICTIM

Bereavement following suicide is frequently associated with many conflicting emotions. Feelings of guilt are the most common with family members wondering if they could have done more to prevent the tragedy. Others feel anger and shame and articulate thoughts such as, 'Why did he do this to me?' Work in this area has shown that the duration and severity of the grief are similar to that with any death but that relatives find the inquest the most distressing aspect of the aftermath.

Despite their initial feelings of guilt, anger and shame, they welcome the support and comfort of others. There is no evidence for an increase in psychiatric illness in the family following suicide although feelings of stigma and shame are common and in particular the method of reporting the suicide by the media and the inquest have been identified as particularly distressing (Harwood *et al.*, 2002).

When dealing with the family it is important to allow them 'space' to ventilate their true feelings. By articulating these they will eventually resolve them as with any other loss. Children are the most vulnerable family members and many will have been living in an environment which was far from satisfactory prior to the suicide. Many adults underestimate the child's capacity to understand and it is important to approach each child individually. Allowing the child time to grieve and answering his questions sympathetically is the most satisfactory approach if he too is not to carry the stigma of the parent's misfortune.

SUMMARY

1. Parasuicide is a behaviour with diverse motivations. The most urgent concern is that of suicide intent.
2. Suicide intent is assessed by direct questioning and where it is high the patient requires hospitalisation to reduce the immediate risk of suicide irrespective of whether illness is present or not.
3. Hopelessness is especially associated with the future risk of suicide.
4. Family and personal crises rather than psychiatric illness are the backdrop against which parasuicide occurs.
5. Attempts at primary and secondary prevention have so far failed.
6. Most completed suicides suffer from psychiatric illness of which depressive illness is the most common but co-occurring disorders such as personality disorder and alcohol abuse are important.
7. There is debate about the role of the doctors in suicide prevention and it is argued that a combined medical and sociopolitical approach is best.
8. The recognition and vigorous treatment of depressive illness is essential.

CASE HISTORIES

Case I

Mr X , a 58 year-old man, was referred as an emergency after he had decided to end his life by letting his car free-wheel down a steep hill which was traversed by a concrete wall at the bottom. He was deterred from completing this by seeing a boy who reminded him of his son as he neared the bottom. He damaged his car because he failed to prevent an impact with the wall although he was physically uninjured himself. He had been having serious financial difficulties for some months becoming bankrupt and with debt collectors pressing him for money. He decided the best way to resolve these problems was by suicide. On further questioning he had impaired concentration, which prevented him from going through his 'books'. His sleep was impaired with both initial and late insomnia. His wife was unsupportive and constantly harangued his employees so that there was a high turnover of staff who felt unable to work while she was involved. Her odd behaviour may have been explained by the fact that she was diagnosed some 4 months later with a frontal lobe tumor. At the time of her husband's referral she did not wish him to have any contact with the psychiatric services even though he explicitly told her of his thwarted intentions. He decided to remain in hospital where a diagnosis of a depressive episode was made, precipitated by financial problems. Tricyclic antidepressants were commenced but in view of his ongoing suicidal ideation a course of ECT was administered with remission in his symptoms and enabling him to examine his business difficulties realistically. He was discharged on an antidepressant and was asymptomatic at follow-up.

Comment

To the unwary his decision to end his life may have seemed the only reasonable way to deal with his difficulties since there was clear evidence of his dire financial problems and his wife was unsupportive. In this patient's case his mental state was preventing him from doing anything about his situation, e.g. going to his accountant and making the decision to declare himself bankrupt. Treating his illness facilitated this. The fear of suicide while awaiting antidepressants to work is a real one and ECT is frequently the most rapid treatment. Such patients must be prescribed antidepressants also as prophylaxis if relapse is to be avoided. This treatment should be continued for about 9 months and sometimes longer if symptoms recur on decreasing or discontinuing the medication.

Case 2

Mr X, a 30 year-old man, was admitted to a medical ward after an overdose of 15 paracetamol tablets following an argument with his homosexual partner who had left him saying their relationship was over. His overdose was impulsive using tablets from his own medicine cupboard. Prior to the row he was asymptomatic although he admitted to being emotionally dependent on his boyfriend. He was found by a friend who unexpectedly called to see him – the door was unlocked. At assessment he saw no hope for the future and still wished to die. He cried frequently during the interview and declared that he would jump from a bridge rather than face life without his lover. He refused admission for psychiatric assessment and was compulsorily admitted in view of the immediate risk of suicide. After 1 week he was calmer and beginning to plan his future without his partner. He agreed to long-term psychotherapy and medication was not prescribed.

Comment

A diagnosis of adjustment disorder along with a subsidiary (axis 2 in DSM IV) diagnosis of dependent personality disorder was made. This gentleman's reaction to his stressful event was extreme and while in a crisis he was unable to plan his future realistically. The suicide potential was considered high in view of his continuing threats and sense of hopelessness. Compulsory admission was therefore justified to prevent him from committing suicide. The absence of a depressive illness might have tempted some to discharge this man home arguing that his problems were situational and outside the realm of medicine. Compulsory admission in these circumstances should not be eschewed if it is life saving.

Case 3

Mrs X was a 39 year-old married woman with marital problems relating to her husband's drinking and infidelity. Two weeks earlier she had been prescribed antidepressants by her general practitioner because of a depressive illness. Her symptoms consisted of early wakening, diurnal mood swing, palpitations, loss of interest and impaired concentration. She did not have any suicidal ideation at the time this medication was prescribed. On the evening of the overdose she returned home to find a note from her husband saying that he had left to live with his new girlfriend. Mrs X went straight to the bathroom and took an overdose of 8 paraceta-mol tablets. She was alone at the time and shortly became frightened that she may have harmed herself permanently. She telephoned her mother who arranged her admission for medical treatment. The psychiatrist felt the general practitioner had correctly diagnosed a depressive illness and that the parasuicide was of low intent and secondary to the recent development with her husband rather than directly due to her depressive illness. Her husband made contact during her hospitalization and decided to return to her and have marriage counselling. Both in-patient and day care were offered but she declined both and admitted regret at the episode of self-harm. She was discharged home and her mother given charge of the medication. Out-patient follow-up and marriage counselling were arranged.

Comment

This case was complex in that suicide intent was low despite the presence of a definite depressive illness. There was the worry that this lady's impulsive behaviour was atypical and related to her pervasive despondency. Despite this concern she did not exhibit any further suicidal ideation and as the crisis which provoked it had resolved and it was considered inappropriate to pursue compulsory admission, she was discharged.

REFERENCES

Durkheim, E. (1951). *Suicide: a Study in Sociology* (translated by J. A. Spaulding and G. Simpson). Free Press, Glencoe, Illinois.

Foster, T., Gillespie, K., McClelland, R. and Patterson, C. (1999). Risk factors for suicide independent of DSM-III-R Axis I disorder. Case-control psychological autopsy study in Northern Ireland. *British Journal of Psychiatry*, **175**, 175–9.

Gairin, L., House, A. and Owens, A. (2003). Attendance at the accident and emergency department in the year before suicide; retrospective study. *British Journal of Psychiatry*, **183**, 28–33.

Gunnell, D., Bennewith, O., Peters, T.J., Stocks, N. and Sharp, D.J. (2002). Do patients who self-harm consult their general practitioner soon after hospital discharge? A cohort study. *Social Psychiatry and Psychiatric Epidemiology*, **37**, 599–602.

Harwood, D., Hawton, K., Hope, T. and Jacoby, R. (2002). The grief experiences and needs of bereaved relatives and friends of older people dying through suicide: a descriptive and case-control study. *Journal of Affective Disorders*, **72**, 185–194.

Hawton, K., Harriss, L., Hall, S. *et al.* (20030). Deliberate self-harm in Oxford, 1990-2000: a time of change in patient characteristics. *Psychological Medicine*, **33**, 987–995.

Henriksson, M.M., Aro, H.M., Marttunen, M.J. *et al.* (1993). Mental disorders and co-morbidity in suicide. *American Journal of Psychiatry*, **150**, 935–940.

Houston, K., Haw, C., Townsend, E. and Hawton, K. (2003). General practitioner contacts with patients before and after deliberate self harm. *British Journal of General Practice*, **53**, 365–370.

Khan, A., Khan, S., Kolts, R. and Brown, W.A. (2003). Suicide rates in clinical trials of SSRIs, other antidepressants and placebo. *American Journal of Psychiatry*, **160**, 790–792.

Kelleher, M. (1996). *Suicide and the Irish*. Mercier Press, Dublin.

Linehan, M.M., Heard, H.L. and Armstrong, H.E. (1993). Naturalistic follow-up of behavioural therapy for chronically parasuicidal borderline patients. *Archives of General Psychiatry*, **50**, 971–974.

McClure, G.M.G. (2000). Changes in suicide in England and Wales, 1960-1997. *British Journal of Psychiatry*, **176**, 64–67.

McDonough, S., Wynaden, D., Finn, M. *et al.* (2004). Emergency department mental health triage consultancy service: an evaluation of the first year of the service. *Accident and Emergency Nursing*, **12**, 31–38.

Owens, C., Booth, N., Briscoe, M., Lawrence, C. and Lloyd, K. (2003). Suicide outside the care of mental health services: a case-controlled psychological autopsy study. *Crisis*, **24**, 113–121.

Suokas, T. and Lonnqvist, J. (1991). Outcome of attempted suicide and psychiatric consultation. Risk factors and suicide mortality during a five year follow-up. *Acta Psychiatrica Scandinavica*, **84**, 545–549.

Suokas, J., Suominen, K., Isometsa, E., Ostamo, A. and Lonnqvist, J. (2004). Long-term risk factors for suicide mortality after attempted suicide—findings of a 14-year follow-up study. *Acta Psychiatrica Scandinavica*, **104**,117–121.

Tyrer, P., Thompson, S., Schmidt, U. *et al.* (2003). Randomized controlled trial of brief cognitive behaviour therapy versus treatment as usual in recurrent deliberate self-harm: the POPMACT study. *Psychological Medicine*, **33**, 969–976.

Van Praag, H.M. (2003). A stubborn behaviour: the failure of antidepressants to reduce suicide rates. *World Journal of Biological Psychiatry*, **4**, 184–191.

Whitley, E., Gunnell, D., Dorling, D. and Smith, G.D. (1999). Ecological study of social fragmentation, poverty and suicide. *British Medical Journal*, **319**, 1034–1037.

Wilkinson, G. (1994). Can suicide be prevented? Better treatment of mental illness is a more appropriate aim. *British Medical Journal*, **309**, 860–86l.

FURTHER READING

Boer, H., Booth, N., Russell, D., Powell, R. and Briscoe, M. (1996). Antidepressant prescribing prior to suicide: role of doctors. *Psychiatric Bulletin*, **20**, 282–284.

Durkheim, F. (1975). *Suicide*. Routledge and Kegan Paul, London.

Crawford, M.J. and Wessely, S. (2000). The Management of patients following deliberate self-harm – what happens to those discharged from hospital to GP. *Primary Care Psychiatry*, **6**, 61–65.

Hawton, K. and van Heeringen, K. (Eds) (2002). *The International Handbook of Suicide and Attempted Suicide*. Wiley, Chichester.

Luoma, J.B., Martin, C.E. and Pearson, J.L. (2002). Contact with mental health and primary care providers before suicide: a review of the evidence. *American Journal of Psychiatry*, **159**, 909–916.

SUGGESTED READING FOR PATIENTS

Lukas, C. and Seiden, H. (1987). *Silent Grief: Living in the Wake of Suicide*. Papermac, London.

McCarthy, S. (2001). *A Voice for those Bereaved by Suicide*. Veritas, Dublin.

Jamison, KR. (1999). *Night Falls Fast. Understanding Suicide*. Picador, London.

Golant, M. and Golant, S.K. (1998). *What to do When Someone you Love is Depressed*. Henry Holt, London.

USEFUL WEBSITES

National Alliance for the mentally Ill: www.nami.org

Self-injury support and information: www.palace.net/~llama/psych/injury.html

Help for those who have attempted suicide and for those bereaved by suicide: www.rdg.ac.uk/Counselling/counselling

USEFUL CONTACTS

The Samaritans
National freephone (UK): 0845 790 90 90
National telephone (Ireland): 01850 60 90 90
Local telephone: .... (fill in your local number)
Email: jo@samaritans.org
Website: www.samaritans.org

8

Anxiety

The term 'anxiety state' is frequently used in clinical practice. Such rubrics are vague and broad, providing little information about the classification of anxiety and are avoided in this text. There is general agreement however that anxiety is a universal emotion, which is unpleasant and associated with psychological feelings of tension and bodily sensations such as palpitations, sweating, etc. The roots of anxiety lie in our phylogenetic ancestry where it served as a warning of danger and threat.

ANXIETY AS A NORMAL RESPONSE

Anxiety is first and foremost the normal response to threat or stress. Thus, prior to an interview or other stressful situation feelings of psychic tension along with somatic symptoms will be described by most people. This anxiety will, in most, improve performance and is colloquially referred to as 'being psyched up'. Any attempt to reduce this anxiety will adversely affect performance and is inadvisable. If however the level of anxiety is excessive then performance will deteriorate. The relationship between anxiety and performance is illustrated by the Yerkes–Dodson curve shown in Figure 8.1.

ANXIETY AS A SYMPTOM

Anxiety can be present in all psychiatric disturbances to a greater or lesser degree. In most of these there is no difficulty recognising that anxiety is secondary. Depressive illness is the exception however and because anxiety is present in up to 70% of those with this illness, especially in the milder or atypical forms, it is frequently misdiagnosed as anxiety and consequently inappropriately treated. Such misdiagnosis is not surprising since there is debate within the body of psychiatry about the separation of these two disorders. On the one hand some believe that both can be clearly distinguished on the basis of their symptoms while the opposing view that they cannot be clearly delineated from each other is supported by findings from therapeutic trials and from natural history studies. When attempting

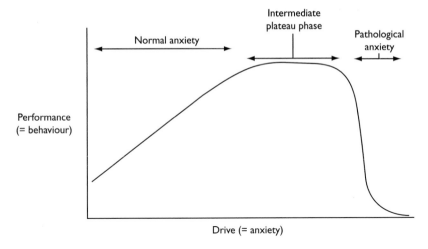

Figure 8.1. The relationship between anxiety and performance (Yerkes–Dodson law). (Reproduced with permission from Yerkes and Dodson, 1908.)

to decide which is primary, age and previous history are essential considerations. Many believe that generalised anxiety (previously termed neurosis) does not occur for the first time in those over the age of 35 and all such conditions should be regarded as 'masked' depressions and treated accordingly.

ANXIETY AS A TRAIT

This refers to the habitual tendency of the individual to be anxious and to worry. It describes a lifelong personality trait and must be distinguished from generalised anxiety (see below), which is a description of an illness. When severe the trait of anxiety may be a manifestation of an anxious or avoidant personality disorder although many with no personality disorder describe themselves as anxious. In addition to persistent worrying and tension the patient with anxiety traits frequently has feelings of social inadequacy, fear of criticism and rejection with a consequent unwillingness to become involved in relationships or occupations. Many patients with this personality disorder develop generalised anxiety also.

ANXIETY AS A DISORDER

Anxiety disorders are classified into three groups – free-floating anxiety now called generalised anxiety disorder (GAD), panic disorder, and phobic anxiety. Indeed some also further divide panic disorder into panic with and without agoraphobia and contend that panic disorder underpins all agoraphobia. This is not common practice and most clinicians regard agoraphobia as separate and hence classify it with the phobias. When anxiety, either as GAD, panic or phobia, is part of depressive illness it is diagnosed as such and treated accordingly, and most patients seen in primary care who describe either GAD or panic are suffering from a depressive illness rather than primary anxiety (see Chapter 6).

As well as uncertainty about the separation of GAD from depressive illness, some authorities also question the validity of panic as a diagnostic entity and point to the instability of the diagnosis with many patients developing other disorders especially depressive illness and alcohol abuse but also agoraphobia and hypochondriasis. Some also argue that panic is nothing more than a severe form of GAD. In spite of these misgivings, which this author shares, the disorder is classified in ICD 10 and in DSM IV.

Epidemiology

Among primary care attendees GAD is found in about 8% although those with serious medical conditions will have much higher levels of secondary anxiety (Wittchen, 2002). There is a 2:1 female excess in GAD seen in primary care but among psychiatric in-patients the ratio is equal. The lifetime prevalence for panic disorder is about 8% although the point prevalence is much lower at about 1% and there is an excess in females. The prevalence of phobias varies with the sampling frame but in the general population an estimated 5–10% of the population have disabling fears although only a minority seek help. Social phobia (social anxiety disorder) has received a lot of attention recently and figures from the US suggest that around 7% of attendees meet the criteria for this condition. For all phobias there is a female excess and all social classes are represented. They begin in adolescence or early adulthood and the young are therefore over-represented. In primary care, GAD and phobias were once thought to represent the commonest psychiatric disorder but they are now believed to take second place to depressive and adjustment disorders.

Aetiology

The aetiology is unknown and various neurotransmitter systems have been investigated including the GABA, α_2-adrenergic and $5HT_{1A}$ systems. Genetic contributions may also play a part since up to 50% of monozygotic twins are concordant for the disorder, especially panic disorder. Cognitive theorists hypothesise that those with anxiety disorders are responding to incorrectly perceived dangers. For phobias learning theory is invoked and it has been demonstrated that the fear response becomes attached to another stimulus through conditioning (see below).

GENERALISED ANXIETY

The core feature of GAD is generalised and persistent anxiety, which is not confined to any one situation. Feelings of nervousness, tension and light-headedness are common and terms such as 'being like a taut wire' and 'feeling like bursting' are often used by patients to describe their feelings. Others include palpitations, sweating, hypersensitivity to noise, headaches and gastrointestinal discomfort. Fears that a family member will have an accident or anxious foreboding (a general feeling of fear which is unfocused) are also common and there may be a tendency to worry about everything. Sleep difficulties, especially initial insomnia are also present. Untreated it runs a chronic course.

PANIC DISORDER

The principal features of panic disorder include the sudden onset of attacks of palpitations, sweating, breathlessness, etc., which overwhelm the patient and are associated with intense feelings of fear. This may lead to the belief that a myocardial infarction or cerebrovascular accident is occurring. Secondary fear of dying, of losing control, or of going mad is common. The crescendo of fear may lead to the person exiting the situation in which the panic has occurred with phobic avoidance developing as a result. The attacks are not related to any particular situation and are therefore unpredictable.

PHOBIC ANXIETY

The aetiology of phobic anxiety is best understood in terms of classical conditioning. It is recognised that many phobias begin after a traumatic event, e.g. fear of dogs after being bitten. Using this model, the bite is the unconditioned stimulus and fear the response. Fear then becomes linked to all dogs (the conditioned stimulus) and may generalise to all furry animals or to some other similar stimulus. In classical theory extinction of the response occurs if the conditioned stimulus is presented repeatedly without the unconditioned stimulus. This is the basis for exposure as a method of treatment. By contrast psychodynamic theory focuses on the displacement of signal anxiety onto a symbolic object or situation. There is no evidence that genetic factors play any part in the development of phobias but personality difficulties such as dependence may be important in the aetiology of agoraphobia and social anxiety. Phobias are classified into five types, described below.

It is important to bear in mind that phobias, panic or generalised anxiety, do not begin for the first time in middle adulthood except as a symptom of a depressive illness and the treatment is then of that disorder.

Agoraphobia

Agoraphobia is the commonest and most disabling of the phobias. It not only includes fears of open spaces but also of being enclosed, of crowds and of leaving home. In its most severe form the sufferer is completely housebound. It is more common in women than men and begins in late adolescence and early adulthood. There is some evidence for a link with dependent personality disorder. Without treatment it runs a fluctuating course and may persist for years being interspersed with episodes of depression which itself may need treatment.

Social phobia

Also known as social anxiety, this disorder was first described as a discrete entity in the 1960s and is next in frequency to agoraphobia. Social anxiety is classified into two types: generalised, in which there is excessive fear in a wide variety of social situations outside the family circle that may include writing or using a key board in public, and non-generalized, in which the anxiety is circumscribed to only one or two isolated situations such as answering the door. Social anxiety should not be confused with shyness, as the latter does not impair function. The simple question 'Do you feel embarrassed in front of others' may point to this diagnosis and further evaluation would be required to make the diagnosis. Similar symptoms can develop as part of a depressive illness. The condition is slightly more common among boys and has its onset in the teen years or earlier. Without treatment its course is chronic and depressive illness may also develop.

Animal phobias

Animal phobias begin in childhood and rarely present for treatment. The sufferers are normal in personality and function well in every other respect. They rarely develop other symptoms such as depression and there is no free-floating anxiety unlike agoraphobia or social anxiety.

Miscellaneous phobias

These include fears of blood and injury, of storms, of heights, of particular forms of travel and a host of other situations. They run a continuous course and begin any time throughout early adulthood. They resemble animal phobias in other respects.

Illness phobias

Illness phobias are different from the rest in that the focus of fear is internal. They include fears of any illness but usually those which are fashionable or in the news.

There is often intense worrying and rumination about the feared disease. They are equally common in both sexes (see Chapter 14).

DIFFERENTIAL DIAGNOSIS

The most common confusion arises in relation to *depressive illness* where anxiety is a prominent feature. The age of the patient along with details of other symptoms of depression will clarify the diagnosis. Generalised anxiety must also be distinguished from *alcohol withdrawal* since patients often conceal the amount they consume and withdrawal symptoms during periods of relative abstinence mimic anxiety and panic attacks. The episodic nature of these will also aid in concealing alcohol abuse as the true cause. *Benzodiazepine withdrawal* also gives rise to psychic and physiological anxiety and unless specifically enquired about may be missed. The *discontinuation syndrome* associated with SSRIs also causes similar symptoms.

TREATMENT

In general no formal treatment is required for normal or for trait anxiety; support and reassurance are necessary although they may be challenged at times by the patient who believes himself to be ill. The temptation to prescribe should be resisted both for philosophical reasons but more importantly because of the risk of tranquilliser dependence. Relaxation techniques should be taught to the chronically tense patient. The treatments outlined below refer therefore to GAD, panic and phobic states.

Psychological

For mild anxiety an *explanation of the cause* and reassurance that the symptoms are not due to organic disease will help the patient from unnecessarily worrying that the symptoms are organic in origin. A common fear is of collapsing during a panic, although this rarely occurs. Other concerns are that heart disease will result from the symptoms or that a severe psychiatric illness will ensue. Usually the relief from such reassurance is temporary and in all but the mildest of conditions more active treatments are needed. Where the symptoms have been precipitated by a known cause, e.g. marital conflict, counselling along the lines outlined in Chapters 12 and 17 is necessary and may be fruitfully carried out in a general practice setting. More psychodynamic or cognitive exploration of the conflicts causing the disorder is not generally within the remit of the GP and secondary referral will be necessary

Behavioural

The next approach to treatment for the general practitioner should be *relaxation techniques*. These are within the competence of every practitioner but demonstrating them to the patient, essential for improving the likelihood of a positive outcome, may require more time than the traditional appointment allows. The general approach is the progressive relaxation of different muscle groups throughout the body and is outlined in Appendix 1 of this chapter. In addition, this approach may be combined with imagery – the use of pleasant images to facilitate and maintain relaxation. Those GPs who are trained in hypnotherapy can also use this to facilitate relaxation.

Practical advice about restructuring the patient's timetable, so as to avoid unnecessary stress, e.g. rushing, is given along with guidance on distraction when tension is developing. This may take the form of exercise such as jogging or deep breathing, of concentrating on the surroundings or of mental activities such as doing calculations, reciting a poem or prayer, etc. The patient may also be advised to avoid coffee or alcohol, at least for a time, since these sometimes worsen preexisting anxiety.

A more sophisticated variant of this is called *Anxiety Management Training* in which the therapist induces anxiety-provoking stimuli and the patient is taught to control his anxiety simultaneously. In addition, insight is given about the abnormal thinking, which leads to tension and ways of controlling the unhelpful thoughts outlined. Cognitive therapy is based on the theory that distorted perceptions of dangers and of situations underpin the anxiety symptoms and by learning to identify these faulty thinking patterns the symptoms can be brought under control. It should only be used by a trained therapist and many community psychiatric nurses are now trained in this therapy making it an invaluable resource for those practices that have close links with community psychiatric services.

For phobias, the treatment of choice is *systematic desensitisation*. First, this involves training in progressive relaxation as described above although there is debate about the necessity for this initial step. Then hierarchies of situations provoking anxiety are constructed followed by graded exposure to these situations. For example, a social phobic may describe answering the telephone as the least fearful, then answering the door, then eating in public, and so on. By counterposing these anxiety provoking stimuli, either in imagination or ideally *in vivo*, with relaxation, the anxiety is extinguished. Throughout the exposure the patient self-monitors the level of anxiety and this is fed back at the end of the session to demonstrate the reduction that occurs with repeated exposure (Appendix 2 of this chapter). Graded exposure beginning with the least fearful situation and systematically working through the hierarchy is generally preferred to flooding. In the latter the patient is allowed to experience extended exposure to highly anxiety provoking stimuli.

These behavioural approaches are time-consuming and for this reason are not used by general practitioners themselves. However, those who have the facility of trained nurse therapists may be in a position to offer this form of treatment. There is some evidence that training a relative to participate in treatment is advantageous as is the involvement of former agoraphobic patients (Tyrer, 1986).

There is evidence linking abnormal marital relationships to the maintenance of phobias, especially agoraphobia. The phobia preserves the delicate balance within the marriage between the dependent patient and a controlling spouse. Treating the phobia may disturb this balance and is sometimes resisted by one or both parties. Before commencing therapy it is essential to assess the commitment of both to this.

Those phobic patients who have personality disorders, especially of passive–dependent types, benefit from additional help with *social skills and assertiveness* as outlined in Chapter 11.

Many patients enquire about *self-help groups* and while there is no conclusive evidence that they are unhelpful, it is possible that they may attract those with low motivation for treatment and those who derive some psychological benefit from maintenance of the phobia. However, many are now incorporating active treatment programmes so as to avoid these problems.

Pharmacological

Over the past few years there is increasing evidence that tricyclic antidepressants are superior to benzodiazepines, not just in depressive illness but also in GAD (formerly termed anxiety neurosis) (Modigh, 1987). This relates to their sedative properties and the onset of effect is usually within a few days, unlike their antidepressant effect, which takes several weeks.

The SSRIs have also found a niche in treating GAD although the starting dose should be lower than the antidepressant dose and titrated upwards thereafter. A disadvantage is that there is often an initial worsening of symptoms and it may take several weeks for a noticeable response. It is recommended that treatment with SSRIs be for at least 8 months with some recommending a duration of up to 18 months.

The benzodiazepines have been the mainstay of treatment of GAD for several decades since they provide rapid symptomatic relief. Due to the risk of dependence their use has waned and ideally they should only be prescribed on an 'as required' basis; if required regularly then this should be for no longer than 4 weeks during which time other pharmacological, cognitive and psychosocial strategies can be implemented. A few patients with disabling chronic anxiety may require long-term treatment with benzodiazepines. In general it is best to use a medium- or long-acting preparation since the short-acting benzodiazepines are more associated with withdrawal symptoms.

Beta-blockers such as propranolol were first reported as successful in treating generalized anxiety in 1966 and since then there have been several studies verifying this. Their anti-anxiety property relates to their peripheral activity and they are therefore most useful in those presenting with somatic symptoms, having no effect on psychic anxiety. There is little to choose between various preparations but propranolol (40–160 mg) or oxprenolol may be preferred because of the paucity of side effects associated with them. Low dose phenothiazines may occasionally be used although this is not the first line of treatment especially now that thioridazine, the most commonly used of this group, is licensed only for use as a second line treatment in schizophrenia. Buspirone, although licensed for the treatment of GAD has not found widespread use in Britain and Ireland due to the delay in onset of effects although it may have a place in the treatment of those with chronic anxiety who fail to respond to other measures.

Panic disorder is treated in a manner similar to GAD with the exception that beta-blockers and buspirone are not useful. The SSRIs are specifically licensed for treating panic disorder and as with GAD there is a delay in the onset of effect and the initiating dose should be lower than that used in depression. Early reduction of medication results in relapse and it should therefore be continued for 6–12 months. The TCAs are also used due to their sedative properties and there is evidence that monoamine oxidase inhibitors (MAOIs) are also effective although they are unlikely to find widespread use because of the potential for serious drug interactions.

Medication has little use in the long-term treatment of phobias with the exception of social anxiety. Paroxetine is the only SSRI which is licensed for its treatment although all the other SSRIs and venlafaxine have shown benefit in individual trials. Beta-blockers may indirectly benefit those with the non-generalised form by reducing tremor and palpitations, as may the benzodiazepines. Musicians often use beta-blockers for performance anxiety.

Overall both pharmacological and psychological treatments produce significant improvement although additional studies are required to demonstrate specific indications and benefits of pharmacological over psychological treatments. For the specific phobias benzodiazepines may be used prior to commencing behaviour therapy to reduce anxiety levels and facilitate engagement with the specific exposure process.

SUMMARY

1. Anxiety may be a normal response to stressful situations but it may occur as a symptom of some other syndrome, e.g. depressive illness, or may be a disorder in itself.
2. Treatment is required only if anxiety is considered to be pathological. Attempts to reduce the normal anxiety response will impair performance.
3. Depressive illness is frequently misdiagnosed as generalized anxiety.

4. In general practice the prevalence of anxiety disorders takes second place to depressive illness and adjustment reactions.
5. Behaviour therapy is the treatment of choice for phobias while cognitive therapy is effective in the management of panic and generalised anxiety disorder and social anxiety.
6. Antidepressants are also useful adjuncts and are significantly better than tranquillisers especially in the management of free-floating anxiety.
7. Behavioural techniques, many of which are within the competence of the general practitioner, are time-consuming and may only be available realistically in practices which have access to those trained in these methods.

CASE HISTORIES

Case 1

Mr X, a 22 year-old student, was referred at the suggestion of his parents because of worries about his impending degree examination. He had always done well and was one of a family of six, all of whom had professional qualifications. He admitted to feeling tense and getting overwhelming feelings of panic when he thought of the volume of work he had to get through. On closer questioning he admitted that he had felt similar tension before exams in the past, all of which he had been successful in. It was explained that his tension was a natural reaction to the pressure he was under and as similar feelings in the past had not incapacitated him, he was not offered any other therapy. He was successful in his exams and returned 2 months after the results still feeling keyed-up and having episodic palpitations, sweating and dizziness. His pleasure from life was normal and he looked forward to his future career with excitement. Appetite, concentration and sleep were normal and he denied feeling depressed although his symptoms 'got him down'. A diagnosis of generalized anxiety was made and his symptoms resolved with instruction in relaxation techniques.

Comment

The decision not to 'treat' at first referral was appropriate although the doctor should have been alerted to the family pressure and expectations, which might render him vulnerable to an ongoing anxiety. Diagnosis and treatment were appropriate when he developed pathological anxiety. For the future, encouragement to distance himself from his family at such times should be proffered along with family intervention to reduce their over-involvement.

Case 2

Mr X, a 52 year-old man with a 6-year history of panic attacks, was referred. These were especially bad in the mornings and in consequence he would wake up early. He had difficulty in beginning his day's work as managing director of his firm and he attributed this to tiredness from the sleep disturbance and from the almost continuous panics. He denied depression but admitted to feeling hopeless about his symptoms ever resolving. He had no previous contact with the medical profession and had a supportive wife and children. He was by nature punctilious. He could not recall any precipitating event or any untoward stresses at the onset of his symptoms. He had earlier been prescribed tranquillisers with some slight improvement in his symptoms. A diagnosis of depressive illness was made and he responded dramatically to a tricyclic antidepressant.

Comment

The age of onset along with the diurnal swing in the symptoms should have been sufficient to make the correct diagnosis initially. Even where depression is denied, there is often a change in intensity of other symptoms, in this case anxiety, throughout the day. Where anxiety is part of a depressive illness, treatment of the former brings only temporary relief.

Case 3

Mrs X, a 28 year-old lady with a lifelong history of fear of meeting people, was referred for desensitisation. Her list of fears, compiled in a hierarchy from most to least disabling were as follows: meeting people who were strangers, meeting people whom she knew, signing cheques in public places, e.g. banks, queuing in the supermarket, eating in public, drinking in public, and speaking on the telephone. This lady had always had this constellation of symptoms with little exception. Her husband was sympathetic but constantly encouraged her to carry out these activities. A diagnosis of social anxiety was made and in vivo desensitisation was commenced, dealing firstly with her fear of the telephone. She was encouraged to hold and use the telephone in the presence of the therapist or her spouse. Immediately beforehand she was instructed to carry out relaxation exercises and throughout the session to take slow, deep breaths. She monitored her own level of anxiety using a simple visual analogue scale and the reduction in her level of anxiety with practice was demonstrated to her. This session lasted approximately 1 hour and until the next appointment she was told to practise this in her own home. At the second appointment a brief period was devoted to rehearsing the making of telephone calls before proceeding to answering the telephone. Initially the spouse made calls from the office next door and while answering it the patient was encouraged to relax as before. Self-monitoring continued and practice in between sessions involved receiving preplanned and then unplanned telephone calls from her spouse. The next stage concerned receiving calls from other persons, e.g. friends and family, to which she was exposed in a graded manner. After 6 hours work she was able to use the telephone spontaneously and without fear. It was decided to progress to the next step in the hierarchy, i.e. drinking in public. Therapy commenced with drinking tea in the presence of the therapist while practising relaxation simultaneously and self-monitoring her level of fear. She then progressed to drinking in front of a few members of staff in the unit dining room. Subsequently she was taken into a city café during a quiet period and later during a busy period. This sequence continued with practice sessions in between until she could go into a crowded bar. To achieve this took 5 hours of therapist time and practice sessions. At this point the patient felt she had achieved her main objectives and requested to be discharged. This was agreed. She has not been referred since nor has she kept in contact. Information from her general practitioner is that she remains free from fear of speaking on the telephone and drinking in public but is still incapacitated by her other phobias.

Comment

This lady illustrates the time-consuming nature of desensitisation. Despite her supportive and sensible husband who was used as the co-therapist and who did not reinforce her abnormal behaviour, she did not persist with treatment. This is a frequent occurrence. At no point was medication used. The use of self-monitoring provides visible evidence for the patient that exposure to the feared stimulus ultimately decreases anxiety (see Appendix 2).

REFERENCES

Modigh, K. (1987). Antidepressant drugs in anxiety disorders. *Acta Psychiatrica Scandinavica*, **76** (Suppl. 335), 57–71.

Tyrer, P. (1986). Ex-phobic volunteers in the treatment of agoraphobic patients. *Bulletin of the Royal College of Psychiatrists*, **10**, 111–113.

Wittchen, H.U. (2002). Generalised anxiety disorder; prevalence, burden and cost to society. *Depression Anxiety*, **16**, 162–171.

Yerkes, R.H. and Dodson, J.D. (1908). The relation of strength of stimulus to rapidity of habit formation. *Journal of Comparative Neurological Psychology*, **18**, 459–482.

FURTHER READING

France, R. and Robson, M. (1986). *Behaviour Therapy in Primary Care. A Practical Guide.* Croom Helm, London.

Marks, I. (2001). *Living with Fear.* McGraw-Hill Education, London.
Wittchen, H.U., Kessler, R.C., Beesdo, K. *et al.* (2002). Generalised anxiety and depression in primary care: prevalence, recognition and management. *Journal of Clinical Psychiatry,* **63** (Suppl. 8), 24–34.

SUGGESTED READING FOR PATIENTS

Marks, I. (2001). *Living with Fear.* McGraw Hill, London.
Page, A. (2002). *Don't Panic. Overcoming Anxiety, Phobias and Tension, 2nd edition.* Gore and Osmeni, Sydney.
Butler, G. (1999). *Overcoming Social Anxiety and Shyness.* Robinson, London.

USEFUL WEBSITES FOR PATIENTS

Anxiety: www.rcpsych.ac.uk/info/help/anxiety/

Social phobia: www.rcpsych.ac.uk/info/help/socphob/

USEFUL CONTACTS

National Phobics Society
Zion Community Resource Centre
339 Stretford Road
Manchester M15 4ZY
Email: nationalphobic@btconnect.com
Website: www.phobics-society.org.uk

Triumph Over Phobia
PO Box 3760
Bath BA2 3WY
Tel: 0845 600 9601
Email: info@triumphoverphobia.org.uk
Website: www.triumphoverphobia.com

Relaxation for Living
'Foxhills'
30 Victoria Avenue
Shanklin
Isle of Wight PO37 6LS
Tel: 01983 868 166

Out and About Organisation
140 St Lawrence's Road
Clontarf
Dublin

APPENDIX 1: DEEP MUSCLE RELAXATION

The patient is seated on a comfortable reclining chair or lying on a couch. The room must be quiet and the doctor aims to convey a feeling of relaxation himself. The whole routine takes about 20 minutes. The therapist begins:

'Anxiety and tension are frequently associated with tense muscles. By using these exercises which I will demonstrate to you, you will be able to distinguish tension from relaxation and you will learn to relax yourself when this tension occurs. We will work through all the muscle groups first tensing them and then relaxing them. We will begin with the right arm. I want you to make a tight fist, bend your wrist and then your elbow up to your shoulder. Get these as tight as you can so that you will be aware of the tension and pain in them. When they are as tight as possible begin to slowly unbend your arm so that it lies beside you, then your wrist, and finally your fist so that your palm is facing downwards. When you hear the word 'relax' let the remaining tension leave your arm so that it feels loose and relaxed.'

Pause for about 10–15 seconds during which the word 'relax' is spoken once.

'I want you to make the fist again and bend your wrist and elbow like you did the last time, but now tensing your muscles even more. When they are as tight as possible begin to slowly relax them concentrating on how different your relaxed arm feels from the tension of a moment ago. Now try to relax your arm, forearm and fingers even more than before.' (Pause). *'Let all the tension flow out through your fingers.'*

This sequence is continued for the other arm and forearm. For the shoulders tension is achieved by extending the neck and pulling the shoulders up round the neck, relaxation by allowing the head to fall forward and the shoulders to drop.

For the forehead the patient is instructed to frown and to tightly shut the eyes. Relaxation is achieved by smoothing the forehead and opening the eyes. The jaws are then clenched and the tongue pressed against the roof of the mouth and then slowly released.

The chin is pressed firmly against the upper sternum and then released. To control breathing a deep breath is inhaled which is then forced out against a fixed diaphragm and closed throat. The patient is then told to note the feeling of pressure in the intercostal muscles. He is then told to expire slowly and to continue to breathe slowly and evenly.

The stomach muscles are contracted and then relaxed while the patient is instructed to concentrate on the feeling of tension and then relaxation. The shoulders and buttocks are pulled together while the back is arched. They are then slowly released so that the patient is limp and heavy. The knees are pushed into extension as far as they will go followed by the ankle and toes being extended as far as possible until a feeling of tightness is noted in the thighs, calves and feet. Relaxation then follows with the knees going into a position of slight flexion and falling slightly apart.

For each of these muscle groups it is important to repeat the exercise so that '*a little more tension than the last time*' is felt. Words like '*calm*', '*relax*' and '*loose*' are used repeatedly.

When the patient is fully relaxed it is useful to ask the patient to conjure up some relaxing picture and to think about this for a few moments. This is followed by a pause of about 1 minute so as to allow the patient to enjoy the feeling of complete relaxation and freedom from tension.

The patient is instructed to carry out these exercises twice each day. When he is fully conversant with them, then they can be modified according to individual needs. The breathing and shoulder/neck routines are especially useful for controlling situational anxiety, e.g. in a queue. For the practised patient the tension routine may be omitted and the instruction to '*relax*' given straight away.

APPENDIX 2: SELF MONITORING

'*I want you to mark off on the line below what your present level of overall tension and anxiety is.*'

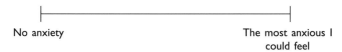

No anxiety   The most anxious I
                                 could feel

Over the period of therapy, the decrease in anxiety will be plainly in evidence and can be utilised in giving the patient insight.

9

Alcohol Abuse

Since various definitions of alcohol abuse have been used, prevalence studies have found a rate of between 5 and 25% for general practice attendees.

In no other area is the distinction between out-patients and general practice patients more obvious than in alcohol abuse. Those seen at out-patient clinics are generally suffering from physical dependence, have numerous social and interpersonal problems and may also have physical complications. Obviously to limit the definition to this group who exhibit the complications of alcohol abuse is to exclude those with milder forms of the syndrome.

One approach is to define alcohol abuse by the quantity consumed and the Royal College of Psychiatrists suggests that consumption of 21 or more units per week (a unit being half a pint of beer or a glass of wine) for men and of 14 or more units for women constitutes at-risk drinking. This has the advantage of being intuitively simple but has the disadvantage of excluding those who develop difficulties with a lower intake and or those who are unaffected by larger quantities. In a clinical setting it is easy to become diverted into a debate about what constitutes alcoholism when dealing with an alcohol abuser. The term 'alcoholic' conjures up the notion of destitutes on skid-row and in the early stages of dealing with the problem its use is likely to impair the process of encouraging abstinence due to resentment at being so labelled.

The alcohol dependence syndrome described by Edwards and Gross (1976) outlines the features of that disorder and includes:

1. The predominance of drinking over other activities.
2. The development of tolerance.
3. Narrowing of the drink repertoire such that the pattern of consumption is unrelated to external events. In the normal drinker there is a variability in the amount consumed, e.g. at a weekend or at a social function more is ingested than usual. This variability is lacking in the person dependent on alcohol.
4. Withdrawal symptoms on stopping alcohol which are relieved by further alcohol.
5. A period of abstinence is followed by rapid reinstatement of dependence if drinking is resumed.
6. Tolerance to the effects necessitating a heavier consumption to produce the same effects.

Unfortunately the debate about where heavy drinking ends and 'problem' drinking or alcoholism begins remains unresolved. The difficulties centre around the issues outlined above but also are culturally determined since what constitutes social or interpersonal harm is arbitrary. Thus, in some cultures social or marital violence may be viewed with tolerance and even as a mark of manhood. The syndromal approach above has the advantage of being free from cultural bias but is likely to be of little use in epidemiological work since its application requires an admission of the problem by the patient.

TYPES OF ALCOHOLISM

Older classifications of alcoholism relied on patterns of drinking and the name of Jellinek is particularly associated with this approach; thus those who had a craving for alcohol were believed to be separate from those who drank in binges or from those who drank to relieve psychological distress. However, over the years it has been shown that there is little justification for retaining these subdivisions since individual patients are not true to type and present with different patterns at different times in their drinking careers. Even the simple classification of alcoholics into primary and secondary, according to whether the alcohol abuse is secondary to some other psychological condition such as depression, or not, is felt to be of little help in terms of treatment and outcome.

SCREENING

Questionnaires

To overcome the problems associated with detection of alcohol abuse or alcoholism a number of screening questionnaires have been popularised. The most extensively documented are the MAST (Selzer, 1971) and the CAGE (Mayfield *et al.*, 1974) questionnaires. These have some value but are dependent on the recognition of alcohol problems by the patient for their diagnostic value. For general practice the CAGE questionnaire is the most useful since it consists of just 4 questions:

- Have you ever felt you should **C**ut down on your drinking?
- Have people **A**nnoyed you by criticising your drinking?
- Have you ever felt bad or **G**uilty about your drinking?
- Have you ever had a drink first thing in the morning to steady your nerves or get rid of a hangover (**E**ye-opener)?

Two or more positive answers point to the possibility of alcohol dependence and to the need for further evaluation.

Laboratory markers

Chemical markers elevated in those drinking to excess include gamma glutamyl-transferase (GGT) (over 45 IU/l) and mean cell volume (MCV) (over 98 fl). A newer test, carbohydrate deficient transferrin (CDT), is believed to have higher sensitivity and specificity than the other measures but is not widely used. Recent studies suggest that in primary care laboratory markers are unhelpful in diagnosing alcohol abuse or dependence and that clinical evaluation combined with a screening questionnaire are best (Aertgeerts *et al.*, 2001).

EPIDEMIOLOGY

Figures based on hospital admission figures are known to be inadequate since many alcoholics do not receive treatment at all. Nevertheless admissions for alcohol problems constitute 10% of all psychiatric admissions in England and Wales and a much higher proportion in Scotland, Ireland and mainland Europe. Attempts at calculating the prevalence of alcoholism on the basis of the numbers with cirrhosis of the liver annually shows that France has the highest prevalence with England and Wales having relatively low rates. It is agreed that this approach is no longer acceptable and it has been abandoned. Indirect evidence for the escalating problem comes from the rising numbers of convictions for drunkenness offences and for drunken driving convictions.

Among primary care attendees a WHO study found that the rates of alcohol dependence and harmful use of alcohol were 2.2% and 1.4%, respectively (Kisley *et al.*, 1995), with men predominating.

AETIOLOGY

The debate about aetiology centres round two arguments – one the illness theory, the other the social learning theory. Until the middle of the last century alcoholics were generally regarded as weak, lacking in moral fibre or in some way degenerate. The work of Jellinek was instrumental in reversing this and in promulgating the view of alcohol dependence as an illness. This became the dominant theory in the 1950s and 60s and is still accepted by many, most notably Alcoholics Anonymous. Regarding alcoholism as a disease serves the purpose of encouraging more humane treatments and stimulating research into this disorder. However, the counter argument is that alcohol abuse does not possess the properties of a disease, i.e. a known cause, course, symptom pattern and response to treatment. Indeed there is some evidence that in the early stages of excessive drinking the process may be reversed by simple counselling. Moreover, since active treatment of established alcohol dependence is generally no more successful than simple advice and since a proportion eventually return to social drinking it can be argued that there is no consistent pattern observable.

The search for the cause amongst those adhering to the disease model centred initially upon the genetic inheritance of alcoholism. There is some evidence from adoptive studies that the sons of alcoholics are more than twice as likely to become alcoholic than the general population and that children adopted into alcoholic families are not at increased risk. Other studies point to a genetic link with unipolar depression. In addition the concordance is higher for monozygotic than for dizygotic twins and heritability is higher for men than for women. It is likely that the inheritance is polygenic. A different approach to causation has focused on a presumed abnormality in alcohol dehydrogenase but the findings are so far unproven.

More recently with our increased understanding of learning and of social theory other causes for alcoholism are now suggested. The social model is generally the one favoured by the medical profession who argue that while the disease model served a useful humanitarian purpose, it has robbed the patient of responsibility for controlling his drinking and changing his lifestyle.

The social learning theory is based upon the acceptability of heavy drinking in our culture and on the ready availability of alcohol at relatively low prices. The evidence for this is the observation that during prohibition admission rates for alcohol related problems declined considerably (even though criminal activity increased). The work of Ledermann, a French demographer, has also lent some weight to this argument by his demonstration of a logarithmic relationship between the average consumption and the numbers of problem drinkers in a community. His methodology has received much criticism but his hypothesis is intuitively attractive and also suggests a means whereby the problem may be controlled, i.e. reducing the *per capita* consumption by formal controls such as stricter licensing laws, heavier taxes on alcohol and a host of other legal restraints.

The role of personality in determining who becomes alcoholic has received some consideration also. The view that there was a particular type of person who became alcoholic has now been disproved, although there is no doubt that those with sociopathic personality disorder are more at risk of developing substance abuse including alcohol dependence than other groups. Also at risk are those who as children had conduct disorders or attention deficit hyperactivity disorder (ADHD).

In recent years the rate of alcohol abuse and dependence amongst women has increased considerably. It is uncertain if this represents a real increase in its prevalence in women or just an increased willingness to admit the problem. There is no doubt however that women are more vulnerable to both the medical and psychiatric complications of alcohol abuse than their male counterparts and are less likely to be counselled about problem drinking when presenting in primary care (Roeloffs *et al.*, 2001). Opinions have varied as to the factors underlying heavy drinking in women and the focus has been on the changing role of women in society although much is inconclusive.

It is apparent that the search for a single cause for alcohol abuse and dependence is naïve. Moreover it must be remembered that many people possess the at-risk characteristics described above but do not become problem drinkers. Our understanding is therefore incomplete.

ALERTING THE GP

It is advisable to have a high index of suspicion of alcohol abuse when certain conditions prevail. These can roughly be divided as follows.

Physical abnormalities

- Pancreatitis
- Gastritis
- Unexplained peripheral neuropathy
- Unexplained abnormalities of liver function
- Raised MCV on haematological testing
- Unexplained chest pain; this frequently accompanies panic attacks (see below)
- Tremors, especially in the morning.

Psychological disturbance

- Panic attacks, especially those which do not respond rapidly to the treatments outlined in Chapter 8; these tend to occur during periods of relative abstinence and represent mild forms of withdrawal symptoms
- Depressed mood, often misdiagnosed as a depressive illness and not responsive to antidepressants
- Marital violence
- General deterioration in self care and social functioning for which there is no obvious psychological explanation such as the presence of depressive illness or schizophrenia.

Other

- Monday morning absenteeism
- Frequent dismissal from jobs
- Repeated drunk driving offences.

TREATMENT

Advice on limiting alcohol intake should be offered to all those whom the GP regards as being a heavy or problem drinker. Research suggests that this advice is frequently taken on board and that such people do not progress to alcohol dependence. For those dependent on alcohol more active treatment methods have been developed and should be offered to the patient who is motivated. There is little point in forcing treatment upon the unmotivated patient although families frequently make such requests. In particular the GP should avoid the temptation to recommend compulsory admission in these circumstances. Only if the patient is an immediate danger to others or to himself should there be recourse to this (see Chapter 18). Usually it is a relative who first seeks treatment for the sufferer who is often both insightless and reluctant. However using Motivational Interviewing (see Maintaining Abstinence below) it may be possible to provide the patient with enough insight into the effect that alcohol is having on his family and health so that he will accept treatment. In addition, encouragement or even pressure from outside may also galvanise an alcohol abuser into seeking treatment and threats of separation or of job loss, for example, may act as powerful motivators.

Detoxification

This is only the first step in achieving abstinence. Many patients especially those seen in general practice request home detoxification. For those who are highly motivated and who have the support of their family this may be possible. Typically a patient would be commenced on chlordiazepoxide or alprazolam in divided doses sufficient to relieve withdrawal symptoms. Chlordiazepoxide may be used in doses of up to 50 mg q.i.d and alprazolam up to 1 mg q.i.d. in hospital patients, but among general practice patients much lower doses are used. Reduction is titrated against the patient's symptomatology and in general detoxification should be complete in about two weeks. There is some evidence to suggest that alprazolam is a more rapid detoxifying agent. Several studies have shown that carbamazepine in doses up to 800 mg per day are as effective as benzodiazepines, although less frequently used. Multivitamin supplements, orally or intravenously, are also prescribed to minimise the risk of Wernicke's encephalopathy or Korsakoff's psychosis. There is usually no requirement to prescribe a hypnotic since the benzodiazepines used for detoxification will aid sleep also. If symptomatic relief of the withdrawal syndrome cannot be brought about without recourse to the full doses detailed above, the patient should be hospitalised.

Unfortunately, some of those who are alcohol dependent lack the motivation necessary to allow such a scheme of management by their general practitioner and in many cases detoxification in hospital becomes necessary. This is done usually using tranquillisers and vitamin supplements as described above but recently an α_2 agonist, clonidine, has also been used (up to 17 µg/kg body weight). Although this helps control sympathetic overactivity, it does not prevent seizures. Heminevrin has also been widely used in detoxification but it is not generally favoured by psychiatrists because of its addictive potential. Whichever drug is used, care should be taken to discontinue it before discharge from hospital.

MAINTAINING ABSTINENCE

Studies of the efficacy of various treatment methods for alcoholism make gloomy reading. Unfortunately, simple advice about abstinence and maintaining it seems to fare as well as the more intensive treatments in all the comparative studies that have been done so far. It is striking that from many different centres the results are similar. In primary care this should be the initial approach with referral to specialist services only required for those who have physical dependence or who fail to respond to medical advice.

A form of therapy called Motivational Enhancement Therapy (also called Motivational Interviewing) is useful in stimulating change and maintaining abstinence. Developed in the 1980s it is directive and patient centred. Its method is to identify conflicts between the goals of the patient and the impact of alcohol abuse on achieving these goals. Other approaches that involve identifying the triggers to excessive drinking, either emotional or environmental, are more appropriate than more broadly based psychodynamic psychotherapy.

Specialist treatment units

Specialist treatment units with intensive group therapy and family therapy were developed in the 1960s. These focus on the patient's alcohol centred lifestyle and encourage changes to this. Self-awareness is considered an important component and the role of alcohol in aiding the patient in dealing with problems such as anxiety, shyness, etc., is identified and corrective measures introduced. Unfortunately the results from these are all dismal and suggest that the financial and training input into these has not proved as efficacious as common sense would have suggested . It has been suggested that there may be special groups of alcoholics, e.g. those recently diagnosed, who derive benefit from such intensive therapy. However, although this has intuitive appeal, it remains to be proven scientifically. Some specialist centres who carefully select patients for their programmes claim long-term success.

Alcoholics Anonymous

Alcoholics Anonymous, together with its sister organization Al-Anon, provides help and support for alcoholics and their families. These groups are based on an illness model and also have a very strong spiritual overlay. The approach is one of self-disclosure which to many is unacceptable. Because of its anonymity there are no data available on its efficacy. For individual patients however it provides support and guidance which is invaluable.

Drug treatment

Disulfiram and citrated calcium carbimide are drugs which inhibit the metabolism of acetaldehyde. The build-up of acetaldehyde causes nausea when alcohol is consumed with it and many patients value this prop to sobriety, at least in the immediate period following detoxification. Disulfiram implants have also been used but their efficacy is uncertain.

Acamprosate calcium facilitates the maintenance of abstinence by stimulating transmission of GABA, an inhibitory neurotransmitter involved in substance dependence. The usual dose is 666 mg t.i.d. but lower doses should be used in those under 60 kg. Liver function should be checked prior to prescription since severe liver failure is a contraindication. It is not useful in the management of detoxification and is recommended in conjunction with counselling, treatment being for about 1 year.

CONTROLLED DRINKING

Up to 15% of those dependent on alcohol return to social drinking following a period of abstinence. The realisation of this formed the basis for the retraining of alcoholics in their drinking habits which became fashionable in the 1970s (Clark, 1976). It consists of video-taped recordings, using simulated bar-rooms, of the patient in this setting. Aspects of his drinking behaviour are noted and fed back to him. These include taking bigger gulps, continually keeping his glass in hand and any other behaviours which could potentially be re-learnt. Agreeing daily limits, keeping a diary of consumption, identifying triggers to over-drinking and developing strategies for saying 'No' are also included.

Follow-up studies have demonstrated the value of controlled drinking and it is no longer dismissed out of hand. While it would be a foolhardy doctor who recommends that an alcoholic return to social drinking, it is likely that in the future the specialist services will be able to assist the GP in identifying the special group for whom this may be possible. Also the possibility of controlled drinking is likely to attract more patients into treatment, particularly those who are not yet dependent but having problems with control.

REHABILITATION

For the chronic or skid-row alcoholic who is homeless the GP will need the assistance of the psychiatric and social services to provide half-way houses and hostels following detoxification. Although this group represents less than 5% of the total presenting for treatment, it represents the greatest treatment and humanitarian challenge. Although many present to casualty departments they frequently default from follow-up.

PSYCHOLOGICAL COMPLICATIONS

Depression

Alcohol abuse is associated with feelings of gloom, despondency and dysphoria. The relationship between alcohol abuse and depressed mood is a complex one. First, the mood change tends to be transient and may be a direct consequence of the central effects of alcohol. In addition, many heavy drinkers have family, financial and marital problems making them unhappy. This may be mistaken for depressive illness. Thus the GP confronted with the alcoholic who complains of depression should withhold antidepressant treatment for at least one month following detoxification as the symptoms tend to subside spontaneously. In the small group who do not improve (less than 10%) (Brown and Schuckit, 1988) antidepressant medication may be required, provided the patient is now abstinent since there may be untoward interactions with alcohol. In general, women are more prone to depressive illness following detoxification than are men and indeed a pre-existing depressive disorder is often present.

Anxiety disorders

As described above, panic attacks frequently occur during periods of relative abstinence. These usually subside when total abstinence has been established. However, social anxiety often manifests itself following detoxification and this is usually a manifestation of a pre-existing disorder for which alcohol may have been used to bring about relief. The treatment of the social anxiety in these circumstances is outlined in Chapter 8.

Other drug abuse

Many alcoholics abuse other drugs in addition to alcohol; in particular benzodiazepines or chlormethiazole prescribed to relieve withdrawal symptoms are common drugs of abuse. It is thus advisable to be circumspect when prescribing to alcoholics and medication should never be prescribed on a long-term basis. The rules governing the prescription of drugs of potential abuse apply as much to alcoholics as to other patients.

Marital and sexual problems

These are a common accompaniment to alcohol abuse. The violence, poverty and unemployment which are associated with alcoholism are common sources of conflict. Unless the patient becomes abstinent there is little point in pursuing marital therapy since any attempts at resolving the conflicts will be sabotaged during periods of drinking. Sexual difficulties, especially impotence are common complications since alcohol increases the desire but reduces the ability to perform sexually. As with marital disharmony, unless abstinence from alcohol is achieved treatment of the sexual problem is doomed to failure.

Pathological jealousy and psychosis

Alcohol abuse is commonly associated with morbid jealousy (referred to as the Othello syndrome). This often improves after cessation of drinking but a minority become deluded about their spouse's fidelity and require treatment as for any other psychotic condition. Occasionally auditory hallucinations (referred to as alcoholic hallucinosis) occur in the context of clear consciousness and must be distinguished from the hallucinations of delirium tremens. These occur either at times of relative abstinence or relative increase in alcohol intake and although improvement occurs once abstinence is established some turn out to be schizophrenic. The treatment is with major tranquillisers.

Delirium tremens

Delirium tremens is the acute confusional state which occurs during withdrawal from alcohol. It lasts up to four days and is accompanied by agitation, visual hallucinations and intense fear. It has a mortality of about 15% due to the electrolyte disturbances which accompany the condition. Emergency treatment with major tranquillisers, correction of the electrolyte imbalance and intravenous vitamin supplements are essential although care must be taken to administer saline rather than dextrose solutions if Korsakoff's syndrome is not to develop.

Brain damage

Brain damage is a common complication of alcoholism and may range from the mild vermian atrophy which occurs early in the history to the more severe amnestic syndrome, often eponymously called Korsakoff's psychosis, and caused by thiamine deficiency. Haemorrhagic lesions in the mammillary bodies, in the thalamus and hypothalamus have been found at post-mortem examination. Korsakoff's psychosis is associated with confabulation, a profound impairment of recent memory, disorientation in time, apathy and impairment of perceptual and conceptual function. It is sometimes preceded by Wernicke's encephalopathy – a condition characterised by nystagmus, peripheral neuropathy, ataxia and confusion. More generalised impairment of intellect may occur and presents with similar symptoms to those occurring in dementia from any other cause. CT scans show generalised atrophy. Wernicke's syndrome is treated with intravenous thiamine while it is prescribed orally in the treatment of Korsakoff's syndrome. Sometimes more focal changes occur such as frontal lobe damage, cerebellar degeneration, temporal lobe lesions and a host of other rarer abnormalities.

Personality deterioration

This is frequently described in alcoholics who often appear to become coarse and aggressive. The debate about whether this is the cause or the result of excessive drinking has aroused much controversy. While it is recognised that personality deterioration can occur both due to the social consequences and due to frontal lobe damage, recent work on personality suggests that psychopathy is a common prodrome of alcohol abuse and tends to be the cause rather than the effect of this.

Suicide

Suicide is a common outcome particularly in chronic, middle-aged alcoholics. It tends to be associated with concurrent depressive symptoms and is often precipitated by interpersonal loss or conflict. Long-term studies have demonstrated that between 7 and 21% commit suicide. Alcohol has also been shown to play a part in the suicides of those taking their own lives in the general population due to its destabilising effects on mood (Goldberg *et al.*, 2001). Moreover, among the parasuicide population alcohol abuse has been shown to be a major problem, with up to 50% of men showing evidence of dependence. In addition alcohol is frequently taken prior to such an attempt.

Both the physical complications and the psychological disabilities associated with alcohol abuse are more prevalent in women than men. Whether this is because women are more vulnerable or because they tend to be secret drinkers and are therefore more chronic, has yet to be clarified. It is essential to be alert to the distress of the alcoholic, particularly at times of conflict, if suicide and attempts at self-harm are to be avoided.

OUTCOME

Little is known about the effects of intervention at the GP level upon alcoholism. However, heavy drinkers who are counselled to cut down their intake have been shown to respond positively to this. The effects of in-patient treatment for alcohol dependence have been studied extensively but unfortunately seem to have little impact on outcome when compared with simple advice. Some centres, such as Hazelden in Minnesota, have demonstrated the effectiveness of intensive counselling but as patients are specially selected on the basis of their motivation, family support and personality these findings may not be generalisable. The confrontational method used in 'Minnesota Model' residential centres is not suitable for all patients and increasingly treatment is based on cognitive–behavioural models. Overall, between a third and a half of those treated continue to have a drinking problem when followed up for several years, and up to 15% have been shown to return to social drinking. Prognosis is best in those with good premorbid personalities and in those who have stable families for support. Untreated, alcoholics have a high mortality and morbidity. Although there is little research available on this group, one study in 1953 showed that 50% continue with their problem until death, roughly one quarter moderate it or become abstinent and the remaining quarter become worse.

PREVENTION

The compulsion 'to do something' whenever a major problem is identified is as evident in relation to alcoholism as to any of the other problems of our modern times. Simple answers to complex problems have been suggested and the question of education about alcohol and its complications is one such simple solution which has been suggested and tried. Unfortunately the evidence so far (and it is extensive) is that while education increases people's knowledge about alcohol it does not affect attitude or behaviour. A number of studies have examined the effects of education programmes on teenagers, on recidivist drunken drivers and groups recruited through advertisements. They confirm the relative ineffectiveness of education programmes in bringing about behavioural change.

Attempts to identify problem drinkers in the workplace are promising but are still in their infancy in Britain and Ireland. The approach is to recognise and provide help for those who may have emotional problems from any cause. Efforts to identify problem drinkers *per se* have proved less successful than a more general and holistic approach to occupational medicine.

A different approach to prevention stems from the observations of Ledermann, outlined above, of an association between the national *per capita* alcohol consumption and the prevalence of alcoholism. Although this hypothesis has been criticised, its application lies in reducing the mean consumption by increasing taxation on alcohol. Other approaches to influencing the *per capita* consumption include tighter control of the conditions under which alcohol is sold and licensing restrictions. This strategy may be no more than a pious hope since the economic effects of such measures may make it prohibitive and some would view them as Draconian and an infringement of civil liberties.

SUMMARY

1. Defining alcoholism by the presence of the physical, social or psychological complications is likely to result in those with milder forms of the syndrome being missed.
2. The controversy over whether it is an illness is still unresolved although both illness and social models have distinct implications for management.
3. The search for a single cause is naïve and current theories of causation focus largely on social and personality factors. Genetic inheritance may play a part in some but the findings are disparate.
4. A number of physical illnesses and of chronic psychiatric disorders, especially panic attacks and resistant depression, should alert the GP to the possibility of problem drinking. Various social and employment difficulties should also increase vigilance.
5. The general practitioner is one of the most successful agents in detecting alcohol abuse.
6. The role of the family doctor in treatment is crucial and he has a central role in counselling the patient and in the detoxification of those who are motivated.
7. Although in-patient detoxification and intensive aftercare by trained personnel has been diligently studied, few centres have shown better results than those obtained from simple advice.
8. Psychological complications of alcohol such as marital and sexual dysfunction as well as depression and anxiety may need treatment when the patient is alcohol-free.
9. Although abstinence is the desired goal for every alcoholic, it is possible that certain sub-groups may, with specialist retraining, return to social drinking.
10. The type of alcoholism, i.e. whether binge or regular drinker, primary or symptomatic, does not affect the prognosis.

CASE HISTORIES

Case 1

Mrs X, a 35 year-old woman, was referred with a recent history of depression. In addition she suffered occasional panic attacks but her general practitioner's main worry was her gross neglect of herself and her house. Prior to this she was a self-employed and successful beautician. She still socialised and met friends regularly for meals but her home had become dirty and she would often lie in bed until noon. Her husband was a businessman and she claimed he was supportive, although this was not felt to be the case by the family doctor. There were no children as the marriage had not been consummated. They had sought help for this but her husband had refused to attend after the first appointment and she had 'reassured' him since then that the problem was hers. There was no definite family history of psychiatric illness but Mrs X thought that a brother may have had a drink problem in the past. She said she drank socially and her husband was also a moderate drinker. Her mother was killed in a fire when she was 14 and she laughed when she received the news. She had a very poor relationship with her parents and she was not close to her siblings. At presentation she complained of constant tiredness, feeling slow in the mornings, waking 2 hours earlier than usual and crying frequently. Suicidal ideas were absent. Attempts to explore her relationship with her husband were always intercepted by comments such as 'He basically cares' or 'He doesn't believe in all of this', etc., and requests to interview him were always blocked in this way. Similarly, questions about her mother's death and her response to it were dealt with in a superficial manner. Antidepressants were prescribed in view of the symptom pattern and the deterioration in self care and she claimed some improvement but the panic attacks continued. In addition she was noted to be tremulous at some interviews but she attributed it to rushing for the appointments. Two months after commencing treatment her husband contacted to tell me that his wife was having visual hallucinations. He admitted that she had been drinking heavily for several months, often beginning at 9 a.m. He also spoke of his own reluctance to admit the problem and that he had known I had asked to see him but had been unwilling. Mrs X was admitted to hospital and diagnosed as suffering from delirium tremens. She had visual hallucinations of mice and for several days was agitated. She was treated in the usual manner with high dose benzodiazepines and intravenous vitamins and made a full recovery. At follow-up 3 weeks later she was free from depression and panics but refused further counselling for her drink problem or her marital difficulties. She also refused disulfiram for prophylaxis. Antidepressants had been discontinued at admission.

Comment

This lady illustrates several interesting points. First, the discrepancy between the severity of depression and her self-neglect was striking. Her failure to show a full response to antidepressants in therapeutic doses along with the persisting panic attacks is a frequent finding in those who are alcohol dependent. Panic attacks tend to occur at times of relative abstinence. She admitted that before her appointments with me she would not drink – hence the tremulousness at interview. Her husband's failure to admit the problem was a reflection of the severe marital difficulties which this couple experienced and is a common pattern in relationships of indifference or hostility. Her excessive drinking was probably due to these and to other unresolved conflicts from her past. In view of these persisting difficulties and her failure to continue in therapy, the prognosis is poor. If, at initial interview, she had admitted the alcohol problem I would not have prescribed antidepressants.

Case 2

Mr X was a 54 year-old hotelier who was referred with depression. He claimed this had begun a few weeks earlier after he had sold a business to which he was particularly attached. His new outlet was being run jointly with his wife and he resented this sharing. His wife felt he was unable to run a business any longer because of his alcohol consumption and when confronted with this at the first interview (he had earlier denied that he drank to excess) he admitted to drinking up to one bottle of spirits each day. He also complained of black moods, sleep disturbance and concentration difficulties. Appetite was impaired and his libido was greatly reduced. He would not agree to in-patient detoxification but agreed to try and abstain himself and to admission if this failed. No medication was prescribed. At the subsequent interview 2 weeks later his wife confirmed his abstinence but he still described depressive symptomatology as above. Disulfiram was prescribed and he was advised to begin to seek outlets and find hobbies. He had no particular interests prior to this. He was seen 3 weeks later and on this occasion his symptoms had resolved completely and he had begun to make changes in his working relationship with his wife. Over the following 3 months he maintained his improvement and continued to accept his drinking problem.

Comment

This patient illustrates the difficulty of handling depression in the alcoholic. This man described typical depressive symptoms but these resolved spontaneously. Although he presented with depression, this was not the primary pathology but was a direct result of alcohol abuse. He requested antidepressants at the second interview and suggested that he had drunk to excess because of depression. A simple rule of thumb is to wait for about one month following detoxification and then decide on the basis of current symptomatology and current stresses whether or not to prescribe. Alcoholics often ascribe causation to depression and this may occasionally be correct. It is more likely however to be a rationalisation. At the second interview he was given advice about his lifestyle since the emptiness and absence of social outlets in his life following detoxification may have been contributing to his gloomy state.

Case 3

Mr X was referred with depression. This had followed a personal disappointment relating to his business as a farmer. He had been gloomy for about 4 months and also described waking early, panic attacks and loss of weight. His wife and family were supportive and confirmed a marked change in his personality since the onset of depression. He was irritable, complained constantly of feeling anxious and had lost all energy and drive. His family described him as a high achiever and an ambitious man prior to this. A diagnosis of depressive illness was made and treatment with antidepressants was commenced. He failed to show any response to dothiepin, clomipramine or lofepramine in doses of between 150 and 200 mg nocte. He said his panics were worse than ever and he began to feel hopeless. In view of the large component of anxiety, MAOIs were suggested. He refused to have them because of the restriction on alcohol. He took a drink each night and although he denied drinking more than this, he felt it was his only remaining pleasure. He was commenced on mianserin in increasing doses up to 90 mg per night and two days later his wife telephoned to say that he had just told her that he had for several months previously been drinking, up to six glasses of whisky each day, to relieve his depression and panic attacks. He had begun to carry a small flask of whisky on his person but now realised how psychologically dependent on it he had become, since hearing that alcohol may be contraindicated if he needed MAOIs. He immediately stopped drinking and his depression and panic attacks resolved within 2 weeks of commencing mianserin. At the time of writing this man has remained free from depression, is drinking normally again and has taken steps to change his lifestyle and develop outlets apart from work.

Comment

The history was indicative of a depressive illness which antedated his excessive drinking – the latter was symptomatic of his depression. The heavy intake of alcohol compounded his depression and he presented as having a resistant depression. His panic attacks were also being compounded by alcohol which brought about temporary relief only. Once alcohol was discontinued his depressive illness responded to antidepressants in the usual way. Insight about his abuse of alcohol occurred when faced with the possibility of having to avoid alcohol completely.

REFERENCES

Aertgeerts, B., Buntinx, F., Ansoms, S. and Fervey, J. (2001). Screening properties of questionnaires and laboratory tests for alcohol abuse or dependence in a general practice populations. *British Journal of General Practice*, **51**, 206–217.

Brown, S.A. and Schuckit, M.A. (1988). Changes in depression among abstinent alcoholics. *Journal of Studies in Alcohol*, **49**, 412–417.

Clark, W.B. (1976). Loss of control, heavy drinking and drinking problems in a longitudinal study. *Journal of Studies on Alcoholism*, **37**, 1256–1290.

Edwards, G. and Gross, M.M. (1976). Alcohol dependence: provisional description of a clinical syndrome. *British Medical Journal*, **1**, 1058–1061.

Goldberg, K.F., Singer, T.M. and Garno, J.L. (2001). Suicidality and substance abuse in affective disorders. *Journal of Clinical Psychiatry*, **62** (Suppl. 25), 35–43.

Kisley, S.R., Gater, R. and Goldberg, D.P. (1995). Results from the Manchester Centre (in Ustun, T.B. and Sartorius, N. (Eds), *Mental Illness in General Health Care*. Wiley, Chichester.

Mayfield, G.D., McLeod, G. and Hall, P. (1974). The CAGE questionnaire: validation of a new alcoholism screening instrument. *American Journal of Psychiatry*, **131**, 1121–1123.

Roeloffs, C.A., Fink, A., Tang, L. and Wells, K.B. (2001). Problematic substance use, depressive symptoms and gender in primary care. *Psychiatric Services*, **52**, 1251–1253.

Selzer, M.L. (1971). The Michigan Alcoholism Screening Test. *American Journal of Psychiatry*, **127**, 1653–1658.

FURTHER READING

Beich, A., Thorsen, T. and Rollnick, S. (2003). Screening in brief intervention trials targeting excessive drinkers in general practice: systematic meta-analysis. *British Medical Journal*, **327**, 536–542.

Chick, J. (1995). Alcoholism: detection and management in general practice. *Primary Care Psychiatry*, **1**, 153–161.

Cutting, J. (1982). Neuropsychiatric complications of alcoholism. *British Journal of Hospital Medicine*, **27**, 335–342.

Jellinek, E.M. (1960). *The Disease Concept of Alcoholism*. Hillhouse Press, New Brunswick, New Jersey.

Kendell, R.E. (1979). Alcoholism: A medical or a political problem? *British Medical Journal*, **1**, 367–371.

Paton, A. and Saunders, J.B. (1981). ABC of alcohol. *British Medical Journal*, **283**, 1248–1250.

Royal College of Psychiatrists (1986). *Alcohol our Favourite Drug*. Tavistock, London.

SUGGESTED READING FOR PATIENTS

Cooney, J.G. (2003). *Under the Weather. Alcohol Abuse and Alcoholism. How to Cope, 2nd edition*. Gill and McMillan, Dublin.

Kelcham, K. and Asbury, W.F. (2000). *Beyond the Influence: Understanding and Defeating Alcoholism*. Bantam, New York.

Royal College of Psychiatrists (1986). *Alcohol our Favourite Drug*. Tavistock, London.

Wilson, M. (1989). *Living with a Drinker*. Pandora, London.

USEFUL WEBSITES

www.alcoholmd.com

Royal College of Psychiatrists: www.rcpsych.ac.uk/info/help/alcohol/

USEFUL CONTACTS

Alcoholics Anonymous
General Service Office
PO Box 1
Stonebow House
Stonebow
York YO1 2NJ
UK
Tel: 01904 644026
Website: www.alcoholics-anonymous.org.uk

Alcoholics Anonymous (Ireland)
109 South Circular Road
Dublin 8
Ireland
Tel: 00 353 1453 8998
Email: ala@indigo.ie
Website: www.alcoholicsanonymous.ie

Health Promotion Unit
General Information Department
Hawkins House
Dublin 2
Ireland
Website: www.healthpromotion.ie

Al-Anon Family Groups UK and Eire
61 Great Dover Street
London SE1 4YF
Tel: 020 7403 0888
Website: www.al-anonuk.org.uk

Al-Anon Information Centre
5 Capel Street
Dublin 1
Ireland
Tel: 00 353 1873 2699

Alcoholics Anonymous

....
(please fill in your local branch number
here)

10

Substance Abuse

Older textbooks emphasised the distinction between drugs that were associated with abuse but that did not cause physical dependence and/or physical symptoms on withdrawal and those that did. This distinction rested on the absence of tolerance and on the occurrence of psychological symptoms only on discontinuation. However, the recent editions of DSM and ICD do not make this distinction to the same extent and most substances are now regarded as causing psychological, behavioural and physical dependence although this blurring of the boundary between physical and psychological dependence is not without its critics. For example, cocaine and cannabis, in the past thought not to be associated with a physical withdrawal reaction, are now listed as among those that display this response. Caffeine and nicotine also cited as addictive substances.

The importance of the distinction is that drugs which produce physical dependence, such as opiates and benzodiazepines, must not be discontinued abruptly while those associated mainly with psychological dependence may be, although craving and other psychological symptoms such as depression and agitation may ensue. For virtually all practitioners the most common substance abuse problems are those of alcohol (see Chapter 9) and benzodiazepines. The legal aspects of drug abuse are discussed in Chapter 18.

One in ten adults abuse illicit drugs in Britain and about one-third of those with psychiatric illness have a comorbid diagnosis of substance misuse. Among adults in the US the lifetime prevalence for abuse of illegal substances is around 6% with an excess in males. Clinically there is a suggestion of a link with personality disorder but this has not been adequately investigated.

BENZODIAZEPINE DEPENDENCE

The popularity of the benzodiazepines lay in the fact that for the first time in the early 60s there appeared on the market very powerful and effective anxiolytics which had none of the apparent drawbacks of their antecedents, the barbiturates. Time has once again become the great leveller and since the first caution that these drugs may also be drugs of dependence, the number of cases of addiction has spiralled. The extent of the problem is unknown since there is no knowledge of the number of regular users. About half of regular users are believed to suffer withdrawal symptoms and these are identical to the classical symptoms of anxiety – hence their continuing prescription in times past since such symptoms were attributed to a recrudescence of the anxiety state which they were being used to treat.

Symptoms of withdrawal and predisposing factors

The typical withdrawal reaction consists of two clusters of symptoms (Table 10.1) corresponding approximately to classical symptoms of anxiety and a more serious group of perceptual, physical and sometimes psychotic symptoms (Petrusson and Lader, 1981). These generally occur within 3 days of discontinuing the drug and are more acute following withdrawal from short-acting than long-acting medication. This is believed to be due to the attenuating effect of the active metabolites of the latter. Symptoms last for a varying period from a few days to several weeks or rarely months.

Table 10.1. Symptoms of benzodiazepine withdrawal.

• Restlessness	• Hyperacusis
• Impaired concentration	• Hypersensitivity to touch
• Tremor	• Hallucinations
• Insomnia	• Delusions especially paranoid
• Anxiety	• Depersonalisation
• Palpitations	• Dizziness
• Nausea	• Fits

Some work has focused also on the type of person likely to develop withdrawal symptoms and while there is no consistent pattern, those with dependent personalities have been shown to feature more than others. The explanation for this may lie in the greater tendency of this group to become chronic users of these drugs or it may be associated with their greater awareness and tendency to complain of withdrawal symptoms. Another feature is the history of dependence on other substances especially alcohol which characterises these patients.

Management

A number of options are available to the general practitioner who is treating a patient wishing to discontinue benzodiazepines. The patient must be told at the outset that some symptoms are inevitable but that these will be minimised by the judicious use of adjunct treatments. In all cases it is essential not to discontinue the benzodiazepine abruptly and it is common practice to change from a short-acting to the equivalent dose of a long-acting drug either before or during the period of withdrawal.

Thereafter gradual reduction, with or without other treatments, is the main approach. This should be done at the patient's pace rather than in any predetermined way since overzealous reduction may result in intolerable withdrawal symptoms with treatment being compromised. The duration of detoxification may vary from a few weeks to several months and indeed some patients fail to be withdrawn completely although continuing to use a benzodiazepine at a much reduced dose.

Several ancillary techniques are available to the doctor although it is not essential to use these.

Tricyclic antidepressants

The tricyclic antidepressants because of their effect on symptoms of anxiety are often used in benzodiazepine detoxification. It is important to realise that many patients receiving benzodiazepines will in fact have an undiagnosed depressive illness, presenting as anxiety and will require suitable treatment for this once detoxification has been completed. Thus, using these antidepressants during detoxification will serve a dual purpose for many patients. Where depression is adjudged to be present the duration of antidepressant treatment will be as usual for depression (see Chapter 6). If depression is not diagnosed and antidepressants are being used solely to modify the withdrawal syndrome they can be discontinued once withdrawal has been completed.

Beta-blockers

Since beta-blockers are established as having an effect on the physical symptoms of anxiety, these may be used to diminish peripheral withdrawal symptoms. The dosage will vary with the degree of symptomatology and is generally in the range used for the treatment of anxiety. They will be used until the benzodiazepines have been withdrawn totally and are then discontinued themselves.

Major tranquillisers

Major tranquillisers will assist in reducing symptoms but the drawback of drowsiness generally precludes their use.

Relaxation techniques

Relaxation techniques are useful either on their own or combined with the above approaches.

Self-help groups

Self-help groups are promoted by many and although these do not necessarily help in controlling symptoms, their benefit lies in the comfort patients find from meeting others with similar problems and in stimulating motivation when this is flagging. As with all self-help groups, the danger of becoming 'stuck' and not moving out of the group to resume normal functioning and the tendency to use the group as an opportunity to endlessly 'discuss' the problem rather than as a stepping stone must be emphasised.

Other drugs

Clonidine, an α_2 agonist, normally used as an antihypertensive, has been successfully used in opiate and alcohol withdrawal. It may have a use in benzodiazepine withdrawal but this has yet to be evaluated. Some recommend the use of carbamazepine although this is almost exclusively in the US. Buspirone, a non-benzodiazepine tranquilliser, is not of benefit in withdrawal.

Prevention

1. The cautious use of benzodiazepines hardly needs reiterating and the advice at present is that they should not be prescribed on a regular basis for longer than 4 weeks. Also long-acting drugs are to be preferred to short-acting ones and flexible rather than regular dosage is recommended.
2. The accurate diagnosis and treatment of depression, especially when anxiety is to the fore will reduce the inappropriate prescribing of these substances.
3. As outlined in Chapter 8, there are many techniques available to the practitioner in dealing with anxiety. Using this broad range of treatments is to be commended.
4. It must be realised that problems of living should not be 'treated' with drugs and a willingness to accept the limitations of medicine in dealing with understandable human suffering is a philosophical stance which has become a medical necessity in view of the iatrogenic problems associated with benzodiazepine over-prescribing.

OPIATE DEPENDENCE

The author recognises that many general practitioners have little contact with opiate addicts in large numbers. However, those working in the inner cities will unfortunately be frequently confronted with this problem and the attendant legal and medical difficulties. In addition general practitioners are increasingly involved in the ongoing management of opiate addicts in collaboration with psychiatric specialists in substance abuse.

The epidemiology of this problem is unknown since there are difficulties inherent in measuring its prevalence, not least being the reluctance of patients to admit the dependence. In an attempt to overcome this uncertainty the Home Office made compulsory the notification of opiate abusers to the Addicts Index in Britain. No such law exists in Ireland. In 1989 there were roughly 9000 registered opiate addicts in Britain. Since the Addicts Index closed at the end of April 1997 there are no current figures from that source. However, the Department of Health publishes information on the number of persons presenting to drug misuse services for treatment in Great Britain and includes those whose main drug of abuse is either heroin or cocaine. In September 2000 there were almost 25,000 heroin addicts (Department of Health, 2002). This huge increase is probably related to the fall in street prices for heroin and the increasing affluence of young people. The fashion in opiates changes periodically and although heroin remains the substance of first choice for most addicts, methadone, pethidine and DF118 have been variously sought after. Most addicts will also abuse other drugs either alone or with opiates and so a combination with hallucinogens, cocaine and others is commonplace.

Social and demographic features

Opiate dependence is largely found in those under 25 and there is an excess of men. Many have histories of non-drug related offences even prior to the addiction and further offences continue in an effort to steal drugs from pharmacies, etc. Other offences such as shop lifting and prostitution are common as the addict attempts to finance the spiralling debt which invariably ensues. Up to 50% are diagnosed with antisocial personality disorder although this behaviour may represent a symptom of opiate addiction rather than an inherent personality disorder. Addicts tend to congregate in the poorer non-residential areas of large towns and cities. Many are unemployed and have few close, lasting relationships outside the drug culture. All social classes are represented.

Presentation

Frequently the addict first presents as a result of pressure from the courts. This inevitably will compromise the patient's motivation and hence the doctor–patient relationship. Opiate addicts should be assessed initially by a psychiatrist specialising in substance abuse and the practitioner who himself attempts to detoxify or otherwise treat an opiate abuser may rapidly find himself attracting patients who wish to have their habit facilitated by him.

Addicts also often present at times of crisis for themselves and this includes weekends, or when money or supplies are not available. In such circumstances it is tempting to prescribe on humanitarian grounds. Again, this is ill-advised and may be dangerous since the patient will often exaggerate his need and death may follow from overdose.

Those who have been prescribed long-term opiates for genuine painful conditions abuse their drugs at times also. Many are not aware of the addiction until withdrawal is attempted while others have a well-developed preference. Detoxification in this group should be carried out on an in-patient basis and while waiting to commence treatment, cautious prescribing, with supervision from a family member and the doctor, can be continued. Close liaison with the prescribing doctor will clarify the issue of the genuine needs of the patient for pain relief. The patient who refuses detoxification, in the absence of a genuine *physical* reason for continuing, should be discharged from the practitioner's care and advised of the risks of continuing dependence.

Pregnancy

Addiction to opiates in the neonate is an increasing problem and about three-quarters of all infants born to addicted mothers experience withdrawal symptoms. The mortality among newborn infants withdrawing from opiates is much higher than among adults, where it is almost never fatal. In addition there is a risk of miscarriage when withdrawal occurs earlier in pregnancy. Maintaining the pregnant woman on low dose methadone (up to 40 mg per day) may be the least hazardous and if a reduction is required it should be carried out slowly and with monitoring of fetal movements. Withdrawal from opiates is least hazardous to the fetus in the second trimester.

The doctor–patient relationship

This is more compromised when dealing with drug abusers, including opiate addicts, than with any other group of patients. The trust, which is central to this relationship, is often lacking since the addict is attending to importune rather than to seek counsel while the doctor may find himself questioning his patient's motives. He may also have to refuse medication, which would bring symptomatic relief – a practice which is alien to the caring doctor. Not surprisingly, many find this difficult and adopt a permissive approach to prescribing. It behoves every doctor when confronted with these issues to bear in mind the function of medicine and the nature of the doctor–patient relationship if the medical profession is not to become guilty of compounding rather than alleviating the problem.

The problem of AIDS in relation to opiate abusers raises further dilemmas for the GP, especially in relation to prescribing, in areas where specialist services for addicts are lacking. The issue centres round whether the continued prescribing of oral or injectable opiates is warranted for those who are unwilling or unable to undergo detoxification and who, by needle sharing, are at risk of contracting AIDS. The pressure that the doctor may feel to acquiesce with the patient's wish for drugs and/or needles must be tempered by the doctor's equal concern that in so doing the patient's motivation may be minimised. Needle exchange only takes place with the agreement of the specialist services and the individual general practitioner should not provide needles if this is requested without such an arrangement.

Recent data from general practice point to the feasibility of providing methadone maintenance treatment in this setting. A recently published study in Britain shows that the frequency of heroin use was reduced from a mean of 3.02 episodes per day to a mean of 0.22 episodes per day, confirmed by urinalysis. Mean numbers of convictions and cautions were reduced by 62% for all crime. HIV risk-taking behaviour, social functioning, and physical and psychological well-being all showed significant improvements (Keen *et al.*, 2003). While this study is positive in its findings, the patients are likely to be among the more stable addicts as those with poor motivation and continuing abuse remain under the care of the secondary services.

Detoxification

Detoxification is most easily carried out in in-patient treatment units but in some circumstances, where the patient has a stable family for support, it may be done as an out-patient. A large number of drug treatment centres now exist in Britain although they are much scarcer in Ireland. These also have community drug prevention teams to help at primary care level in the detection and early treatment of this addiction. Detoxification is most commonly done by substituting methadone for the other opiates which the patient has been using. Care must be taken lest the doctor unwittingly overdoses the patient since patients do not generally have an accurate record of their opiate consumption and may exaggerate it for the purpose of procuring extra. It is best to titrate upwards against the emergence of withdrawal symptoms rather than the reverse. Having established the lowest dose to prevent withdrawal symptoms, dose reduction begins and this is then titrated downwards against the withdrawal symptoms, the objective being to minimise these. In general, short-acting substances such as heroin produce brief but intense discontinuation symptoms while long-acting opiates lead to a relatively mild but more prolonged withdrawal phase, although when an opiate antagonist such as naloxone or naltrexone are used the reaction can be severe.

Using methadone for detoxification the process takes about 2–3 weeks. An alternative is to use clonidine (Gold *et al.*, 1982), beginning with a test dose of 10 µg/kg/day orally and then increasing to 17 µg/kg/day (in two divided doses) if there is no hypotension. This is then decreased gradually over a 10-day period. It is the central α_2 agonist action which is believed to inhibit the withdrawal syndrome. Alternatively lofexidine, also a central α_2 agonist, can be used instead of clonidine if postural hypotension is problematic.

Subsequent to detoxification the patient must be encouraged to change his lifestyle, which has usually centred upon procuring drugs. Many patients describe missing the ritual of searching and of injecting more than the drug effect and will often describe a void in their life. Counselling must be directed towards satisfying recreation, finding a job if possible and towards building a trusting relationship with the therapist (GP, psychiatrist or counsellor) since the recovering addict will continue to be vulnerable at times of crisis.

Opioid antagonism

Following detoxification the opioid antagonist naltrexone can be used to maintain abstinence since it blocks the agonistic effects of opiates, especially euphoria, making continuing abuse less likely and ultimately leading to extinction of the behaviour due to the absence of any psychological rewards. The initial dose is 25 mg increasing to 50 mg the following day. However it can cause severe withdrawal symptoms if the patient is still physically dependent and should only be instituted when detoxification is fully completed. A period of 7–10 days opiate-free confirmed by urinalysis is required. If there is a risk of occult abuse a naloxone challenge test should be performed. However, there is no mechanism to compel the person to comply with this treatment so high levels of motivation are required.

Harm minimisation and the general practitioner

For those unable to maintain abstinence the alternative of prescribing methadone and/or needle exchange should be considered. Decisions about dosage, etc., are made by the specialist services but increasingly general practitioners are becoming involved in prescribing to the stabilised addict. Once the patient shows signs of wanting to increase the dose or of return to crime, referral back to the addiction services is indicated to re-establish stability. However, there are ethical concerns about some aspects of harm reduction. These include the possibility of the use of injectable heroin for those who will not or cannot be maintained on methadone with the related requirement for the provision of legalised injection rooms as in Holland and Australia.

Morbidity and mortality

The physical consequences of opiate addiction stem probably from the use of contaminated materials and dirty needles. These include thrombophlebitis, hepatitis, muscle contractures, finger gangrene and AIDS. Thrombophlebitis may result in veins becoming permanently damaged and these should be examined not just in the antecubital fossa, but also in the arms and forearms, the ankles, neck and fingers. The social consequences include poverty, repeated crime both petty and serious, prostitution (homosexual and heterosexual) and loss of family and friends. Opiate addiction is not associated with any particular psychiatric syndrome although depression is often described during detoxification. This does not usually require treatment and improves spontaneously. The mortality among opiate addicts is 30 times higher than in the general population and is from accidental overdose and from suicide. Follow-up studies indicate that up to 20% have died after 10 years and 33% are abstinent. The concomitant abuse of cocaine is a poor prognostic indicator.

AMPHETAMINE (AND RELATED SUBSTANCE) ABUSE

Amphetamine was discovered in 1887 and was marketed in the 1930s as an over-the-counter treatment for nasal congestion. Within a few years reports of abuse began to appear. Amphetamine sulphate, the most common preparation, is easily synthesised in home laboratories although a stronger version, methylamphetamine ('ice') is also available and its effects are said to last much longer. Amphetamines are often used on their own but they may also be abused in conjunction with opiates and while they are associated with some physiological changes such as fatigue, headaches, muscle cramps, profuse sweating and insatiable hunger when withdrawn, the main discontinuation symptoms are emotional in nature. These consist of profound craving for the drug, severe depression, often suicidal in intensity especially associated with methylamphetamine abuse, lethargy, nightmares and either agitation or psychomotor retardation. For the patient's safety hospitalisation is advised during this period. Symptoms begin within a few hours of discontinuation, peak within two days and resolve within a week usually.

In the early 1960s most abusers were women who had been prescribed these drugs for obesity or depression. Today, they are mainly men and are similar to opiate addicts – in fact amphetamine abuse now seldom occurs in isolation and amphetamines are often abused to counteract the dysphoria many opiate addicts experience in the aftermath of a 'buzz'.

The immediate effects of amphetamines are to reduce fatigue, decrease hunger, improve concentration and heighten awareness in association with an intense feeling of bodily pleasure. In some users an amphetamine psychosis can occur with paranoid delusions, hallucinations in multiple modalities, and thought disorder. Consciousness is clear and in the acute phase is indistinguishable from schizophrenia. However, when the symptoms are chronic, amphetamine psychosis lacks the affective flattening and poverty of speech characteristic of chronic schizophrenia. It is uncertain if amphetamine psychosis occurs in those who are predisposed to schizophrenia or if it is sporadic. The treatment is as for any acute psychosis and if chronic symptoms supervene maintenance treatment will be necessary as for schizophrenia. Occasionally high dose amphetamines may produce life-threatening cerebrovascular accidents and focal neurological signs.

Methylene dioxymethamphetamine (MDMA) or 'Ecstasy' is a party drug, used socially, which rapidly induces energy, alertness, and euphoria. Adverse effects include severe headache, tension in the jaw and teeth grinding, panic attacks and elevated blood pressure. After use irritability, depression and insomnia are commonly described and then fade after 2–3 hours. Occasionally hallucinations and paranoid ideation may occur and paranoid psychosis has been described with high doses, as have abnormalities of gait and nystagmus. Seizures, renal failure and cardiovascular accident have also been documented. Malignant hyperpyrexia with disseminated intravascular coagulation can also result from dehydration but rapid rehydration can cause circulatory overload and death. Occasionally MDMA may be combined with fluoxetine to enhance its effects, believed to result from a massive release of central serotonin. Although not physically addictive, it can induce psychological dependence. Treatment is symptomatic and most users presenting to the medical services do so for control of psychotic symptoms or for the treatment of acute dehydration.

Khat (pronounced COT) is derived from a plant of the same name and can be bought from greengrocers in East London, where it is imported from the Horn of Africa. Nowadays, it is chewed or made into a tea and used by immigrants from Somalia, the Yemen and Ethiopia. Its active ingredients, cathinone and cathine are stimulating and are class C drugs under the Misuse of Drugs Act. In other countries it is more strictly controlled by law. Similar in effect to amphetamines, it increases alertness and reduces appetite. It also induces a feeling of calmness but regular use results in insomnia, anxiety and anorexia. Chewing the leaves results in intense thirst and produces a strong aroma. It may lead to irritability, violence and craving along with depression on discontinuation.

COCAINE ABUSE

Although less common than opiate addiction, there were 2000 cocaine addicts receiving treatment in Britain in 2000. The acute effects of cocaine are generally similar to amphetamines but tactile hallucinations, with a sensation of insects crawling beneath the skin, referred to as formication, are common although less so than delusions. Cocaine acts as a stimulant and because it produces a sudden feeling of euphoria (a 'rush' or 'flush') it may be used repetitively. 'Crack' is an extremely potent form of cocaine that can induce intense craving after only a few experiments. With both forms of cocaine, usually smoked or snorted, paranoid delusions and episodes of psychosis are frequent, occurring in up to 50% of abusers. The risk of violence or homicide associated with cocaine has led to its legal recognition as a class A drug (under the Misuse of Drugs Act, 1971) along with opiates.

As with amphetamines, cocaine withdrawal is not associated with a physical withdrawal syndrome but it can produce a profound depression, termed a 'crash'. This is usually short lived and terminates in less than a day although when the abuse is severe the withdrawal may be prolonged for several days. In-patient care during withdrawal is not mandatory since these drugs may be discontinued without physical withdrawal symptoms but it is advisable due to the associated depression. Moreover, cocaine is frequently abused alongside opiates and opiate detoxification may need to be carried out concurrently. With long-term snorting, cocaine users are subject to ulceration of the nasal mucosa. No one treatment has been shown to be effective in reducing the withdrawal symptoms although dopamine agonists such as bromocriptine have been tested with varying results. Management of acute psychotic episodes is as for any psychotic episode.

HALLUCINOGENS

Lysergic acid diethylamide (LSD) is the most popular of this group of drugs and is a class A controlled drug. It is usually taken by mouth and the first effects are felt 30–90 minutes after ingestion. These include dilated pupils, sweating, increased heart rate and high blood pressure. Perceptual disturbances including vivid visual hallucinations, heightened senses of colour and auditory changes are common. Sensory inputs are blended (synaesthesiae) so that sounds may be seen and colours felt! Thought processes are distorted and thinking becomes illogical and with a magical quality to it. During the peak of the experience there may be a loss of personal identity which some regard as a quasi-religious experience while others become terrified with feelings of impending insanity and loss of control. Vivid recollections of the past and delirium are sometimes present and distractability is marked. The acute symptoms fade in about 6 hours but residual symptoms, e.g. distractability persist for up to 24 hours. When these symptoms induce fear and panic in the patient they are referred to as 'bad trips'. These may present to the general practitioner and treatment is as for any acute psychosis. They require prompt treatment since bizarre accidents can ensue. 'Flashbacks' are another adverse feature of LSD abuse and can occur for up to one year after the last episode of abuse. These too should be treated with major tranquillisers. Occasionally a psychosis, schizophrenic in type, may supervene and a 'psychedelic syndrome' with inert and passive behaviour has been described in chronic users.

Psilocybine is the active ingredient in 'magic mushrooms' and has effects similar to those of LSD. It is an occasional drug of abuse.

SOLVENTS

These include glues, petrol, nail varnish remover, etc., and their abuse is confined to children and teenagers. Most strikingly, these usually come from emotionally deprived backgrounds. The general action of solvents is as a central nervous system depressant. Tolerance develops although the withdrawal symptoms are mild. The initial effects, occurring after a few minutes and lasting for up to a few hours, resemble alcohol intoxication with euphoria followed by depression. Occasional psychotic episodes have been reported. With prolonged inhalation cardiac arrhythmias and loss of consciousness may occur. Chronic abusers may develop hepatic or renal damage and aplastic anaemia has been reported. Delirium or irreversible dementia may develop with persistent use and the associated behavioural disturbance may require symptomatic control with major tranquillisers. Benzodiazepines should be avoided since they may further increase the risk of respiratory depression. Solvents may be discontinued without a physical withdrawal syndrome but there is some evidence that solvent abusers frequently progress to alcohol abuse. Long-term management should centre round the family pathology rather than the solvent abuse in isolation.

CANNABIS

This is now a class C controlled drug in Britain. Within minutes of smoking the subject is relaxed and experiences perceptual distortions although these are not as severe as with the hallucinogens. Sexual arousal occurs and energy increases. Heavy use can cause cannabis intoxication with a heightened awareness of colour, sound and detail. Time also appears slow and there may be feelings of detachment and out of body experiences. Skill such as driving and using machinery are impaired for up to 12 hours after smoking. Either elation or depression can occur in those subject to mood swings. Expectation and ambience is also thought to contribute to these responses. Psychotic reactions have been described although much less commonly than with hallucinogens. The aetiological role of cannabis in long-term psychosis, although subject to doubt, would now seem to have been resolved with the finding of Arseneault *et al.* (2004) that cannabis use is one of the factors interacting with others to provoke schizophrenia and that the incidence of schizophrenia could be reduced by 8% at a population level if cannabis use was eliminated. The role of cannabis in causing an 'amotivational' syndrome, characterised by self-neglect and apathy, remains unresolved between those who argue that this is a direct result of cannabis use and those who believe that it reflects traits present prior to drug abuse. Cannabis detoxification does not require in-patient treatment and is unlikely to occupy much of the practitioner's time since use of cannabis is generally sporadic and recreational. Acute psychotic episodes require sedation in the usual way. This use of cannabis by those with a pre-existing psychosis considerably destabilises their condition.

OTHER DRUGS

Nicotine

It is unclear whether nicotine produces a pharmacological or psychological dependence. Unlike other substances that are abused nicotine intoxication has not been described. There is no doubt that craving occurs and this coupled with the relaxing effects of nicotine make stopping difficult. Social factors contribute to smoking initiation and to its maintenance by encouraging the use of cigarettes in some environments. Moreover, those whose parents or siblings smoke are more likely to do so themselves since they act as role models. Claims have been variously made for the success of hypnotherapy, of chewing gum impregnated with nicotine, transdermal nicotine (patches) and for group and cognitive therapy but the results are inconclusive when studied scientifically. The optimum treatment remains advice from the general practitioner and nicotine replacement. However, up to 50% of those who discontinue smoking permanently do so without any professional help.

Heminevrin

This drug is occasionally abused especially by alcoholics for whom it may have been prescribed during detoxification. It produces a physical withdrawal syndrome and should be gradually reduced in those who are dependent. This may be avoided by cautious prescribing and it should not be given for longer than 10 days. Its former popularity in alcohol detoxification has waned considerably in recent years and with its declining use, the problem of dependence should decline also.

Barbiturates

Once common, barbiturate dependence is now rare and confined mainly to established opiate addicts. These drugs should not be suddenly discontinued because of the risk of fits. The addict should be prescribed a long-acting barbiturate, e.g. phenobarbitone 50 mg t.i.d. and this is then decreased, usually under anticonvulsant cover over a period of a few weeks. Ideally this should be carried out in an in-patient setting. If fits supervene they should be controlled in the usual way with a short-acting barbiturate or with diazepam intravenously.

Methaqualone

Methaqualone is abused mainly by young people and is often preferred to barbiturates in opiate abusers for its euphoriant and hypnotic effects. The risk of pharmacological dependence is still unclear but in view of the possibility, gradual reduction is indicated.

Other drugs of abuse are *analgesics* such as paracetamol and glutethimide. The former is associated with mild feelings of pleasure, peptic ulceration, anaemia and in severe cases analgesic nephropathy. Withdrawal headaches combined with denial of the problem make this difficult to detect and treat. Glutethimide withdrawal causes a delirium tremens-like syndrome and in overdose is highly dangerous. It should not be prescribed.

LABORATORY INVESTIGATIONS FOR DRUGS

The presence of drugs in the body may be detected by either urine or blood analysis. Techniques involving saliva and hair sampling are not widely available. The

Table 10.2. Metabolic profile of common drugs of abuse.

Drug	Half-life (hours)	Unchanged drug in urine
Phenobarbitone	100	25%
Chlormethiazole	5	5%
Amphetamine	12	3%
Methylamphetamine	9	43%
Cocaine	1	4%
Diazepam	48	?
Heroin	0.5	0%
Morphine	3	5%
Methadone	15	4%
Codeine	3	?
LSD	3	1%
Cannabis	30	?4%

usefulness of a particular test depends on being aware of the drawbacks of the method as well as the metabolism of the drug.

A negative finding does not exclude the possibility that illicit drugs have been taken; it merely confirms that the concentration in body fluids was not high enough or that the half-life of the drug was too short to allow detection when the sample was taken. In particular heroin and cocaine have short half-lives. The half-lives of the commonly abused drugs are shown in Table 10.2. False positive results have also been described and interpretation of results must be made in conjunction with clinical and historical information rather than as an end in itself. For example, repeated negative testing for opiates is significant in a patient claiming to be dependent and requesting methadone. In addition some drugs, for example heroin, are metabolised before any excretion in urine occurs thus making detection of the parent substance impossible by urinanalysis. On the other hand, over 40% of methylamphetamine is excreted unchanged in urine making urine testing particularly valuable when assessing the consumption of this drug.

When a urine sample is provided it is important to ensure that it has actually been provided by the patient since abusers of illicit drugs can substitute samples. Not only will regular sampling assist in building up a picture of the patient's drug misuse over time but the threat of spot checks can have a deterrent effect.

SUMMARY

1. Benzodiazepines are the most common drugs of dependence after alcohol.
2. During withdrawal the patient can usually be treated without recourse to hospitalisation.

3. Benzodiazepines should not be discontinued abruptly. About 50% of long-term users suffer withdrawal symptoms. These resemble anxiety but occasionally a more severe reaction may occur.
4. There is no information about the best approach to management but the addition of a tricyclic antidepressant is beneficial in some cases. Propranolol is also used to alleviate the physical withdrawal symptoms. It is best to change from a short-acting to a long-acting benzodiazepine before or during withdrawal.
5. Opiate dependence is increasingly managed in primary care once the initial psychiatric assessment has been completed and a treatment plan devised.
6. Reduction in cannabis abuse would significantly reduce the incidence of schizophrenia.
7. Amphetamines, cocaine, and LSD are not drugs of physical dependence and they may be discontinued without fear of a physical reaction. Hospitalisation may be required to counteract the psychological complications of withdrawal.

CASE HISTORIES

Case I

Mr X was a 30 year-old married man who was referred for benzodiazepine withdrawal having been prescribed a short-acting one 3 years earlier after his wife had a miscarriage late in pregnancy. This was the first pregnancy in the marriage and although they had only been married less than a year were very excited about the prospect of parenthood. His wife miscarried at 22 weeks and Mr X was extremely upset. He arranged a religious burial ceremony for the baby and within a week began to have panic attacks. He went to his GP complaining of anxiety, depression, insomnia and anorexia and was prescribed a short-acting benzodiazepine. He continued to take this for about 2 years but on hearing of the risk of dependence tried without success to discontinue it himself. In the intervening 2 years he felt gloomy and had stopped going out initially because of lack of interest but subsequently due to panic attacks. When seen at the clinic a diagnosis of benzodiazepine dependence and of depressive illness was made and he was commenced on a tricyclic antidepressant. He began to obtain some symptomatic relief from his depression after 3 weeks of treatment at a dose of 100 mg nocte. At this point the first reduction in the benzodiazepine was made while increasing the antidepressant to 150 mg. Subsequently he underwent monthly reductions in benzodiazepine until he could no longer tolerate further changes in dosage. At this point he was changed to diazepam, a long-acting benzodiazepine and reduction continued thereafter until it was discontinued. At no time did the patient require admission to hospital and overall the reduction occurred over a 6-month period. Subsequently antidepressants were continued for a further 9 months.

Comments

This gentleman when he first approached his GP should have been either advised that his symptoms were part of his grief reaction or else given a benzodiazepine for a short time with close monitoring. Two features should have alerted the GP that his reaction might be potentially serious – first, the man was inordinately upset at his wife's miscarriage and, secondly, arranging a burial ceremony is unusual. In the light of these the subsequent depressive illness was not unexpected. His symptoms of anxiety were part of this condition, which had gone unnoticed and untreated. It is common for patients to cope with the initial reductions in benzodiazepines, probably because they are highly motivated at the outset and later experience more difficulty. Changing to a long-acting drug is associated with fewer withdrawal symptoms because of the cumulative effects of the active metabolites. There is also more flexibility of dosage.

Case 2

Mr X was referred by his family practitioner because he was demanding increasing amounts of opiates for back pain. He had been involved in a road accident 3 years earlier and having had his vertebrae fused continued to complain of pain. His wife was taught while in hospital to administer the opiate injections and thereafter he attended his GP who prescribed these drugs under the instruction of his orthopaedic consultant. His GP felt that he was deceiving him about the severity of his back pain and having confronted him he admitted this. Mr X was admitted for detoxification and this was successfully carried out using clonidine. Throughout his stay in hospital he remained repentant and motivated and although he still described some back pain agreed that it was not constant nor did it interfere with his day-to-day activities as he had suggested. His reason for taking opiates was for euphoria. Prior to discharge he was referred back to his consultant for further consideration of his analgesic requirements.

Comment

Cases such as this are difficult since the doctor is totally dependent on the accuracy of the patient's history when making decisions about treatment. The iatrogenic addict is often not recognised and the patient who complains of constant pain despite 'successful' prior treatment should alert the prescribing doctor to the possibility of opiate abuse.

REFERENCES

Arseneault, L., Connon, M., Witton, J. and Murray, RM. (2004). Causal association between cannabis and psychosis: examination of the evidence. *British Journal of Psychiatry*, **184**, 110–117.

Department of Health. (2002). *Statistics from the Regional Drug Misuse Databases*. Department of Health, London.

Gold, M.S., Pottash, A.L.C. and Extein, I. (1982). Clonidine: Inpatient studies from 1978 to 1981. *Journal of Clinical Psychiatry*, **46**, 35–38.

Keen, J., Oliver, P., Rowse, G. and Mathers, N. (2003). Does methadone maintenance treatment based on the new national guidelines work in a primary care setting? *British Journal of General Practice*, **53**, 461–467.

Petrusson, H. and Lader, M.H. (1981). Withdrawal from long-term benzodiazepine treatment. *British Medical Journal*, **282**, 643–646.

FURTHER READING

Keen, J., Oliver, P., Rowse, G. and Mathers, N. (2003). Does methadone maintenance treatment based on the new national guidelines work in a primary care setting? *British Journal of General Practice*, **53**, 461–467.

SUGGESTED READING FOR PATIENTS

Pryor, W. (2003). *The Survival of the Coolest*. Clear Books, London. (This book deals with heroin addiction.)

Ling, W., Smith, D.E. and Wesson, D. (1994). *Prescription Drug Abuse and Addiction. Answering Your Questions*. Hazelden Publishing and Educational Services, USA.

USEFUL WEBSITES

National drugs helpline: www.release.org.uk

Cannabis: www.cannabis.net

Cocaine abuse: www.nlm.nih.gov/medlineplus/cocaineabuse.html

Ecstasy: www.ecstasy.org

National Institute on Drug Abuse's information on heroin (USA): www.drugabuse.gov/ResearchReports/Heroin/Heroin.html

Benzodiazepine addiction, withdrawal and recovery: www.benzo.org.uk

USEFUL CONTACTS

**Standing Conference on Drug Abuse
(SCODA)**
32–36 Loman Street
London SE1 0EE
Tel: 020 7928 9500

Aid for Addicts and Family (ADFAM)
(Address as for SCODA)

The Drug Treatment Centre Board
Trinity Court
30 Pearse Street
Dublin 2
Ireland
Tel: 00 353 1 6488 700
Email: info@dtcb.ie
Website: www.addictionireland.ie

11

Personality Disorder

Personality disorder is a diagnosis usually made by psychiatrists. However, it is important that general practitioners also recognise those with this diagnosis since its co-morbidity with other psychiatric disorders worsens the response to treatment and prognosis. It is also associated with unplanned surgery attendances (Moran *et al.*, 2000).

Recent years have seen a burgeoning literature on various aspects of psychiatric disturbance in general practice. Noticeably few of these have included data on personality disorder. One of the reasons for this omission is the absence of a treatment for abnormalities of personality which has regrettably diminished rather than stimulated interest. There have also been problems of measurement which have militated against the valid and reliable assessment of personality status. A more fundamental difficulty has been the controversy surrounding the number and categories of personality disorder (this is described in more detail below since it has implications for clinical practice). The diagnosis of personality disorder is one which should be made with caution since it often alienates service providers such as psychiatrists and psychologists. Conjuring up images of difficult, dependent or at times violent people, it has a stigmatising effect even in the presence of axis 1 disorders such as anxiety or depressive disorders. For this reason it is essential that the diagnosis is made only when the doctor is certain that the traits are of lifelong duration and lead to significant social as well as personal suffering. In spite of the significant impairment associated with it, personality disorder is excluded from the present mental health legislation in Britain as justifying compulsory treatment except for 'dangerous, severe personality disorder' (DSPD) which it is proposed will allow for detention and compulsory treatment even when crimes have not been committed. The newly enacted Irish legislation does not include personality disorder either as grounds for compulsory treatment.

CATEGORIES OF PERSONALITY DISORDER

The nosological status and the categories of personality disorders vary between continents and even sometimes between individual psychiatrists. The explanation lies in the derivation of these from subjective clinical opinion. Ideally this should be a starting point from which to attempt to prove their validity (existence) rather than assuming them to be immutable. This task has been hindered largely by lack of interest. Also the absence of adequate definitions would cause even the most basic of attempts to founder. So vague have been the descriptions of these categories that the level of agreement between psychiatrists in clinically diagnosing personality disorders is only around 30%. In the USA the problem of definition has been overcome by using rigorous criteria to facilitate accuracy of diagnosis. However, the number of categories identified in the USA has increased now to 11, adding to the complexity of validation and even these have been the subject of much criticism with many claiming that these are arbitrary epithets rather than scientifically validated disorders.

The principal categories identified in European psychiatry (ICD 10) are as follows.

Obsessional or anankastic personality

This refers to the predominating traits of punctiliousness, order, punctuality, perfectionism and rigidity. Lack of spontaneity, a dislike of surprises and sometimes indecisiveness are also found. Such people thrive in areas that require order and regulation but because of inflexibility they often alienate others. Occasionally, obsessive–compulsive disorder may supervene.

Passive–dependent or asthenic personality

Shyness, worrying, inability to make decisions, emotional dependence and low self-esteem characterise this group. In older parlance such people were often described as 'inadequate' but judgemental terms such as this are no longer acceptable in the modern psychiatric lexicon.

Histrionic (hysterical) personality

This refers to those who are shallow, flirtatious, self-centred, attention-seeking, dramatic and childish in behaviour. Unfortunately this label is frequently applied without adequate evidence and it is also used as a term of opprobrium (Thompson and Goldberg, 1987). There is no relationship with the condition known as hysteria and the association is phonetic not clinical.

Paranoid personality

Paranoid personalities are those who are suspicious of the motives of others, have difficulty trusting and in consequence make few close relationships. They respond poorly to justified criticism and are sensitive to the extent that they easily take umbrage. This may lead to difficulties with friends and colleagues. Paranoid psychosis may supervene when the suspicion becomes psychotic in intensity.

Schizoid personality

This is associated with coldness, a desire to be alone and to shun people, few relationships and often an interest in the eccentric. There is no definite evidence of a relationship to schizophrenia although earlier work suggested this association. It is probable that the features were a manifestation of early illness rather than of persistent personality type.

Cyclothymic personality

These personalities are those who are subject to swings of mood from depression to happiness. The swings are not related to circumstances and are never severe enough to require hospitalisation. Duration is usually a few days. Recent work suggests that this does not belong to the personality disorder category but is a subclinical form of bipolar disorder. Treatment with mood stabilisers has been tried with success (Akiskal *et al.*, 1977).

Sociopathic or psychopathic personality

This is associated with antisocial behaviour, impulsivity, emotional coldness and an absence of guilt. Alcohol abuse is sometimes associated.

Anxious personality

The anxious personality is tense, self-conscious and avoids relationships unless there is the certainty of acceptance. Some also call it the avoidant personality. It must be distinguished from generalised anxiety and from social anxiety disorder.

Impulsive personality

The impulsive personality is characterised by poor emotional control, unpredictable moods and argumentative behaviour. Forward planning is absent and decisions are often made which are subsequently regretted. A number of terms are often used clinically including 'immature' and 'borderline'. The former is a term of opprobrium and has no place in clinical practice. Borderline personality disorder is contentious (Tyrer, 2002) and while it is a frequently used description in the USA and has a vast body of associated research, the view of many is that it is no more than another label for either sociopathic or hysterical personality (Kroll *et al.*, 1982). This disorder is associated with chronic feelings of boredom, intense relationships which alternate between over idealisation and hostility, impulsiveness and emotional instability.

Personality change following a catastrophic experience

It is well recognised that periods of extreme stress such as being in a serious accident or following a severe psychiatric or medical illness can bring about a change in personality that persists even after the primary illness has been success-fully treated. In order to make this diagnosis the features must persist for more than two years with no prior history of personality disorder, and it presents either as persistent withdrawal, disinterest and lack of trust in people or with dependence and making excessive demands on others.

Organic personality disorder

This diagnosis is made when there is permanent personality change following brain injury, usually head injury.

Uncertain categories

The American system of classification also describes a number of additional categories that are not included in the European system of classification. Schizotypal personality disorder is regarded among European psychiatrists as a variant of schizophrenia and classified in that section of ICD 10. However, American psychiatrists view it as a personality disorder since such people appear to others as distinctly odd and strange. They often demonstrate magical thinking but also have great difficulty describing their interpersonal problems, as their speech is often metaphorical and circumstantial, requiring interpretation. They may claim clairvoyance and describe illusions and derealisation.

Narcissistic personality disorder is also included in DSM IV but not in the European classification. Persons with this disorder view themselves as unique and self-important. They see themselves as cleverer than others and they appear self-absorbed. Special treatment is expected and they often present as boastful. European psychiatrists, treating a person with these features, would make a diagnosis of histrionic personality disorder. Passive–aggressive personality disor-der, also not classified in ICD 10, is characterised in DSM IV by covert obstructive-ness and stubbornness to mask underlying aggression. Depressive personality disorder is characterised by persistent pessimism, gloom and unhappiness. The content of conversation is negative and dreary and there is little joy in the person's demeanour.

DANGEROUS, SEVERE PERSONALITY DISORDER (DSPD)

Under government proposals in England and Wales those deemed to have 'danger-ous, severe personality disorder' (DSPD) may be subject to a compulsory treatment order with detention in a unit specialising in the treatment of this condition. It is envisaged that this will reduce the threat of violence posed to the public by this group, who will present from three sources – those leaving secure hospitals, some leaving prison and some people in the community. It is estimated that 300–600 people will be so designated. However, the proposals have provoked controversy, from civil rights groups as well as psychiatrists, who point out that this legislation will result in the committal of those who have yet to commit a crime. In addition, as the prediction of future violence is unreliable, many more are likely to be incarcerated than are predicted by the Home Office. The necessary legislation is yet to be enacted.

PERSONALITY ASSESSMENT

Clinical methods

First, the general practitioner must attempt to *separate lifelong traits from current symptoms*, e.g. the apathetic, quiet patient with a depressive illness will give the impression of having a passive–dependent personality unless the doctor makes specific enquiries about the patient's usual behaviour. The assessor should begin by a simple statement such as, 'I'm trying to find out what sort of person you have been throughout your adult life. I know you may be different now because of your problems, but I want you to remember how you were before you became ill'. The traits and behaviour which the GP assesses must therefore be persistent over a number of years.

Secondly, the doctor must be aware of the common *sources of bias*. It is well recognised that male doctors diagnose attractive women as having hysterical personality disorder, especially if they are distressed. Similarly men are frequently labelled as psychopathic on inadequate grounds. Social class also contributes to bias, with personality disorder being diagnosed more frequently in lower socioeconomic groups.

Thirdly, *a single abnormal trait does not constitute a personality disorder*. The prosaic adage that 'nobody is perfect' should be borne in mind before the patient is labelled as being personality disordered. Thus a patient who describes himself as always being tidy and conscientious may not necessarily have an obsessional personality disorder unless other abnormal traits are also present. The threshold for this diagnosis should be high and unless the trait is causing problems to those who come into contact with the patient such labelling should be withheld.

Fourthly, information about personality is best obtained from *informants*, although there are few data on which informants are the most reliable. This is especially true when dealing with somebody who may be alcoholic, depressed or psychotic. Either because of deliberate obfuscation or lack of insight these categories of patients are unreliable.

Fifthly, personality disorder does not protect against psychiatric illness. A person with a sociopathic personality disorder may become clinically depressed and require treatment for this. 'Either/or' thinking may lead to treatable disorders being neglected and subsumed under an all-embracing rubric of personality disorder. Such practice will only increase the suffering of those already incapacitated by their personality. It is thus important to attempt to assess personality even when the doctor is certain that a mental state diagnosis such as depressive illness is present.

There are a number of attributes that should alert the doctor to the possibility of a personality disorder. These include frequent changes of job, an inability to sustain long-term relationships and multiple partners, excessive dependence on others for help with day-to-day decisions that may lead to self-referral to multiple counsellors or frequent utilisation of voluntary sector services.. Multiple episodes of self-harm, petty criminality and substance abuse and those who decompensate into anxiety or depression during transition periods whether this involves emotional change, such as bereavement, or physical changes, such as moving house, may also have a personality disorder. A history of sexual abuse in childhood is a known risk factor as is a history of disruptive behaviour in childhood. Finally patients who GPs describe as 'difficult' may have a personality disorder diagnosis (see p. 157).

Schedules

Many schedules have been developed for measuring abnormalities of personality. Among the earliest was the Rorschach Ink Blot test, which used the patient's interpretation of ink blots to develop a comprehensive understanding of the psychodynamics of the patient's personality. This is not widely used today since there was no standardisation of the test. Still used is the Minnesota Multiphasic Personality Inventory (Buros, 1972) but its use is limited by the time it takes to administer and by the interpretation of scores; it may also be contaminated by current psychiatric disorder. The Eysenck Personality Inventory (Eysenck and Eysenck, 1969), favoured because it is easily administered, has been widely used in general medical research. It describes the patient's personality on dimensions which are labelled neurotic, introversion–extraversion and psychotic. The dimensional concept is difficult to grasp and there is also concern about the particular dimensions chosen. The scores in each dimension have been shown to be unreliable and to change as intercurrent illness changes. Some schedules have overcome the problems of older ones which made no attempt to distinguish between symptoms of illness and enduring traits of personality and which obtained information from the subject only. Other schedules include the Standardised Assessment of Personality (Mann *et al.*, 1981) and the Personality Assessment Schedule (Tyrer and Alexander, 1979). These consist of a series of questions about individual traits of personality and information is collected from informants only in the former and from both subject and informant in the latter. These schedules have considerably enhanced research in this area although they are cumbersome to use. A recent schedule, the Standardised Assessment of Personality Abbreviated Scale (SAPAS) (Moran *et al.*, 2003) consists of eight items from the Standardised Assessment of Personality (SAP) (Mann *et al.*, 1981) and may prove feasible for use in everyday clinical practice.

There is no simple or rapid technique for assessing personality and even with schedules such as those described above the interview is lengthy and is only as reliable as the information obtained. Questions with 'hidden' meanings such as those used in popular magazines have more commercial than scientific appeal. Thus clinical assessment remains for the present the only viable method available to the general practitioner.

EPIDEMIOLOGY

Studies in general practice have consistently shown that about 5% of patients with psychiatric morbidity have personality disorder diagnosed by their general practitioner as the primary diagnosis. When assessment is made using an interview schedule this rises to around 26% (Patience *et al.*, 1995) and most of these patients will also have an illness diagnosis, e.g. passive–dependent personality disorder and generalized anxiety. In general, the incidence of personality disorder is higher in urban than rural general practices because of the attraction of the anonymous city for those who are chaotic and disturbed. Personality disorder is slightly more common in men than women and the obsessional, sociopathic and passive–dependent types are the most common.

In the general population personality disorder is found in about 13% of people and is most frequent in men (Casey and Tyrer, 1986). Moran *et al.* (2000) confirmed a prevalence of 24% among consecutive general practice attendees for any personality disorder General practitioners identified 27% of attendees as having a personality disorder but in this study those identified by the general practitioners were generally not the same as those identified by the research psychiatrist, suggesting that different constructs were being used by general practitioners and psychiatrists to identify personality disorder.

THE 'DIFFICULT PATIENT' AND THE GENERAL PRACTITIONER

The patient with a personality disorder rarely presents for help with this and more usually presents only when a crisis or some intercurrent illness/problem supervenes. Treatment of the presenting problem is called for first. This may involve crisis intervention, pharmacotherapy, social manipulation or a combination of these. However, the personality disordered patient will often pose additional problems that require special consideration. Recent evidence from Schafer and Nowlis (1998) found that patients identified as 'difficult' by family practitioners had unrecognised personality disorder when compared to control patients and that dependent rather than antisocial or borderline type predominated in this group.

Non-compliance is a frequent difficulty and the doctor has to carefully explain the necessity for taking prescribed treatments. In psychiatry this will often manifest itself as the patient wanting non-drug treatments even where this is indicated or failing to take medication that has been prescribed. It is important, while respecting the patient's understandable worries about drugs, to stress the value of the chosen approach. The doctor who is using counselling will experience non-compliance when the patient fails to follow simple instructions or makes what initially appear to be plausible excuses for not doing so, e.g. during marriage counselling the patient may make the excuse of being too tired to go out with the spouse as agreed in the sessions. There may of course be alternative explanations, other than personality disorder, for resistance to treatment. The explanations proferred by the patient may be genuine, or confronting the issue in counselling may be too painful at that time. These must be borne in mind but if non-compliance continues indefinitely and despite explanations to assuage the patient's concerns about the chosen therapy, this diagnosis must be considered. In the event of non-compliance, treatment must be suspended until motivation is more obvious.

Manipulation is another problem frequently associated with personality disorder. This may be overt, as when the patient asks for extra time off work even though there is no indication for it, or more subtle, as when the doctor gets drawn into subterfuge, e.g. a patient constantly complains about aspects of her marriage but yet refuses to discuss this openly with her spouse. A patient requested the author to contact her husband ostensibly about another matter and then to discretely raise the marital problem. It is easy to understand the tendency of the caring doctor to carry out such requests especially if he feels that the situation can be helped. However, before this course of action is followed the doctor should bear in mind the nature of the doctor–patient relationship of which mutual trust and openness is an essential ingredient. The manipulative patient may also visit different doctors and give contradictory accounts of previous treatments. A common problem is the 'playing off' of consultant against general practitioner and when in doubt this should be clarified, on the spot if necessary. A patient whom the author was seeing for an eating disorder and alcohol abuse asked permission to drink in order to stimulate her appetite. Permission was withheld. The following day she went to her general practitioner with this request also and failed to mention that she had discussed it only the previous day. He promptly contacted me to clarify our respective positions and to ensure consistency in the advice we gave this patient.

Blaming the doctor is a frequent and powerful technique used by the difficult patient. The patient whose request for admission to hospital, for drugs or for other inappropriate treatment is not acceded to may threaten self-harm or may lay the blame for any consequences at the doctor's feet. Such threats must not be dismissed since patients do harm themselves when angry. The risks of these threats must be assessed taking into account the patient's past history, their family support and the danger for future therapy of colluding with the patient's maladaptive behaviour. When in doubt the advice of a colleague should be sought and at times that of the defence organisation also.

Flattery is frequently used to win the approval of another and words of gratitude are appreciated by the doctor no less than anybody else. However constant expressions of indebtedness need to be treated warily since they may indicate that the patient feels a special affinity with the doctor over and above the usual doctor–patient relationship. In some forms of therapy especially the 'talking therapies' it may dupe the doctor into believing that the patient is being helped whereas no progress is in fact being made. The doctor who has been propitiated may also find it difficult to be objective about the patient and may become over-involved.

Dictating terms, such as the wanting to be seen at special times or demanding certain treatments, etc., will often be exhibited by patients who are demanding in their personal lives also. It is common practice to acquiesce to such demands initially since they often seem reasonable but the doctor must be aware that other inadmissible requests may follow. This may cause considerable friction and at its most extreme the patient may accuse the doctor of refusing treatment. Such a *modus operandi* is clinically and therapeutically crippling to the doctor and the patient may have to be confronted about this.

Frequent visits or calls are perhaps the most demoralising since they are often at unsocial hours and the outcome may be unsatisfactory. Obviously when these are requested to control panic attacks or to deal with the actively suicidal they must be followed-up with appropriate emergency intervention. Those which are to dispel various persistent hypochondriacal worries are more difficult since there is the inevitable fear that there is an organic basis for the symptom. Rather than refuse to attend when the 'emergency' presents the doctor should afterwards draw up a 'contract' with the patient regarding this behaviour. For instance the patient may agree to desist from such emergency calls in return for a regular agreed appointment with the doctor to explore personal difficulties. The patient's family may need to be involved in reaching this decision also since they are sometimes the instigators of such requests. It is tempting also to arrange yet another physical investigation so as to 'do' something even though there are inadequate grounds or it has been done previously. The temptation should be resisted since this may reinforce the illness behaviour and the patient advised that the matter will be discussed in less compelling circumstances – the doctor may then if necessary give the patient a specific appointment for further discussion.

TREATMENT

There is little optimism about the management of the personality-disordered patient. Even for those receiving dynamic psychotherapy the results are disappointing. Among general practitioners the scope is even narrower than for their psychiatric colleagues. The impediments to successful treatment include lack of motivation, poor insight and unreliability. The tendency for some patients to become over dependent on the therapist or to see themselves as passive agents in the process also militates against successful treatment. In general, treatment is behavioural and focuses on specific problem areas. For the general practitioner this is the only practical approach.

Social skills are useful for those who are shy and lacking in social confidence. Many centres, both lay and medical, now run social skills groups and the doctor would do well to have details of those run locally. The GP himself can do much to help by providing simple tasks for the patient such as rehearsing answering the door or the telephone. The patient can be advised to write what he will say and then to record it on tape for the next visit when constructive criticism and advice about the next stage will be provided. Suggestions about voice pitch, speed, etc., and demonstrations by the doctor himself take little time and are often very effective in bolstering self-confidence. Information about posture, eye contact, and body language can be incorporated into other sessions. Ideally a group setting should be sought once these very basic skills have been acquired since the aim of easy social intercourse will probably not be achieved otherwise.

Encouraging a positive self-image requires a different strategy. Discussion should concentrate only on the patient's positive attributes and listing these will focus attention on them. People with low self-esteem often fail to meet their own practical needs, have an exaggerated tendency to put others before themselves and are often taken advantage of. They should be encouraged to say 'no' to the undue demands thrust upon them and to regularly reward themselves with treats. Assertive training courses are often available in the local community as well as from the psychiatric services. Those run locally should be assessed before patients are referred lest they are being run by groups with their 'own agenda'. The GP can encourage rehearsal of basic assertiveness, e.g. returning items to shops. An understanding relative or friend may be of great assistance in facilitating the practice sessions and in providing positive feedback to the patient about self-worth.

Dealing with emotions such as anger or frustration is often a problem for those with personality disorder. There may be either a tendency to suppress emotion as with the passive-dependent person or to exhibit uncontrollable violence (towards self or others) in the sociopath. Teaching the appropriate display and control of such emotions is fraught with difficulty because of the danger of decompensation. This requires special skills in behaviour therapy and should not be attempted by the general practitioner. There is, however, cautious optimism for this treatment method in some patients.

Problem solving techniques are helpful for those who react adversely to every-day stresses and have been used with some success in those responding by overdosing, wrist-cutting, etc. Again, this form of behaviour therapy requires special skills which are now available in the psychiatric service.

Drugs have little part to play in the management of personality disorder. There is a suggestion that lithium is helpful in aggressive behaviour but this remains to be evaluated more fully. Lithium has been more successfully used in cyclothymia. Antiepileptic drugs such as phenytoin and carbamazepine have also been used but their value is yet to be established. Many patients with personality disorder request and are prescribed drugs especially benzodiazepines to help cope with the problems of living which they face. This should be discouraged since the risk of dependence is all too obvious in those with long-standing disturbance. Some of the benzodiazepines also have a propensity to release aggression and in those with antisocial personalities may worsen the problem.

IMPLICATIONS OF THE DIAGNOSIS

The received wisdom relating to the association between personality and illness has been questioned. In general there is no consistent association between person-ality disorder and mental state diagnosis with the possible exception of alcohol abuse. The latter is frequently associated with sociopathy. The association between schizophrenia and schizoid personality is questionable as is the assumed relation-ship between type of depression and personality. That is not to suggest that in *individual* patients personality abnormalities do not predispose to illness, but it does suggest that the study of personality in itself will not contribute to our under-standing the aetiology of specific psychiatric disorders.

The relevance of personality disorder to the general practitioner lies not in the treatment of this condition which is time-consuming, intense and best carried out in specialist settings, but in the effect personality has on the outcome of concomi-tant psychiatric disorder and on response to treatment. Psychiatric illnesses have a poorer prognosis when premorbid personality is abnormal and response to medication is adversely affected by abnormal personality. Not only is there more contact with the psychiatric services but there are more frequent visits to the general practitioner, symptoms are slower to resolve and functioning more impaired in the long term (Casey and Tyrer, 1990). It is apparent that assessing personality is of more than esoteric interest and that it has important prognostic implications.

It is to be hoped that in the not too distant future formal assessment of person-ality will be standard practice for the family doctor. He is, after all, in an ideal position to provide accurate information since in most cases he will be familiar with the patient prior to the onset of illness and over a period of several years. It would benefit the patient and those involved in treatment, whether specialist or generalist, if this information could be formulated concisely.

IMPULSE AND HABIT DISORDERS

There are a group of patients with impulsive behaviour and habit disorders, characterised by failure to resist an impulse that is usually ego-syntonic but often harmful. There is increasing tension prior to committing the impulsive act, with a sense of pleasure or gratification once it has been completed. These disorders are variously viewed as personality disorders or as mental state diagnoses or as overlapping into both groups.

Intermittent explosive disorder

As the name suggests, this disorder consists of intermittent bursts of aggression that are out of proportion to any precipitating social stress and triggered by minor conflict. Individuals or their relatives usually describe the episodes as 'spells' or 'attacks'. Associated with the violent outbursts are feelings of tension, relief after the episode followed by remorse. Many describe racing thoughts and an energy surge during the event followed by lowering of mood and decreased energy. Most have a lifetime comorbidity for a mood disorder, including bipolar disorder. In general, the age of onset is in adolescence and men predominate by a 4:1 ratio although some women describe similar symptoms premenstrually. In view of the favourable response to mood stabilisers many believe that it may be linked to bipolar disorder. There is little research on this disorder.

Pathological gambling

The essential feature of pathological gambling (PG) is a chronic and progressive failure to resist impulses to gamble, with the behaviour leading to much damage to personal and family life. Efforts to stop or resist gambling generally fail, and the behaviour shows some resemblances to an addiction. Deprived of the opportunity to gamble, the person becomes restless and irritable and over time there is an increase in the size and frequency of the stake required to achieve the desired level of excitement. In pathological states the gambling will persist even in the face of mounting debts, marital break-up or other legal problems. Some gamblers steal to maintain their habit. PG is a serious problem and may be associated with other addictions, particularly alcohol and tobacco, but there may also be disturbed eating, sleeping, sexual and relationship problems, as well as impaired function at work. Some present with depression or following an overdose.

PG is not rare: a survey in Australia gave a prevalence of 0.25% and surveys of prison populations show that around 10% of prisoners are pathological gamblers. It is probably more common and more obvious among men, who indulge in horse and dog racing, with which dramatic losses soon become apparent. Women prefer bingo and football pools in which morbid patterns are less obvious because losses are smaller and spread over longer periods of time.

The condition begins in adolescence for males and later in life for females. It waxes and wanes but tends to be chronic. The aetiology in unknown and theories abound. There are suggestions that gambling will at least temporarily help people switch out of negative internal mood states such as feelings of loneliness or other forms of dysphoria. The obvious self-destructive nature of the behaviour has provoked much analytical speculation, but there is little scientific study of the problem. There may also be social pressures including early exposure to gambling. Learning theorists point out that the usual sequence of repeated gambling losses with occasional random wins provides a pattern of intermittent reinforcement, the most potent schedule for conditioning. In this respect a big win is thought to be particularly hazardous, and the financial reinforcement of winning prolongs the habit. Recent evidence suggests that a mixture of biological and psychosocial factors is relevant to the development of this condition. Personality disorder, mania and childhood attention deficit hyperactivity disorder (ADHD) are considered risk factors also.

Various treatment approaches are offered, encompassing most known types of psychotherapy. Counselling and support for the family may also be helpful. Both psychodynamic psychotherapy and aversive behavioural therapy have been attempted, but neither claim much success. Most gamblers find the notion of complete abstinence abhorrent, but a few may accept the wisdom of a moratorium for a few months. Recent work suggests that cognitive-behaviour therapy may be helpful along with a 12–step group programme. Among the more severe cases there is usually a disturbed appreciation of the value of money, and in these instances it is wisest for all the family income to be paid into an account over which only the spouse has control. Gamblers Anonymous, which uses the Alcoholics Anonymous model, allows both the patient and spouse to share information about their struggles with the morbid impulses and provide mutual support. There is a little more optimism on the pharmacological front with preliminary studies suggesting a role for naltrexone, either as monotherapy or in combination with an SSRI. Also, lithium and valproate have been used with some success. Clearly, this will be a fruitful area for research in the future.

Trichotillomania

Trichotillomania is defined as the irresistible urge to pull one's hair. This is often associated with subsequent rituals, such as mouthing the hair afterwards, or even ingesting it (trichophagy). Most subjects report a state of tension before pulling.

The hair-pulling is not described as painful, but subjects report tingling and pruritis in the affected areas. As well as the scalp, the eyebrows, eyelashes, beard and pubic hair may be involved. Hair-pulling tends to occur during states of relaxation – while sitting down watching television, reading, studying, etc.

The aetiology of the disorder is not understood and some regard it as being driven by a desire to self mutilate, others as arising from impaired early relationships and others believe it to be biologically determined reflecting inappropriately released motor activity. The repetitive nature of the hair-pulling suggests a link to obsessive–compulsive disorder (OCD).

The disorder occurs in around 1% of new psychiatric referrals, and usually presents to dermatological clinics initially. The onset is typically in childhood and adolescence and there is a marked female preponderance. Depression and substance abuse may lead to exacerbations, but are not thought to be causal. The differential diagnosis is mainly with alopecia areata.

In management behavioural strategies appear to be the most useful. These involve asking the patient to practice some alternative motor response such as grasping or clenching the hands for three minutes, which competes with the urge to pull hair. The behavioural regime relies on identifying situations where the habit takes place, commonly while reading or watching television, and response prevention is attempted in these situations. Relaxation exercises may help. Another component of the behavioural regime is 'over-correction' or positive attention, requiring the subject to brush or comb their hair or repair eye make-up (for eyelash pullers) after each episode of hair-pulling. Drugs such as cloimipramine or an SSRI may also be helpful in view of the possible link to OCD. While both behaviour therapy and drug treatment may offer some relief in the short term, little is known about relapse rates or long-term outcome but a recent longitudinal study found a poor prognosis even with psychiatric treatment.

ADULT ATTENTION DEFICIT HYPERACTIVITY DISORDER

This disorder is incorporated into this chapter since personality disorder is a common complication of severe, untreated attention deficit hyperactivity disorder (ADHD).

ADHD is one of the most common psychiatric disorders of childhood. Until recently most child psychiatrists believed that ADHD improved in adolescence and disappeared in adulthood. In the 1990s follow-up studies of children with ADHD have shown that this is not correct and that 25% still met the criteria in early adulthood with the proportion falling to 8% by the late 20s. 60% have at least one disabling symptom as adults, 33% have antisocial personality disorder and in 16% substance abuse is a complicating factor. Extrapolation from the British and US studies suggests that 0.5–1% of the young adult population has this disorder although studies are few in number. The paucity of follow-up studies until recent years has meant that adult psychiatrists have little experience in managing this disorder in adults, resulting in a lack of services for this patient group. This is important because many will have been treated as children only to be denied on-going treatment when adulthood is reached while others will be undiagnosed as children and have no possibility of receiving a diagnosis and treatment in later life.

There is no evidence that environmental factors such as parental attitudes, deprivation, toxins or pre- or perinatal complications are responsible for ADHD. Monozygotic twins show a 50% concordance and adoption studies confirm the increased concordance for ADHD in the biological rather than the adoptive families of child sufferers. In addition MRI studies have found abnormalities in the corpus callosum and caudate nucleus although these findings require replication. Blood flow studies have also pointed to abnormalities in the prefrontal cortex, an area concerned with attention processes.

The core features of the disorder are hyperactivity, poor ability to maintain attention and poor impulse control. The disorder is classified into three broad groups – the inattentive form, the hyperactive–impulsive form or the more common combined type. To make the diagnosis the features must be present even before school age, should be pervasive rather than sporadic and should give rise significant impairment. ADHD is a chronic and often severe psychiatric disorder but generally improves by the late teenage years. In a very small proportion it continues into adult life with serious consequences for employment, relationships and general emotional well-being. Since impulsivity is one of the features of ADHD the condition is often associated with a poor work record and multiple jobs. Hyperactivity also reduces the ability to attend meetings and engage in concentrated work for long periods. The domineering and noisy behaviour of many sufferers lead to poor peer relationships and rejection both in childhood and adulthood. As a result long-term, stable relationships are difficult. Aggression may be associated with violent crime and imprisonment. Many develop depressive and anxiety disorders and substance misuse is a complicating problem as is antisocial personality disorder.

The pharmacological treatment is usually with methylamphetaine; in Ireland this is not licensed for adult use although it is available in Britain for this purpose. However, for those who have developed alcohol and personality problems, the use of methylamphetamine is not recommended due to the risk of abuse and interaction with other substances. Other pharmacological treatments include clonidine and tricyclic antidepressants, especially cloimipramine and imipramine and desipramine.. Psychological treatments are required both for the patient and for family members. Behaviour therapy is used to establish a reward and punishment system to help the young adult accept their disorder but also to take responsibility for their behaviour. Studying techniques can assist in optimising concentration. When complications such as alcohol abuse arise these should be treated in the usual way.

The earlier the disorder is recognised and treated the better the prognosis since this will reduce the adverse effects on relationships and the attention difficulties that are related to poor academic performance. The inattentive subtype also carries a better outcome. Adverse effects such as personality disorder, impaired relationships and substance abuse are more persistent and continue into middle life often leading to crime and imprisonment.

SUMMARY

1. When assessing personality it is essential to separate symptoms of current disorder from persistent traits of personality.
2. Informants are necessary to obtain objective information about personality.
3. Personality disorder frequently co-exists with psychiatric illness.
4. Obsessional, passive–dependent and antisocial types are the most common.
5. There is no link between any psychiatric disorder and any specific personality disorder with the exception of alcohol abuse which is often associated with antisocial personality.
6. Treatments are psychological and behavioural and are in their infancy.
7. The importance of personality lies in the effect it has on the outcome of mental state disorders – the presence of an abnormal personality adversely affects prognosis.
8. Personality disorder is a stigmatising diagnosis and should be made with caution.
9. ADHD once thought to be exclusively a disorder of children, is now believed to continue into adulthood in a small proportion of patients.

CASE HISTORIES

Case I

Mr X was 35 when admitted to hospital following an overdose. For 6 months previously he had been feeling depressed since beginning his new job. He was a successful businessman and had rapidly progressed up the management ladder to become one of the directors of his firm. He was 'head hunted' 9 months earlier for a post in the public relations and marketing side of his firm. He reluctantly accepted the post with persuasion from his wife. His hesitation stemmed from his introspective and reserved manner. He had few friends preferring to spend his time at home rather than socialising. He had no hobbies except watching television – he rarely read and showed no interest in sport or in the arts. He was meticulous and organised and found the flexibility of having to travel at short notice difficult to cope with. His wife was ambitious for him and felt that his drive and high standards suited him to his new post. His first overdose occurred after his firm had bought him a set of golf clubs so that he could make local business contacts. On admission after the overdose he had initial insomnia, impaired concentration and marked suicidal ideation. His symptoms improved within 2 days without any pharmacological treatment. He was advised that he was unsuited to his present post and he decided to ask for a change. This was procured and he maintained his improvement at the time of writing.

Comment

Mr X had an obsessional (anankastic) personality which had been of initial benefit to his career resulting in him being sought out for promotion. His reserve, limited imagination, as evidenced by his hobbies and inflexibility made him unsuited to the specific demands of his new position. Being emotionally inhibited and having an ambitious spouse he felt unable to confide and chose to persist in his unhappy state. Finally, unable to tolerate the stress of his predicament he overdosed. Changing his job to one which suited his personality resulted in an improvement in his well being. Diagnostically there was some initial uncertainty about the mental state (axis 1) diagnosis – the possibility of a depressive illness was considered but ruled out in view of his spontaneous improvement when removed from the precipitating stress. The axis 1 diagnosis was therefore an adjustment reaction, and the axis 2 diagnosis a personality disorder of obsessional type.

Case 2

Mrs X was referred with a 9–month history of feeling sad, tearful, with both initial and late insomnia. She had lost interest in her usual activities and concentration was impaired. She felt unable to cope, especially with her husband. The marriage had always been bad and she had been unhappy for many years but she described a recent change in her emotional state. Her husband frequently undermined her in public and had refused any sexual contact with her for several years saying she was unattractive. She had always been shy and diffident and felt unable to assert herself especially with her husband, but also with others. Prior to her marriage her colleagues at work would sometimes take advantage of her and she felt too shy to deal with this. She was financially secure and had supportive parents. She stayed with her husband because she was fearful of being without him and recognised her emotional dependence on him. She blamed herself for some of the difficulties and often said 'I mustn't be a very nice person to live with'. She had few friends of her own and her social life centred around her husband and his business associates.

Comment

This lady has an axis 1 diagnosis of depressive illness and axis 2 diagnosis of personality disorder, passive–dependent type. The differential diagnosis was of an adjustment disorder but the recent change in her mood state, which she clearly described clarified the diagnosis and she responded to a tricyclic antidepressant. Her husband refused to attend for marital therapy and indeed denied there were any marital difficulties. When she had returned to her pre-illness level of functioning, help with assertion was offered and she readily accepted this. The image-making effects of posture were outlined and in the early sessions she was encouraged to improve this (she usually sat with her head bowed and her legs sprawled). She was advised to find some outlets, separate from those of her husband and she joined a local charity. Finally the responses she would make to her husband when he became verbally abusive were rehearsed and she practised between sessions using a tape-recorder. She gained enough confidence to threaten to leave him and she also sought legal advice. Finally she asked him to leave for a period and only agreed to have him back if he agreed to marital therapy. At the time of writing he is considering this and she is having ongoing assertiveness training. There would have been no benefit from beginning this therapy prior to her symptomatic improvement since her disinterest and poor concentration would have made the exercises between sessions difficult for her. In addition, it was essential to see this lady's basic personality and the image she projected when well. The confounding effects of depression therefore had to be eliminated before specific therapy for her abnormal personality was offered.

Case 3

Mr X, aged 38, attended the clinic at the request of his girlfriend with whom he was living for the previous 2 years. The relationship had always been strained because of his emotional coldness and his unusual interest in Eastern religions. This occupied much of his home life, to the extent that he would spend all his spare time reading and meditating and refuse to visit family or friends. He told his girlfriend that he had no need of people and suggested that she leave him if he was not behaving as she expected. He had no friends and rarely associated with his workmates. He had never been married and prior to meeting his current girlfriend had only one brief relationship, lasting 3 months when he was 20. At interview rapport was difficult and Mr. X presented himself as a cold but self-sufficient man. He said the only reason he remained in the relationship was because he wanted to avoid a row but admitted that he felt little for his girlfriend. His childhood had been happy but he was regarded by his teachers as unusual since he preferred to play alone. Both parents were dead and he had been fairly close to them but had moved out of home when he was 20 visiting them at holiday time only. He had little contact with his siblings. Mental state examination was normal.

Comment

An axis 2 diagnosis of personality disorder, schizoid type was made. There was no mental state/ axis 1 diagnosis. The couple was offered help for their relationship difficulties but this was declined by Mr X who felt little could be done. With the patient's permission Mr X's girlfriend was informed of the diagnosis and advised of the absence of any known treatment. The lack of motivation is not surprising in view of the detachment and emotional coldness found in those with schizoid personality disorder. This also militates against any therapeutic relationship which is essential to successful treatment.

REFERENCES

Akiskal, H.S., Djenderedjian, A.H., Rosenthal, R.H. and Khani, M.K. (1977). Cyclothymic disorder: validating criteria for inclusion in the bipolar affective group. *American Journal of Psychiatry*, **134**, 1227–1233.

Buros, O.K. (1972). *The Seventh Mental Measurements Yearbook*. Gryphon Press, New Jersey.

Casey, P.R. and Tyrer, P.J. (1986). Personality, functioning and symptomatology. *Journal of Psychiatric Research*, **20**, 363–374.

Casey, P.R. and Tyrer, P. (1990). Personality disorder and psychiatric illness in general practice. *British Journal of Psychiatry*, **156**, 261–265.

Eysenck, H.J. and Eysenck, S.B.G. (1969). *Manual of the Eysenck Personality Questionnaire (EPQ)*. University of London Press, London.

Kroll, J., Carey, K., Lloyd, S. and Roth, M. (1982). Are there borderlines in Britain? A cross validation of US findings. *Archives of General Psychiatry*, **39**, 60–63.

Mann, A.H., Jenkins, R., Cutting, J.C. and Cowen, P.J. (1981). The development and use of a standardised assessment of abnormal personality. *Psychological Medicine*, **11**, 839–847.

Moran, P.A., Jenkins, R., Tylee, A., Blizard, R. and Mann, A.(2000). The prevalence of personality disorder among UK primary care attendees. *Acta Psychiatrica Scandinavica*, **102**, 52–57.

Moran, P., Leese, M, Lee, T. *et al.* (2003). Standardised Assessment of Personality – Abbreviated Scale (SAPAS): preliminary validation of a brief scale for personality disorder. *British Journal of Psychiatry*, **183**, 228–232.

Patience, D.A., McGuire, R.J., Scott, A.I.F. and Freeman, C.P.L. (1995). The Edinburgh Primary Care Depression Study: personality disorder and outcome. *British Journal of Psychiatry*, **167**, 324–330.

Schafer, S. and Nowlis, DP. (1998). Personality disorders among difficult patients. *Archives of Family Medicine*, **7**, 126–129.

Thompson, D.J. and Goldberg, D. (1987). Hysterical personality disorder. The process of diagnosis in clinical and experimental settings. *British Journal of Psychiatry*, **150**, 241–245.

Tyrer, P. (2002). Practice guidelines for the treatment of borderline personality disorder: a bridge too far. *Journal of Personality Disorder*, **16**, 113–118.

Tyrer, P.J. and Alexander, J. (1979). Classification of personality disorder. *British Journal of Psychiatry*, **135**, 163–167.

FURTHER READING

Schwenk, T.L. and Romano, S.E. (1992). Managing the difficult physician–patient relationship. *American Family Physician*, **46**, 1503–1509.

SUGGESTED READING FOR PATIENTS

Bramson, R.M. (1986). *Coping with Difficult People ... in Business and in Life*. Simon and Schuster Sound Ideas, New York.
Lindenfield, G. (1992). *Assert Yourself*. Thorsons, London.
Walker, A. and Gunderson, J.G. (2001). *The Courtship Dance of the Borderline*. iUniverse.com, ISBN 0595197124.

USEFUL WEBSITE FOR PATIENTS

Personality disorders: www.mentalhelp.net

12

Marital Disharmony
and its Management

In the last 20 years there has been a dramatic increase in the number of divorces, with over 40% of marriages now ending in divorce in those countries where liberal divorce laws exist. A similar proportion of children are directly involved with parental divorce. Not surprisingly the services providing counselling to those marriages in distress are overburdened. Many couples turn to such agencies as Relate (in Britain) and Accord (in Ireland) for assistance although this is often in the late stages of marital disharmony despite the evidence for the efficacy of couple therapy (Shadish and Baldwin, 2003). Some couples are reluctant to go to these voluntary bodies since they frequently have personal knowledge of the counsellors who are usually chosen from their local community. They prefer instead to seek the help of other professionals especially the general practitioner.

THE CONTEXT OF MARITAL DIFFICULTIES

Marriages between those of different social, religious or cultural backgrounds are at obvious risk due to misunderstandings about expectations, values and habits. The 'workaholic' husband is also included in this category as his career takes precedence over the needs and expectations of his family.

Marriages where there is an intellectual gap between the couple, especially where the woman is the more intelligent of the two, are at risk since the other partner may feel, and indeed may be, undermined. Differences in outlets and interests may be apparent and become a cause of conflict. The man whose main hobby is dart playing is unlikely to entice his poetry-loving wife into his world and vice versa.

Those marriages which are contracted due to pregnancy or at a young age are likely to become problematic as both partners mature and develop their own identities.

The changing role of women creates problems for many marriages especially when this restructuring occurs during the marriage. A man with traditional views of the role of each within the marriage may become embittered and hostile.

The arrival of the first baby may for some be a time of readjustment as the husband becomes less central to his wife's life. In addition the demands made by a baby may lead to tiredness, loss of libido and irritability, all of which are likely to impinge upon the husband and create tension within the relationship. Similarly the later years of a marriage may become fraught when the children have left home and their modifying influence has gone. This is especially a problem where couples have had difficulties and have stayed together for their children's sake.

The presence of psychiatric illness in one partner is a common and obvious cause of marital tension. Less acknowledged are the effects of recovery from a chronic psychiatric illness upon a marriage. Chronic disorders require readjustment in the well spouse. Having achieved an equilibrium which allows the marriage to continue, any upset to this such as follows recovery may lead to major marital difficulties (see below).

Pre-existing personality disorder, alcohol abuse or pathological jealousy will rapidly place a relationship under pressure as will infidelity.

PRESENTATION OF THE PROBLEM

It is most frequently the woman who seeks help initially. The explanation for this is probably that women have a greater ability to express their emotions and also have more contact with the general practitioner than do their spouses (Doss *et al.*, 2003). The manner of presentation varies but is generally one of the following.

The spouse may present *overtly complaining of marital conflict* and seeking help for this. In the author's practice this is uncommon except in those patients who have a long-standing knowledge of, and trust in, their family doctor.

The patient who attends for *frequent consultations* for relatively minor symptoms, either physical or psychological, should be questioned about the state of the marriage since such a manner of presentation is frequent (Law *et al.*, 2003).

Overt *psychological symptoms* are commonly described. These include feelings of depression, anxiety or general distress. While it would be wrong to 'maritalise' all emotional problems it is important to enquire about the marriage during the course of any psychiatric history. Moreover if the marital problems stem from the impact that the depressive illness has on the relationship, improvement will occur once treatment has been initiated (Whisman, 2001)

Sexual problems may occur in those with marital disharmony, usually frigidity and anorgasmia in the woman and loss of libido in the man. Where the sexual problem is considered to be secondary to a marital problem the management is of the latter rather than of the former. If the sexual difficulty is primary, sex therapy must be instituted (see Chapter 13). Only by a very comprehensive history of the marital relationship and sexual behaviour can this be clarified.

Presentation with *physical consequences of violence* may occur but is relatively uncommon since the injured spouse usually feels humiliated and is reluctant to expose the injuries. However, the person who presents with evidence of physical assault for which no adequate explanation has been found should be questioned closely and sympathetically about the possibility of marital violence.

Conduct disorders in the offspring of the marriage may be evidence of marital problems. Thus the child who is excessively violent or clingy, or the child who is refusing school or bed-wetting may be the product of an unhappy marriage.

BEGINNING THERAPY

There are several approaches to family therapy of which Systemic Therapy is the most commonly used. Associated with the name of Selvini Palazzoli *et al.* (1978), it was developed in Milan in the early 1980s. It is based on the theory that marital problems arise within the dynamic of the couple, family or extended family, which is regarded as a system in itself, rather than from within the individual. Other approaches include Structural Therapy (Minuchin, 1974) with its emphasis on family types (enmeshed/disengaged) and correct hierarchical structures and boundaries, and Strategic Therapy (Haley, 1976) which focuses on helping families through the life-cycle stages.

Do both spouses need to attend?

The spouse presenting with the problem will commonly tell the doctor of his or her fear that the partner will resent exposure of the problems and may request help for the marriage without the partner attending. In exceptional circumstances this may be possible, e.g. if the presenting party is extremely passive and for that reason taken advantage of by the other. Some sessions of assertiveness training may be all that is necessary in these circumstances. This however is unusual and it is always advisable for the other spouse to attend since the problems involve both. In some circumstances with the permission of the presenting partner it is appropriate to contact the other spouse by letter. This may take the form of a request to attend in order that both sides of the difficulties can be considered, and explaining that so far the therapist has only heard one side. Such a request is often met with acceptance and once the initial feelings of threat have been overcome therapy can begin.

How many therapists?

There is no agreement on this issue and for most general practitioners more than one therapist is not feasible. For those who are in a position to provide a second therapist advantage should be taken of this. Not only does it reduce the possibility of collusion between therapist and one or other of the pair in therapy but a co-therapist also provides a useful springboard for subsequent discussion of sessions. Finally, it is important that therapists have adequate supervision in order to explore the issues that are arising during therapy including transference problems.

Clarifying the possibilities

At the beginning of therapy it is important to clarify the aims and possibilities of the treatment on offer. Many couples expect that by just presenting themselves at the session their marriage will magically be healed. This has to be dispelled and the importance of them working at it has to be emphasised.

Motivation

The therapist must thus examine the motivation of the couple to improve their relationship and the willingness of both to participate actively in the sessions and in the tasks assigned to them. The capacity and willingness to change must be stressed. Many couples fear that therapy will lead to one or other being blamed and prompt reassurance that this has no part to play should dispel these misgivings. Some spouses are unsure of their role in therapy and may attend believing that they have come to provide information about the 'sick' partner. Their equal part in the process of therapy must be clarified.

Facilitation

The therapist must explain that he cannot of himself save the marriage but is a facilitator in the process of resolving the difficulties. Thus any blame for the failure of the marriage cannot be apportioned to the therapist. Moreover the therapist should explain that his task is not to save the marriage or to make decisions about the future of the relationship but to assist the couple in doing so. Thus the realistic expectations which the couple should have of the sessions must be specified at the outset.

Identifying the problems

This is the next step before therapy can begin and failure to do this will result in floundering with little being achieved. It is useful to provide a checklist for the couple and the areas of difficulty along with the degree of difficulty should be specified in each of the major areas. These should include:

- Sexual
- Roles/independence
- Financial

- Communication (verbal/non-verbal)
- Religious values and expectations
- Spare time
- Children
- Friends and relatives

Details

At the outset specify the number of sessions, the place at which they will be held and the duration of each session. Inevitably marital therapy takes longer than the ordinary consultation and it is best that such sessions be conducted at the end of surgery. Specifying the number of sessions in advance is also a stimulus to the couple to work at the tasks given them by the therapist.

THE SESSIONS

Bolstering

The positive attributes of each partner should be identified by the other early in therapy since these will improve mutual self-esteem. Many couples complain that they feel their spouse takes them for granted or has lost sight of the qualities which they possess. A session devoted to emphasising these will help redress this view. Where no qualities are forthcoming the spouse can be asked to identify the aspects which first attracted them to the other.

Communication

Stage 1

Without exception those with marital difficulties say that they have ceased to communicate with their spouse or when they do so that arguments supervene. It is thus essential to facilitate communication again and this may take several sessions. It may be necessary initially to specify a time each day when discussion can take place – this may only be a few minutes but may be vital. Later the couple should be encouraged to spend more time alone, e.g. going out once per week. Those in difficulty frequently go out in groups, with friends, thereby further limiting the possibility of discussion. Unless specific enquiry is made about this the therapist may be unaware of the extent of the silence which exists.

Stage 2

Once some communication has been re-established the couple should be encouraged to verbally express positive feelings. There is a prevailing view that 'actions speak louder than words' and this is frequently used to defend the stance that verbal expressions of regard are not necessary. The need to be positively valued is universal and requires words as much as actions. The expression of positive feelings may be especially difficult for the male partner and it may be necessary to begin in a simple way by making positive comments about meals, appearance, etc. Later more personal emotions may be expressed.

Stage 3

Where arguments are a problem in communication the therapist should prohibit discussion of any potentially inflammatory topics and may actually have to specify neutral topics. At times, subjects as bland as the weather or television may be the only ones that are prescribed. As the couple progress more emotional areas may be touched on, initially during the session and at home for a specified time after the sessions. Guidance can be given to avoid inciting arguments using role-play; the therapist may model a manner of speaking or a gesture which may provoke an argument and in turn can provide examples of alternatives which the couple can rehearse in sessions if necessary. Where arguments have occurred a careful examination of the verbal and non-verbal cues which led to it may be necessary. Where a couple are unable to talk at all without arguing it may be necessary to have practice sessions of listening and answering without interruption.

Contracting

The aim of therapy is to arrive at compromises in the areas in which difficulties have been identified. Dealing with each area in turn will facilitate the working out of these. The therapist must ask the couple to be specific in their requests. A request that financial responsibilities should be shared is too broad and must be made more specific, e.g. telephone bill to be paid by husband, etc.

Each partner selects one particular item of difficulty described by the other and agrees to change this. A reciprocal agreement is made by the second spouse to modify an undesirable behaviour in return for this. For example the woman may complain that her husband never puts the children to bed while he may say that his wife never greets him in the evenings. Both may agree to simultaneously change these behaviours and each is contingent upon change in the other. Some recommend a less Procrustean approach and suggest that the reward can be varied and taken on goodwill, e.g. the reward may be a drink instead of a kiss and may be given at various times. Whichever approach is used the principle is that the rewards extinguish the undesirable behaviour and the new patterns become consolidated and permanent.

Time is spent working out the contingencies in the various spheres of difficulty until the couple is satisfied that they have arrived at an acceptable arrangement.

WHEN TO DISCONTINUE THERAPY

Initially the therapist will have specified the number of sessions. It may be impossible to limit the number in this way as the complexity of the problem unfolds itself and in particular if the couple are changing and are shown to be deriving mutual benefit from therapy. However, the couple who continue to attend but are making no progress should be advised to terminate therapy. This is frequently met with pleas of 'We are just beginning to come to grips with our problems' or some such ruse. The therapist should be cautious of being seduced by this since the couple may be using the sessions to avoid making a final decision about separating. Even where one partner is making a unilateral attempt to change there is little point in continuing if this is not reciprocated.

During therapy one of the couple may indulge in acting-out behaviour, e.g. overdosing to manipulate change. If change does occur as a result it is unlikely to be sustained since it probably based on fear. This partner may need brief individual therapy before marital therapy can proceed.

Occasionally couples become angry and focus this on the therapist. This may be indicative of frustration and anger lying dormant in the marital relationship. Provided the couple can express these feelings to each other in an acceptable manner at the sessions, therapy can continue. Failure to do so or persistent outbursts of this type compromise the mutual regard and trust between doctor and patient(s) which is part of any therapeutic relationship. The couple should be recommended to seek help elsewhere.

COMMON PITFALLS

Reassurance

It may be comforting to the therapist to reassure the couple that all will be well but it is not necessarily accurate. Reassurance doled out in a perfunctory manner is unhelpful and frequently serves to diminish the effort the couple put into their marriage. Reassurance should be given sparingly and appropriately. The couple who have marital problems after seven or eight years of marriage should not be reassured that they are going through a 'seven year itch' – to do so would be to diminish the gravity of their difficulties. On the other hand to reassure the couple who are arguing at times of temporary financial difficulties may be helpful.

Collusion

It is common for the therapist to unwittingly take sides in marital disputes. This frequently occurs with the member of his or her own sex. However the therapist should be vigilant and emotionally detached from the problems of the couple. To do otherwise would compromise therapy and lose the trust of one or other spouse. In a similar vein the doctor who becomes emotionally over-involved with the couple and takes their problems upon his own shoulders will rapidly burn out and will cease to contribute actively to the sessions.

Comparison with therapist's own marriage

Using one's own marriage as the yardstick against which to measure difficulties is fraught with danger. Not only is it unacceptable to impose one's own values on another couple but it may also be dangerous for the therapist himself since he will inevitably begin to see the motes and beams in his own relationship. Each couple deserves to be considered in their own right and separate from the expectations which the doctor may have of his own marriage. Thus a couple may wish to have a traditional marriage with the female partner working at home and the male partner working outside the home. Such role boundaries may be unacceptable in the therapist's own marriage. To bring the therapist's expectations of roles into the sessions will inevitably cause the sessions to founder.

Interpretation of behaviour

Glib interpretations of the behaviour which the therapist observes within the marriage do not serve any useful purpose and may distance one or both of the partners from therapy. Thus choosing how and when to make interpretations about the behaviour which the therapist observes in the marriage has to be done sensitively. The therapist who tells the passive, indecisive spouse that her behaviour invites her over-bearing husband to be excessively controlling may be correct, but would be mistaken if this observation was made in a joint session as it might give the impression that the man's approach to his wife was acceptable. On the other hand, to do so when seen on her own may be helpful if accompanied by advice on how to overcome this behaviour pattern.

Impatience

Impatience is not an uncommon feeling in the therapist and the general practitioner may be especially vulnerable to this since he is trained in rapid consultation and in a system of health care which demands speed. If the doctor feels unable to cope with the slower pace he should not attempt this intervention. Equally the couple who want their problems resolved speedily should at the outset be disabused of this.

Passive v. active approach

There is in some quarters a view that all that is required of the therapist in 'talking' therapies is to sit back and listen. The opposite is the case and being attuned to the verbal and non-verbal cues of the couple as well as actively guiding the sessions are the skills which must be acquired (see Chapter 17 on Counselling).

SHOULD THERAPY EVER BE REFUSED?

It is rare that marital therapy would not have something to offer and it is seldom contraindicated. There are problems however for which marital therapy may not be the best option. In particular, where one spouse has a psychosis which is causing the conflict the best approach to management is treatment of the psychosis. A similar caveat exists in regard to alcohol abuse and treatment of this condition is the first line of management although marital therapy may be required later on to overcome some of the resentment which has resulted from this. Those who are pathologically jealous do very badly, and in most circumstances are not amenable to treatment. The spouses of such people frequently seek advice on how to deal with their plight. They should be advised against trying to prove their 'innocence' although few find this advice acceptable. Where the jealousy has led to physical violence or to infringements of privacy, e.g. following the spouse, separation may be indicated. Physical abuse also carries a poor prognosis and protection orders may be more appropriate than marital therapy.

MENTAL ILLNESS AND MARRIAGE

The prevalence of psychiatric illness in both husband and wife is higher than would be expected by chance. A number of suggestions have been put forward to explain this phenomenon. One is that shared environmental stresses such as poverty might render a couple vulnerable. Another is that ill people select each other as spouses, the 'assortive mating' hypothesis. The possibility that if one partner is ill and in contact with the psychiatric services the other will be referred early is described as the 'accelerated referral' theory. So far the data to support any of these theories are inconclusive and the most credible view is that the stress of having an ill spouse puts increasing pressure on the other until illness supervenes. In general where the husband is initially ill the probability of the wife becoming ill is higher than where the reverse prevails. Also where one partner is ill the roles and social relationships of the couple are constricted rendering the other more vulnerable to emotional disturbance.

Where prolonged and severe mental illness has been present the well spouse frequently devises a method of coping and adapting to this. When the illness is treated and the partner has recovered the remaining spouse may then have difficulties readjusting to the new role and relinquishing the old one which had developed over the years. Resentment often occurs and sentiments such as 'After all I've had to cope with, he seems not to be even aware of it' are frequently expressed. This is particularly true after recovery from a chronic depressive illness or some such disorder. The doctor must be aware of the possibility of this and give time for these feelings to be voiced without judgement.

It must be stressed that mental illness and marital difficulties are not synonymous. Many couples have gross marital conflict without ever developing any psychiatric disorder. Some on the other hand have emotional problems which serve to bind them more closely. This may happen with agoraphobia where the well spouse functions best when the other is housebound and dependent (Hafner, 1977). Although the roles in such marriages may be very abnormal by conventional standards, attempts to treat the phobia may be met with resistance and frank hostility (see Chapter 8). Similar difficulties arise with dominant–passive pairings.

SUMMARY

1. Marriages are at risk if there is a difference in educational or social background, if the marriage has been precipitated by a pregnancy, if the couple is young, or where personality or emotional problems exist. Other factors contributing to this vulnerability include changing roles within the marriage or the adjustment required during transition periods, e.g. following childbirth, retirement, etc.

2. The woman most commonly presents with the problem. The difficulties may be openly admitted or may present covertly with other emotional complaints, e.g. depression, with the physical consequences of violence or with frequent visits for minor ailments.

3. The expectations of the couple and their motivation must be discussed before therapy begins. On no account should the therapist take responsibility for saving the marriage and it must be specified from the outset that the success of therapy depends on their commitment.

4. The first stage in marital therapy is to assist the couple in communicating and in acknowledging their positive attributes. Then areas of conflict are defined and it may be necessary to assign tasks to help in overcoming these difficulties and in re-establishing more appropriate behaviour.

5. The therapist should avoid reassurance that the marriage will survive the problems, should not use his own marriage as a yardstick and should be cautious not to take sides. Interpretations of behaviour should usually be avoided.

6. Therapy should be terminated either when the specified number of sessions has been reached or earlier if the assigned tasks are not being carried out, or if either spouse shows signs of lacking motivation.

7. The effects of chronic psychological disturbance upon psychological well being and upon marriage must not be overlooked and where the male partner is ill the female is particularly at risk. When long-standing disorders are treated successfully the marriage may deteriorate since the change in roles consequent upon this may upset an established balance. Attention should be given to this during and after such treatments.

CASE HISTORIES

Case 1

Mrs X sought help for herself and unknown to her husband because of his physical violence to her. He hit her at least once each week and had been doing so for years. His violence was unrelated to alcohol and always occurred when his wife tried to prevent him from going to see his girlfriend. He had numerous affairs throughout their 20 years of married life and although she had considered leaving him when she first discovered this, decided to remain in the marriage for the sake of their children. She was financially independent and her children were now in their late teens. The discovery that he was having an ongoing affair despite his denials prompted her to seek help. She agreed to ask her husband to come to therapy and he agreed to this. He was seen on his own initially and told the therapist of his wife's nagging, of his disinterest in his wife and the relationship and although he denied an affair initially, admitted it when confronted directly. He told the therapist that he did not intend finishing the affair and that he would only agree to remain in the marriage if his wife agreed to their living separate lives. He agreed to tell his wife of this request and she initially said that she was willing to try and accommodate him in this way provided the violence stopped. Both of them were requested to discuss with each other the details of this arrangement and at the following interview both had agreed that this was an impractical and an impossible arrangement. No further appointments were offered and Mrs X accepted that her husband's lack of motivation and his unrealistic expectations precluded therapy.

Comments

This couple illustrates the unrealistic expectations of many who assume that motivation can somehow be instilled in the errant partner. Apart from this man's violence, his unwillingness to compromise and his expectations that they could live independently made therapy impossible. Many spouses ask if living separate lives under the one roof is viable. This is invariably impossible since the emotional distance that is required to live as flat-mates is absent. What the spouse is really hoping is that this arrangement will somehow assist in overcoming their difficulties. If this couple had not arrived at the conclusion they did in relation to their living arrangements they would have been requested to discuss its advantages and disadvantages in company with the therapist so that misapprehensions could be corrected.

Case 2

Mr and Mrs X were referred because Mrs X had tried to run away from home with their three children one week earlier. She had returned within a few hours saying she had nowhere to go. She said that for 3 or 4 years she had been feeling fed up in the marriage. Her husband was rarely at home and spent all his time starting business ventures, most of which were successful. She had wanted to look for work but her husband had objected saying she should be at home to answer the telephone and take his business calls. Mr X said that he felt his wife did not care for him or indeed for the family since she refused to do 'family' things such as picnics at weekends. He denied forbidding her to seek work and at her request he was about to set up a business for her. They rarely talked together and he felt excluded from her life. In particular he was upset that she had stayed out until 2 a.m. with friends on a few occasions recently without forewarning him and he had gone in search of her fearing an accident. Both agreed that they wished their marriage to remain intact and spoke of their feelings for each other when they married. They agreed that they spoke very little of these nowadays. A series of six sessions, lasting 50 minutes each were offered and the couple agreed. At the end of the first session Mrs X agreed to go out on Sunday afternoons with her husband and children while he agreed to take care of the children one evening each week when she went out with friends. The next session took place 2 weeks later and the intervening period had seen an improvement in their relationship. The second session was spent discussing Mrs X's desire for a job and she agreed that her husband was setting up a business for her but she felt he was delaying this. He agreed that he was delaying because of his wife's apparent lack of interest in the project and her failure to look at plans for the premises or even the financial arrangements. Both agreed to spend time together discussing these details and that by the next appointment the final arrangements would have been set in motion by her husband contingent upon her becoming involved in the meantime. They also agreed to continue the behaviour pattern which had been established at the previous session. At the third session Mrs X had fulfilled her part of the 'contract' and the opening of the business was imminent. At this session they requested termination of therapy since their relationship had improved so much.

Comment

It will be noted that no attempt was made at apportioning blame or establishing how the misunderstandings had arisen. Intervention was practical and task-oriented. It would be wrong to 'prescribe' too many tasks at each session since invariably these would not be carried out or would be forgotten about. Each new behaviour in one spouse was contingent upon changed behaviour in the other. Couples commonly desist from therapy after a few sessions since improvement in one area inevitably leads to improvement in others. Sessions lasting 50 minutes may seem lengthy and marital therapy can be conducted with briefer interviews although the total number may need to be increased.

Case 3

Mr and Mrs X presented for marital therapy because of violence which had been part of their marriage for 4 years. Mrs X was now threatening to leave. Her husband had been involved in an accident and, although not seriously injured, had been emotionally disturbed at the time and began drinking heavily then. He currently drank about 10 pints of beer each night and more at weekends and the violence occurred when he was drunk or when she would try to stop him going to the pub. Prior to the accident they had a good marriage. This couple was told that detoxification was indicated in the first instance for Mr X. He agreed to this and following discharge entered a treatment programme for recovering alcoholics. There was no evidence of depressive illness or current post traumatic stress disorder. Simultaneous to entering the programme for alcoholics he and his wife commenced marital therapy since she felt very bitter and angry with him. She was encouraged to articulate these feelings to her husband, but only in the sessions. Discussion of her feelings was forbidden at other times. Mr X agreed that he had to win back his wife's trust and both contracted to go out together every 2 weeks and to have a holiday together in the summer. At subsequent sessions Mrs X agreed that her husband was indeed making an effort and she was feeling closer to him than she had for many years; Mr X was happy that his wife was not referring to their previous problems or in any way blaming him, although he accepted that he was to blame. Therapy was suspended with the agreement of the couple since the relationship had improved dramatically and Mr X remained alcohol-free and motivated.

Comment

Beginning therapy without first treating the alcohol problem would have been foolhardy and if Mr X had refused this then marital therapy could not have been offered. Even where the marital problem seems to have predated the alcohol abuse, it is essential to first deal with the latter since it may affect insight and be an additional contributor to the difficulties. Once detoxified it is common for resentments and mistrust to come to the fore. Help in resolving these should be part of the therapy for alcohol problems. These sessions do not usually need to be task-oriented and a supportive, non-directive role is preferred to give the couple the 'space' in which to mend their marriage. If this fails a more practical approach may then be required.

REFERENCES

Doss, B.D., Atkins, D.C. and Christensen, A. (2003).Who's dragging their feet? Husbands and wives seeking marital therapy. *Journal of Marital and Family Therapy*, **29**, 165–177.

Hafner, R.J. (1977). The spouses of agoraphobic women. *British Journal of Psychiatry*, **131**, 289–294.

Haley, J., (1976). *Problem Solving Therapy: New Strategies for Effective Family Therapy*. Jossey-Bass, San Francisco.

Law, D.D., Crane, D.R. and Berge, J.M. (2003). The influence of the individual, marital and family therapy on high utilizers of health care. *Journal of Family and Marital Therapy*, **29**, 353–363.

Minuchin, S. (1974). *Families and Family Therapy*. Harvard University Press, Cambridge MA.

Selvini Palazzoli, M., Boscolo, M., Cecchin, G. and Prata, G. (1978). *Paradox and Counterparadox*. Jason Aronson, New York.

Shadish, W.R. and Baldwin, S.A. (2003). Meta-analysis of MFT interventions. *Journal of Family and Marital Therapy*, **29**, 547–570.

Whisman, M.A. (2001). Marital adjustment and outcome following treatments for depression. *Journal of Consulting and Clinical Psychology*, **69**, 125–129.

FURTHER READING

Dixon, P. (1995). *The Rising Price of Love*. Hodder, London.

Skynner, R. and Cleese, J. (1983). *Families and How to Survive Them*. Methuen, London.

USEFUL WEBSITE FOR PATIENTS

Education for couples and families: www.smartmarriages.com

USEFUL CONTACTS

RELATE
Herbert Grey College
Little Church Street
Rugby
Warwickshire CV21 3AP
UK
Tel: 0845 456 1310
Website: www.relate.org.uk

ACCORD (formerly Catholic Marriage Advisory Service)
Central Office
Columba Centre
Maynooth
Co. Kildare
Ireland

....
(Fill in local branch telephone number)

13

Sexual Disorders

Sexual disorders may be categorised into three groups: sexual dysfunction, sexual deviations and gender identity problems. In no other area of psychiatry is it more important to understand the patient's moral and religious attitudes, since treatment will founder if practices are suggested which are contrary to the patient's personal ethic.

SEXUAL DYSFUNCTION

Prevalence

There are no accurate figures on the epidemiology of sexual dysfunction but it is more frequently admitted to by women and up to 15% of married women have complete failure to achieve orgasm. Impotence and premature ejaculation are the most frequent problems in men, while among women lack of enjoyment predominates. Erectile dysfunction increases with increasing age and is present in up to 20% of men under 60. Sexual problems in both partners are found in up to one-third of those attending sex clinics.

Causes

Predisposing factors are multifarious and include poor sex education, childhood sexual or other physical abuse, repressive upbringing, unrealistic expectations of sex and personality problems. These must be distinguished from factors which precipitate sexual dysfunction and in this category are childbirth, interpersonal stress and infidelity, depressive illness, ageing, physical illnesses or reactions to them, e.g. mastectomy. Finally, once the difficulties have arisen several aspects of the patient's life and relationship maintain them. These include performance anxiety, guilt, unsympathetic partner, ongoing psychiatric or physical illness and personality difficulties especially negative self-image.

History taking

This is the first and obvious step to dealing with a sexual problem and this should be obtained separately from each partner. Some 'secrets' may be disclosed but there is no need to insist on total disclosure of items which do not concern the present problems, e.g. previous sexual contacts, sexually transmitted diseases, etc. Specific enquiry should be made about the sexual and emotional relationship prior to the onset of difficulties. The attitudes of both partners to their bodies and to sex should be explored as should any taboos either of a religious or cultural nature. Details of illnesses and medications should also be obtained and the circumstances leading up to the present problem must be explored in detail. Having obtained this information the doctor must decide if the problem is a sexual or a relationship one since treatment and the agency providing it will be dependent upon this. Physical causes, especially neurological disorders, must be ruled out and alcohol abuse must also be considered.

Before embarking upon treatment it is essential to consider the following points.

1. Is the problem treatable? If the difficulty has a physical cause then sex therapy is unnecessary unless it is being reinforced by secondary performance anxiety. If the couple are not motivated treatment is probably precluded although in some circumstances it may be possible, e.g. vaginismus.
2. Do I have the expertise? Unless the general practitioner has suitable training in sex therapy it is unwise to embark upon it since failure to effect a response may reinforce the couple's anxiety and sense of hopelessness.
3. Do I have the time? Sex therapy is time-consuming although not so much as other behavioural treatments. Weekly or fortnightly sessions are considered the best frequency and unless a commitment can be given to meet this the couple should be referred elsewhere.
4. Can I empathise with the couple? The doctor trying to treat a couple whose moral or personal scruples he regards as silly or primitive is not in a position to offer help since he is unlikely to have the flexibility to adapt the techniques to the couple's needs.
5. If the therapist feels an attraction to one or other of the couple he may not be able to undertake therapy since he will tend to work through his own fantasies in therapy.

The main disorders of sexual function are listed in Table 13.1.

SENSATE FOCUS

This technique originally developed by Masters and Johnson is the backbone of treatment and is used as an adjunct in most dysfunction disorders. Sexual intercourse or mutual masturbation are banned in order to reduce performance anxiety

Table 13.1. Sexual dysfunction.

	Female	Male
Desire phase	Low interest	Low interest
	Excessive interest	Excessive interest
	(nymphomania) – rare	(Don Juanism) – rare
Excitement phase	Impaired arousal	Impotence
Orgasm phase	Anorgasmia	Premature ejaculation
		Failure of ejaculation
	Vaginismus	
	Sex phobia	Sex phobia

and to remove the goal of achieving orgasm. The homework may be practised at different times of the day and in different rooms of the house according to the wishes of the couple. The number of sessions devoted to each stage is also dependent on the couple and their response at each stage.

In the *first stage* one partner is instructed to touch and caress all parts of the other's body except the genitals and breasts. The other concentrates on the pleasurable feelings and gives feedback on their enjoyment. Each partner does this on two to three occasions per week and turns are taken at initiating the process. Some couples may find this artificial or even threatening. When the former occurs they should be reassured that this is temporary and an explanation provided about the rationale for this approach. If the technique is too threatening then simpler non-sexual behaviours such as holding hands or touching when clothed may be necessary before this first stage is tried.

The *second stage* is an extension of the first and each gives more directive feedback on the pleasurable sensations and guides the other's hand to maximise this. Many couples break the ban on intercourse during these early stages. It is important to stress its importance since anxiety may be increased again especially if intercourse was unsatisfactory.

When the couple have overcome their anxieties and self-consciousness about non-genital contact they can proceed to *stage three* or genital sensate focus. As before the aim is to increase pleasure without orgasm. Each partner touches the other lightly and gives feedback as in the earlier stages but also includes the breasts and genitalia. Creams and lotions may be used to increase sensitivity and to prevent soreness of the genitalia and nipples. If an erection occurs the caressing should stop until it has diminished and then restart again. Masturbation to orgasm or ejaculation must be avoided.

The *fourth and final stage* is not reached until each can be relaxed and aroused. The penis is inserted in the vagina with the woman in the superior position for control. Containment of the penis and enjoyment of this without movement is the initial aim and this should be practised over several sessions. Finally movement leading to climax is allowed.

SPECIFIC DISORDERS

Vaginismus

Vaginismus can usually be treated successfully but initially the attitudes of the woman to sex and the genitalia must be explored. Some discussion of these may be necessary before proceeding further. If negative attitudes are found their cause must be explored and resolved using psychotherapy if necessary; this can run in tandem with the sensate focus method outlined above. Diagrams of the female genital organs are shown to the woman and she is encouraged to touch her own genitalia, if necessary in the surgery. A mirror may be used to facilitate this. The next stage is to encourage her to put one finger into her vagina and when this has been achieved, two. If this fails a vaginal examination by the therapist may help and the patient can try again under supervision. Graded dilators can be given to be inserted either by the patient or her partner. Finally, the use of a tampon during menstruation should be encouraged. Lubricants can be of use if the vaginal mucosa is dry. Relaxation exercises should also be taught since tension may occur in the limbs with each new stage. *Always have a female member of staff present during intimate procedures* and obtain permission from the patient at each stage having first given an explanation.

Dyspareunia

Dyspareunia has many causes, some physical, some psychological and some due to technique. Physical causes should be resolved as appropriate. If the woman is menopausal then the use of a lubricant jelly or oestrogen cream can greatly reduce the discomfort. The psychological causes include lack of interest or vaginismus and will be considered separately. Faulty technique with *impaired arousal* is perhaps the most common cause and the use of jelly coupled with an explanation of the physiological and anatomical basis of arousal can be beneficial. Reading suitable manuals may also help and a list is provided at the end of this chapter. The use of sexual fantasies and erotic material may be necessary initially but should be suggested with sensitivity since they may be greeted with horror by some couples. Women with dyspareunia should be advised to adopt the female superior or lateral positions during intercourse.

Impaired sexual interest

This may be due to poor technique or limited foreplay. Sexual inhibitions of a more general nature and a poor emotional relationship with one's partner may also be responsible. Depressive illness is a common cause of loss of libido and should be borne in mind since sex therapy would be of little benefit for this. When these causes have been ruled out and the impaired interest is a primary condition, sex therapy should concentrate on the sensate focus technique. This may be combined with the use of erotic images, words or pictures to stimulate libido.

Orgasmic dysfunction

Orgasmic dysfunction is usually managed by a masturbation training programme to be used by the woman alone if this is acceptable to her. If not, all the stimulation may be provided by her partner. This should be combined with the sensate focus exercises. Once the woman, who has agreed to a masturbation programme, can achieve orgasm on her own, she can guide her partner during the sensate focus approach in which 'teasing' the clitoris, i.e. stimulating and then discontinuing, increases the level of arousal. Combining vaginal containment with clitoral stimulation can increase the likelihood of orgasm. Some women may go on to have orgasm without clitoral stimulation (coital orgasm) while others may not. Clitoral orgasm is not inferior and is the normal method of achieving orgasm for many women. Thus the woman who can have an orgasm only in this way should be reassured. Failure to achieve orgasm despite these techniques may necessitate the use of a vibrator as a temporary measure and this should be explained to the reluctant couple.

Erectile dysfunction

This is a disorder that, more than any other is likely to be secondary to some underlying physical or psychiatric disorder. Diabetes mellitus and neurological disease must be ruled out. It may also occur after prostatectomy. Depressive illness, anxiety, either generalised or performance related, alcohol and recreational drug misuse are the most common psychological conditions associated with impotence. It is a common side effect of most antidepressants and for this reason it is often one of the last symptoms to resolve in those with depression. Treatment consists of lifestyle change where appropriate, e.g. reducing alcohol, etc. However, the availability of medications such as the phosphodiesterase type-5 inhibitors has greatly facilitated the management of impotence. The newer drugs such as tadalafil, vardenafil and apomorphine take effect more quickly than sildenafil, the first such drug available. They are contraindicated in those taking nitrates for angina as dangerous hypotension may result.

The use if the sensate focus technique may also help but since many men become preoccupied by the erection and its size this may lead to further anxiety. The couple should be encouraged to concentrate on the feelings rather than the physical results. It is also useful to advise the man to try not to have an erection – this use of paradoxical intention increases its likelihood. The use of fantasies and erotic material can be added if necessary and if acceptable to the couple. Once an erection has been achieved the teasing technique of starting then stopping stimulation can be used. This further increases confidence until insertion takes place. This should be brief initially with the period of containment gradually increasing until ejaculation takes place.

Premature ejaculation

Premature ejeculation can be successfully treated using the sensate focus combined with the start–stop or squeeze technique. For the success of this it is important that the man be able to identify the point at which ejaculation is about to take place so that caressing the penis can stop. This stopping and starting should be carried out a few times in each session before ejaculation is allowed. In the early sessions this will be extravaginal. Later the penis can be inserted in the vagina and when the man signals that ejaculation may occur his partner lifts herself from him until arousal has decreased. This should happen three or four times before ejaculation in the vagina occurs. If the start–stop technique fails then squeezing the penis just below the glans inhibits the ejaculatory reflex.

Ejaculatory failure

This may be situational with emission occurring normally during masturbation but not during intercourse. This is easier to treat than total failure of ejaculation. The use of sensate focus coupled with creams and lotions to increase sensitivity is usually successful. Initially ejaculation will occur outside the vagina but as treatment progresses the man should place his penis at the vaginal entrance and later in the vagina itself and continue thrusting until ejaculation occurs. If there is complete failure to ejaculate the man may need an individual masturbation training programme until this is achieved, followed later by the sensate focus technique.

Sexual phobia

Sexual phobia is treated by exploration of the cause and systematic desensitisation. This a rare complaint and requires specialist treatment.

HOMOSEXUALITY

It is rare for homosexuals to seek treatment nowadays and homosexuality is not classified as a psychiatric disorder but the doctor is often asked for advice by uncertain young men and women about their sexual orientation.

Classification

Several types have been identified in the literature and these include the following.

Situational homosexuality

This occurs in situations where the company of the opposite sex is prohibited or difficult, as in boarding schools and in prisons. It is more common among men than women and most return to normal heterosexual behaviour. A few are pseudo-homosexual (see below).

Pseudohomosexuality

Pseudohomosexuality refers to those who are homosexual by default. Their behaviour is secondary to conflicts about relationships with the opposite sex whom they fear. Such men are shy and timid and benefit from social skills and assertiveness training.

Developmental homoerotic activity

This refers to homosexual behaviour driven by curiosity rather than sexual orientation. This occurs principally in teenagers and is transient. It is not prognostic of adult homosexuality. In later years some may wonder if in fact this indicated a homosexual preference and reassurance about this can be given with confidence.

Bisexuality and ambisexuality

Bisexuals and ambisexuals are functional with either sex. The former are homosexual but resort to heterosexual behaviour to avoid stigma while the latter truly have no preference.

Idealogical homosexuality

Ideological or political homosexuals are a recently identified group whose motivation is political. It is associated with aggressive denial of the need for or of an attraction to the opposite sex. Conflicts are also denied but they often emerge as their relationships fail to resolve them. A good description of this is given in *Birds of Passage* by Bernice Rubens (1981).

Preferential homosexuality

This is what is commonly referred to as homosexuality and this group will be considered in more detail below.

Aetiology

This is unknown and theories have variously suggested a hereditary cause, an intrauterine abnormality of neuroendocrine function or difficulties in the upbringing and family relationships. This latter has received most attention and in particular overprotective mothers and absent or hostile fathers have been implicated in male homosexuality, while female homosexuals have been shown to have poor relationships with their mothers. The role of genes has been suggested by some investigators. Since many children have abnormal family relationships and do not become homosexual these theories must remain tentative. As yet there is no satisfactory explanation.

Prevalence

Kinsey *et al.* (1948, 1953) in their study of homosexual behaviour found that almost 40% of adult males had a homosexual experience by the age of 45 and 4% were exclusively homosexual throughout their lives. The equivalent figures for women were 15% and 4%, respectively. Recent studies suggest a slightly lower prevalence of exclusive homosexuality.

Features of homosexuality

Homosexuality refers to erotic thoughts and feelings towards members of the same sex whether or not they are acted upon. There is no evidence that homosexuality is associated with any one personality type and the whole range of personalities including those with no personality disorder are represented. There is some evidence for an increased risk of suicidal ideation and deliberate self-harm, especially in young homosexual and bisexual men but this seems to be independent of sexual orientation and linked to depressed mood and unsatisfactory friendships (van Heeringen and Vincke, 2000). A few homosexual men adopt effeminate mannerisms and likewise some lesbian women behave in a masculine way although this is not universal. Male homosexuals tend to be more promiscuous than their female counterparts who are more monogamous. Some are transvestites, but the majority are not. Paedophilia is rare and this group will be described separately. As middle age approaches some experience loneliness and depression due partly to stigma and partly to the absence of confidants. This is less common among female homosexuals who frequently form lasting and confiding relationships.

Myths

A number of false beliefs about homosexuality need to be dispelled.

- Close friendships between the same sex are *not* indicative of homosexuality.
- Homosexual behaviour is not indicative of homosexuality (see classification).
- Effeminate behaviour in men or masculine behaviour in women is not indicative of homosexuality.
- Homosexuality is not regarded as an illness and falls outside the illness model as does alcoholism or personality disorder. Its aetiology is probably related to cultural and environmental factors rather than to any process. Some have suggested that it can be regarded as an illness (Kendell, 1974) but this is now

disputed. However, as with alcohol abuse (see Chapter 9), it can be associated with other emotional problems and each patient must be individually considered in the context of his or her culture, ethics and needs.

Treatment

Although homosexuality is not regarded as an illness sometimes there are requests for therapy to change sexual orientation. More commonly the presentation is with a psychiatric disorder such as depression. (i) The doctor must attempt to decide if the patient is a preferential homosexual. Questions about the content of sexual fantasises, erotic feelings and practices should help elucidate this. (ii) The personality of the patient should be assessed since those who are timid and inhibited may need help in overcoming these difficulties as described in Chapter 11. In particular this would be important for those who belong to the passive (pseudohomosexual) group described above. (iii) Those who are homosexual and who are distressed by this knowledge may need individual psychotherapy in coming to accept their orientation. The person should be referred to a trained psychotherapist and may also need spiritual help. (iv) When depressive illness or other psychiatric condition supervenes, often the result of relationship problems, these should be treated in the ordinary way and counselling offered to help in resolving the problems. (v) A small group may request specific treatment to achieve a heterosexual orientation and these should be referred to the specialist services. Psychoanalysis and aversion therapy have been used to try to effect change in sexual orientation but without much success. Treatment should focus on avoiding situations that stimulate homosexual thoughts and feelings and seeking to maximise the opportunities to meet the opposite sex.

SEXUAL DEVIATIONS

Fetishism

Fetishism refers to the use of inanimate objects to achieve sexual arousal. Most fetishists are heterosexual. There is a gradation from acceptable fetishism to grossly abnormal behaviour. It is common for men to be aroused by stockings but uncommon for shoes to be used for this purpose. The epidemiology is unknown. Treatment is required for gross forms of the behaviour and should be given by a specialist.

Voyeurism

This is defined as sexual arousal obtained chiefly by observing the sexual activity of others. The prevalence and aetiology are unknown although most are heterosexual and male. Their social and interpersonal skills are usually lacking and many are isolated and lonely. There is no convincing evidence for the superiority of any one treatment although general measures aimed at improving self-esteem and social skills may be useful.

Paedophilia and ephebophilia

Paedophilia is the condition of being erotically attracted to or indulging in sexual activity with prepubertal children. This attraction to or activity with post-pubertal children is termed ephebophilia (Lolita syndrome). In some cultures ephebophilia is tolerated, but western norms generally regard it with distaste although it is not listed as a disorder in DSM. Some researchers differentiate paedophilia and ephebophilia both functionally and aetiologically. Both are largely confined to men and there is no exact information on their prevalence although the popularity of pornography involving children suggests that they are not rare. The aetiology is unknown and primary paedophilia must be distinguished from secondary paedophilia described as occurring in those with severe mental illness or brain damage. Within the primary paedophile group there is a distinction between personality disordered paedophiles (sexual psychopaths) who have no concern for their victims and may be aggressive to them and those paedophiles who, although lacking insight into the damage their behaviour can cause, are 'kind' to their victims.

The treatment of sexual abusers is difficult and there is a high recidivism rate. Therapy is intensive and lengthy and based on cognitive principles. It should only be offered by those specifically trained to work with this group of patients.

Sexual abuse

Child sexual abuse refers to the acts perpetrated by paedophiles and the exact prevalence is not known due to variations in definition and in reporting. Moreover different populations exhibit differences in prevalence. A study of sexual abuse in those under 13 found that sexual intercourse occurred in 6.1% of the adult female psychiatric out-patient population while the corresponding figure for general practice attenders was 0.8% (Palmer *et al.*, 1993). For all types of sexual contact, e.g. sexual kissing/hugging, fondling, etc., the figures were 33% and 22.5%, respectively. For those whose abuse began after the age of 13 the figures for intercourse were 12.2% and 4.2% and for all sexual contacts 30.4% and 10.8%, respectively. The corresponding figures for men were lower (Palmer *et al.*, 1993, 1994).

Consequences of child sexual abuse

It is now acknowledged that victims suffer serious long-term emotional consequences into adult life although this is not universal. One of the factors which protects against these effects is the presence of a supportive mother and the extent to which the child is believed. The age of the abuse, its duration and extent have also been identified as influential. A challenge for researchers working in this area lies in disentangling the effects of abuse from deprivation, both physical and emotional, which often co-occur and the evidence to date is conflicting. The inter-generational transfer of abuse is one adverse consequence for which there is some evidence, although it is not inevitable. A recent study found that one-third of abused children become habitual abusers in adulthood, another third do not and a final third abused under extreme stress (Oliver, 1993).

Child sexual abuse is known to be a risk factor for a multiplicity of psychiatric disorders (Spertus *et al.*, 2003), including personality disorder, especially border-line type, dissociation disorder, alcohol abuse and eating disorders. Attempts to relate sexual abuse to specific disorders have foundered and it is best viewed as a general risk factor for most disorders. Sexual dysfunction, particularly vaginismus and frigidity, is also associated with sexual abuse in childhood, as is early sexual activity and promiscuity.

Disclosure

When an adult discloses sexual abuse to a general practitioner there is often uncer-tainty about how to handle this information. First, the doctor should ascertain if the person wishes to report the matter to the police and offer support if this is the decision. If the person does not wish to do this, the doctor must try to establish whether the perpetrator is a risk to children and if there is concern about this possibility then the doctor may breach confidentiality in order to ensure the safety of minors by informing the relevant child protection authorities.

In general those who spontaneously report sexual abuse to their doctor are telling the truth and should be believed. The delay in coming forward with this information may stem from shame, from fear of not being believed or from a dread of the emotional pain that accompanies disclosure. The decision to make this matter known may have been stimulated by a number of factors including media coverage or some personal event such as the birth of a child and the understand-able desire to prevent the abuse being repeated. The victim should be encouraged to talk through the events and their effects and it may be appropriate, if agreed, to refer the patient to the specialist services or to the Rape Crisis centre for further counselling.

Sometimes the disclosure will have come about as a result of 'therapy' to uncover childhood traumas. Alternatively the person may describe little more than a 'feeling' of having been abused and in these circumstances caution is advised since fragmentary memories or vague beliefs of having been abused may be unfounded.

Recovered memory (see Chapter 17) is the term that that been applied to the recovery after prolonged amnesia of memories of sexual abuse in childhood. The victims are generally women in middle life who have recovered such memories during therapy, usually for depression, and who then accuse elderly relatives of the abuse. Those who support the idea of recovered memories argue that most adult problems are the result of 'robust repression' of childhood sexual abuse. Some disagree that memories of repeated sexual abuse can be repressed and term this 'False Memory Syndrome'.

The response in Britain has been for the Royal College of Psychiatrists (1997) to issue guidelines to its members (Brandon *et al.*, 1998). In summary, these reject the concept of massive repression and failed to find evidence that repeated sexual abuse in childhood could be totally forgotten only to emerge many years later. The guidelines strenuously caution on the use of 'repressed memory therapy' including hypnosis, regression therapy, drug mediated interviews or suggestion.

The risk of false memories can be reduced if doctors advise patients against embarking upon any therapy to 'recover' such memories since very long periods of total amnesia for traumatic events are rare. Moreover the danger of seeking to explain all emotional problems in adulthood as due to hidden sexual abuse should be regarded as simplistic and patients embarking on recovered memory therapies should be strongly advised to seek a second opinion. Any person reporting sexual abuse in childhood should be treated with support and sympathy but when there is a claim of lengthy amnesia then extreme caution is required. Unfortunately once created, false memories are held with conviction and often lead to endless suffering for all concerned.

Treatment

Depressive illness may emerge during therapy and indeed details of abuse may only be disclosed during treatment for an existing depressive disorder. Care must be taken in reaching this diagnosis since in many the distress will be an understandable response to painful recollections rather than indicative of depressive illness. Sexually abused patients are prone to self-destructive acts such as repeated wrist cutting but admission to hospital is generally not helpful, reinforcing this behaviour which may subsequently be used to delay discharge. Therapy should focus on the abuse and on attitudes to self and others as a result. It is only recently that evidence has emerged for the effectiveness of therapy, at least in some patients, although it is lengthy and fraught with difficulties such as deliberate self-harm and intense emotional interactions.

Sadism and masochism

Sadism and masochism are defined as disorders in which either the inflicting of pain or the experience of pain are used to obtain sexual pleasure. Their prevalence is unknown and there is no proven treatment. Where serious crimes have been committed by sadists the risk of further offences cannot be underestimated. Other rare deviations include necrophilia and bestiality.

GENDER ROLE DISTURBANCES

Transvestism

This is the repeated dressing in the clothes of the opposite sex. This is not always associated with sexual arousal but the two may coexist. Homosexuality is much less common among male than among female cross-dressers. There is no gender identity problem although this behaviour is frequently confused with transsexualism. Transvestites feel entirely male or female according to gender. The prevalence is unknown as is the aetiology. There is no evidence for a genetic transmission or for hormonal abnormalities. Treatment if requested will necessitate referral to the specialist services where behavioural and psychotherapeutic approaches are used.

Transsexualism

Transsexualism is characterised by the belief that the true gender of the sufferer is characterised not by the anatomical but by the psychological gender. Thus the anatomical male feels he is in reality a female and vice versa. Many feel trapped by their gender and relentlessly seek corrective surgery. It is a rare condition often beginning in early childhood and affects roughly 1/35,000 males and 1/100,000 females. Most transsexuals do not regard themselves as homosexual and insist that their relationships are heterosexual. Many have a history of cross-dressing as a means of looking and behaving like the preferred sex. Impaired social adjustment is common. In some, surgery can be beneficial and requests for this are not usually acceded to unless a full psychological assessment has been made and the person has lived successfully as a member of the opposite sex for 2 years. Attempts to try to change the patient's conviction about his gender are rarely successful. Since the majority of patients do not meet the stringent requirements for surgery, treatment is supportive rather than specific in nature. Many develop depressive illnesses and parasuicide is frequent. The suicide rate may be increased although this is uncertain.

SUMMARY

1. The prevalence of sexual dysfunction is unknown but impotence and ejaculatory failure are the most common in men, and low sexual interest the most prevalent in women.
2. The sensate focus technique is the basis on which specific treatments for sexual dysfunction are built.
3. There are many causes for sexual dysfunction but a physical aetiology has to be ruled out in all patients as do relationship problems where the appropriate intervention is marital therapy.

4. Homosexuals rarely request treatment. The general practitioner may be asked for advice about homoerotic activity in relation to sexual orientation.

5. Isolated homosexual acts are considerably more frequent than exclusive homosexuality and most are part of developmental exploration.

6. Sexual deviations are less common and if presented to the general practitioner will invariably require referral to specialist services.

7. The prevalence of sexual abuse varies with the definition but all studies have reported a higher prevalence among women than men. The psychological consequences are many and require specialist treatment.

CASE HISTORIES

Case 1

Mr X was a 23 year-old clerical student who was referred for counselling regarding his sexual orientation. He decided to study for the priesthood at 18 immediately after he had left secondary school. He felt he had made the right decision and was due to be ordained 9 months from the time of referral. He had requested the appointment himself as he had worries that he may be homosexual. He had always been shy and had few friends of either sex. His fears about homosexuality arose when he was 16 and had indulged in some homosexual activity with a boy of the same age. He did not particularly enjoy these encounters and felt that perhaps he should have discouraged the advances made by his fellow student. He recalled being fearful of refusing because he believed that 'everybody did it' and he was unsure about how to say no. While at school he had two girlfriends and although he found it difficult to talk to members of the opposite sex he enjoyed their company and liked looking at and thinking about girls. At present he described fantasies of women and would have erections when watching women undress in films or on television. He was not currently attracted to men and was horrified by the thought that he may be homosexual. This young man was reassured that he was definitely heterosexual.

Comment

This man was typical of those who fear that isolated homosexual acts in adolescence are indicative of homosexuality. He was by nature shy and lacking in confidence and both of these probably made it difficult for him to refuse the sexual advances of his peer. His attractions and fantasies were directed to women and he was easily reassured that he was heterosexual. He was encouraged to explore his reasons for choosing the priesthood as a profession in view of his shyness with women. This he agreed to do with his supervisor.

Case 2

Mrs X was referred with low sexual interest of 3 years duration. This had begun after she and her husband temporarily separated. This had been provoked by his alcohol abuse. When drunk he would insist on sex irrespective of her wishes and at times would beat her if she tried to thwart him. They had now returned to live together again and he had sought and received help for his drink problem. Despite this his wife still resented his sexual advances. She had decided of her own volition to seek help since she now felt she owed it to her husband in view of his changed behaviour. Initially both were seen together and sexual intercourse banned while some basic marital therapy was instituted. This ban removed the pressure from Mrs X while at the same time further improving their overall relationship. Both were encouraged to spend time alone talking each evening and were encouraged to go out together once each week. Both responded positively to this approach and after three sessions non-genital contact was encouraged. They agreed to hold hands and to kiss each other good night. Mrs X found this easy to accept and thereafter the sensate focus approach was introduced. After three sessions, prior to genital contact being allowed they had intercourse satisfactorily and at follow-up this progress was maintained.

Comment

This lady's sexual problem derived from her poor relationship with her husband. Once he had taken steps to resolve it, her commitment to the marriage improved and the initial sessions were devoted to consolidating this without any sexual pressure. When she felt ready the simple approach outlined above resulted in a return to a satisfactory sexual relationship also. When the sexual problem is temporary, e.g. following childbirth or marital problems, it is common for intercourse to occur early in the sensate focus programme. In all cases it is essential to progress at the speed of the couple and not be enjoined by rigid timetables.

Case 3

Mrs X was referred because of non-comsummation of marriage after one year. She was 28 and was otherwise happily married to a supportive husband. Prior to marriage they had not attempted intercourse for religious reasons and she became aware of her problems on her honeymoon. Both were seen separately at the first appointment and she described having been sexually abused as a child. She had never disclosed this to anybody except her husband. It was decided that she needed individual therapy initially and she was seen on six occasions for psychotherapy during which she worked through her feelings about the abuse. At this point she requested that she and her husband should now proceed to joint therapy and this was arranged as she seemed to have come to terms with her past. The sensate focus approach was used in conjunction with self-exploration and dilators. She responded well to non-genital contact and to the use of dilators but once penetration of the vagina was suggested the difficulties recurred. Therapy was restarted with non-genital contact and proceeded more slowly than before to the stage of vaginal containment. This was faciliated by a vaginal examination during which she was taught relaxation exercises. Sexual intercourse was successfully achieved 8 months from the time of first referral.

Comment

Where there is a definite emotional cause for the problem this must first be explored and resolved if possible. Failure to do so does not necessarily preclude treatment but makes it more difficult and less likely to succeed. Where the progress from one stage to the next is too rapid treatment is likely to founder as it did initially with this couple.

REFERENCES

Brandon, S., Boakes, D., Glaser, D. and Green, R. (1998). Recovered memories of childhood sexual abuse: Implications for clinical practice. *British Journal of Psychiatry*, **172**, 296–307.

van Heeringen, C. and Vincke, J. (2000). Suicidal acts and ideation in homosexual young people: a study of prevalence and risk factors. *Social Psychiatry and Psychiatric Epidemiology*, **35**, 494–499.

Kendell, R. (1974). Concept of disease and its implication for psychiatry. *British Journal of Psychiatry*, **127**, 305–315.

Kinsey, A.C., Pomeroy, W.B. and Martin, C.E. (1948). *Sexual Behaviour in the Human Male*. Saunders, Philadelphia.

Kinsey, A.C., Pomeroy, W.B., Martin, C.E. and Gebhard, P.H. (1953). *Sexual Behaviour in the Human Female*. Saunders, Philadelphia.

Oliver, H.E. (1993). Intergenerational transmission of child abuse: rates, research and clinical implications. *American Journal of Psychiatry*, **150**, 1315–1324.

Palmer, R.L., Colemen, L., Chaloner, D., Oppenheimer, R. and Smith, J. (1993). Childhood sexual experience with adults. A comparison of reports by women psychiatric patients and general practice attenders. *British Journal of Psychiatry*, **163**, 499–504.

Palmer, R.L., Bramble, D., Metcalf, M., Oppenheimer, R. and Smith, J. (1994). Childhood sexual experience with adults: adult male psychiatric patients and general practice attenders. *British Journal of Psychiatry*, **165**, 675–679.

Royal College of Psychiatrists' Working Group on Reported Memories of Child Sexual Abuse. (1997). Recommendations for good practice. *Psychiatric Bulletin*, **21**, 663–665.

Rubens, B. (1981). *Birds of Passage*. Hamish Hamilton, London.

Spertus, I.L., Yehuda, R., Wong, C.M., Halligan, S. and Seremetis, S.V. (2003). Childhood emotional abuse and neglect as predictors of psychological and physical symptoms in women presenting to a primary care practice. *Child Abuse and Neglect*, **27**, 1247–1258.

FURTHER READING

Bancroft, J. (1983). *Human Sexuality and its Problems*. Churchill Livingstone, Edinburgh.
Hawton, K. (1985). *Sex Therapy: A Practical Guide*. Oxford University Press, Oxford.

SUGGESTED READING FOR PATIENTS

Sanford, L.T. (1991). *Strong at the Broken Places; Overcoming the Trauma of Childhood Abuse*. Virago, London.
Stones, R. (2001). *Understanding Sex and Relationships: Overcoming Common Problems*. Sheldon, London.

USEFUL WEBSITES FOR PATIENTS

Impotence: www.impotence.org

Dyspareunia: www.sexwithoutpain.com/dyspareunia.html

14

Other Disorders

OBSESSIVE–COMPULSIVE DISORDER

Obsessive–compulsive disorder (OCD), once thought to be a rare disorder, has been shown to be more common than was previously thought, affecting about 2–3% of the population. A word of caution must be extended against the lay use of the word 'obsessed' which is generally used to describe being preoccupied by some issue or worry. This is quite a different usage from the medical meaning of the term.

Once thought to have its origins in abnormalities of the Freudian defence mechanisms, its putative causes have now moved definitively to the biological sphere. Brain imaging studies, whether functional or structural, have found a decrease in size of the caudate nuclei and also abnormalities to the frontal lobes and the cingulum. Studies of serotonergic function have found differing results but an abnormality of this system is suggested by the superior effect of serotonergic drugs over other neuroleptic agents in treating OCD. Family studies of OCD show that 35% of first-degree relatives of OCD patients themselves have the disorder although whether this is genetically or environmentally determined is uncertain.

The predominant symptom is of a subjective compulsion to carry out some action or to dwell on some thought or abstract subject (ruminations). Resistance to the ruminations or compulsions occurs in the early stages of the illness but frequently disappear as it becomes established. Obsessional rituals may take the form of handwashing, touching doors, carrying out routine behaviours in a certain order, etc., with cleaning, avoiding and checking rituals the most common. The carrying out of the rituals often leads to obsessional slowness. Sometimes the behaviour may be preceded by an obsessional rumination, e.g. repeated handwashing following thoughts of contamination. The content of ruminations may vary from a preoccupation with words, or numbers, or ideas about the origins of the world to intrusive blasphemous or sexual thoughts, or to violent images. The patient is aware that these are his own thoughts and can therefore be distinguished from thought insertion which is a psychotic symptom seen in schizophrenia. Ruminations are especially distressing to the patient since many feel that they augur madness. Associated symptoms include anxiety, depersonalisation and secondary depression.

There is no doubt that some sufferers have obsessional premorbid personalities with the typical features of punctiliousness, perfectionism, rigidity and cautiousness. However most of those with obsessional personalities do not develop OCD.

Obsessional symptoms are seen most commonly, not in obsessive–compulsive disorder, but as part of a depressive illness or sometimes in schizophrenia also.

Differential diagnosis

Schizophrenia

The main diagnostic difficulty lies in distinguishing obsessive–compulsive disorder from schizophrenia since the obsessional symptoms frequently resemble passivity feelings or thought insertion. Obsessional symptoms are described by the patient as eminating from within rather than being due to outside forces, and this or similar statements should clarify the diagnosis.

Depressive illness

Since obsessional symptoms often occur in depressive illness, care must be taken to exclude this condition.

Obsessional personality disorder

Those with obsessional personalities often have rituals, which resemble obsessive–compulsive disorder. The distinction lies in the severity and intrusiveness of the symptoms (see Chapter 11).

Management

Optimum treatment is a combination of pharmacotherapy and behaviour therapy although pharmacotherapy is almost always required indefinitely, even when behavioural techniques have also been used. Several antidepressants have been shown to be effective in the treatment of OCD, even in the absence of depression. In particular the tricyclic clomipramine and the SSRIs fluoxetine, paroxetine and sertraline have been found to bring about a dramatic relief of symptoms although recommended doses of the SSRIs are much higher than those used in treating depression (Kaplan and Hollander, 1995).

Ruminations are the most difficult to manage and for these a behavioural procedure called thought stopping is used, where the patient is instructed to ruminate, then to stop the offending thought and change to a more appropriate one. The switching may be facilitated by pulling on an elastic band attached to the wrist or by some other method, designed to distract. This is practised several times in the session until the patient has learned to control the ruminations. For obsessional rituals, response prevention is the method of choice. Gently restraining the patient from carrying out the action will initially cause anxiety to increase and an overwhelming urge to ritualise but eventually this urge will decrease and with it the rituals. Obsessional fears of contamination are best dealt with by exposure to dirt and desensitisation.

Occasionally depression supervenes during behaviour therapy and this may need treatment with antidepressants. Where the symptoms are part of another condition such as depressive illness or schizophrenia the management is of the underlying condition.

Prognosis

At its most severe this is an extremely disabling condition. For this reason, before the advent of behaviour therapy, leucotomy was on occasions used when all else failed. Behaviour therapy combined with anti-obsessional medication has radically altered the prognosis and now up to 70% of those treated can expect to improve. Those with obsessional personalities or those whose symptoms are chronic have inevitably a poorer outlook but the intensity of symptoms may fluctuate even in this group.

CONVERSION AND DISSOCIATIVE DISORDERS (FORMERLY HYSTERIA)

This is the most controversial of psychiatric disorders and its demise has been both recommended and welcomed by many, being a diagnosis that is made much less frequently than in the past. The term hysteria is no longer used; instead it has been classified into two subcategories – conversion disorder and dissociative disorder. Notwithstanding this change, the older term is occasionally used in several contexts:

1. It is often used as a term to describe a demanding, difficult patient. This usage is incorrect.
2. The patient with hysterical symptoms is frequently thought to be feigning the symptoms. Hysteria is *not* synonymous with pretending symptoms and patients who present with feigned illness should be described as malingering (see below).
3. A melodramatic, superficial person who is often manipulative. This is a description of hysterical personality disorder. There is no relationship between hysteria (conversion or dissociative) and hysterical personality disorder.
4. Temper tantrums, falling on the floor and showing generally disruptive behaviour is described as histrionic, rather than hysterical, and can occur in many conditions. It is frequently indicative of severe depression or of a cerebral organic process.

5. When non-organic physical symptoms (such as paralysis, blindness, fits, etc., referred to as conversion symptoms, or non-organic amnesia and fugue states, referred to as dissociative symptoms) are present they are referred to as hysterical symptoms. These usually arise when there is major psychological trauma but they may augur serious brain disease such as dementia or be symptomatic of depressive illness.

6. When multi-system physical symptoms, with no organic basis, are present the term St Louis or Briquet's hysteria was used. This condition is now called somatisation disorder.

Hysterical symptoms (5, above) are common although conversion and dissociative disorder are not and the symptoms are more usually part of a depressive or organic state than indicating a primary hysterical disorder. The prevalence of conversion and dissociative disorders is difficult to ascertain but is probably about 3–6/1000 and is more common in general medical settings than in psychiatric clinics. It is extremely rare for these disorders to begin for the first time after the age of 35 although when the symptoms are part of another condition they may occur at any time. Conversion and dissociative disorders are more common in those of low intelligence.

Aetiology of conversion and dissociative disorders (hysteria)

Psychoanalytic theory is central to their aetiology although in clinical practice the cause is often obvious and is not always buried deeply within the psyche, as theory would suggest since insight is often gleaned once the connection between cause and symptoms is explained to the patient. For example a person subject to a major trauma fails to remember anything associated with it including his/her own personal details. As a result a fugue or wandering state may occur. Similarly, with conversion disorder the symptoms have important symbolic significance for the patient, e.g. a teacher under stress may develop aphonia. Biological studies are inconclusive with some early genetic studies finding a familial incidence but later work has failed to find any concordance in twins.

Conversion disorder

The prevalence of this condition is uncertain and one study suggests an annual incidence of 22/100,000. Among some groups such as those with learning disabilities, those with low educational status, military personnel and rural people conversion disorder is more common than in the general population. The male:female ratio may be up to 1:5 and among men it is more commonly associated with occupational or military accidents. Most cases of acute conversion disorder present to neurologists but ultimately they are treated by the psychiatric services although when the symptoms are chronic they will inevitably be presenting to their general practitioners.

Physical symptoms

Physical symptoms include motor abnormalities such as paralysis, tremor, gait disturbance, tics, aphonia, fits, etc., and sensory symptoms such as anaesthesia, deafness and blindness. In such patients reflexes are normal, there is no muscle atrophy unless disuse has been present for a long time, the sensory deficits do not conform to any nerve distribution and all symptoms diminish when the patient's attention is diverted. Despite these differences the distinction from true neurological dysfunction can be difficult and every attempt must be made to rule this out. In the past multiple sclerosis was frequently misdiagnosed as hysterical. Occasionally the symptoms may spread to a number of people in the vicinity of the primary sufferer causing epidemic hysteria. In particular young women in closed communities such as schools, convents, etc., are the group most frequently afflicted and the commonest symptoms are fainting and dizziness.

La Belle Indifférence refers to the patient's lack of concern about their incapacitating symptoms and was once believed to be the hallmark of hysteria. However, it is not always present and it may also be a feature of those with organic illness who adopt a stoic attitude to their condition.

Differential diagnosis

Organic disorders

These must be ruled out, especially where neurological symptoms dominate the picture. Cerebral lesions such as tumours, dementia or infections may release conversion disorders and must also be excluded.

Malingering

Malingering, or the fabrication of symptoms for the purposes of external gain such as financial rewards following an accident or to avoid punishment, must also be ruled out since the management of this 'condition' is very different from that of conversion disorder. The distinction is often difficult since the malingerer will rarely admit the nature of his symptoms.

Conversion symptoms

These are more commonly a manifestation of depressive illness or schizophrenia than of primary conversion disorder and every care must therefore be taken to eliminate these conditions as the cause. One guide is the age of the patient, already mentioned. A further guide is the presence of precipitating stressors – their absence rules out conversion disorder and although a stressor is necessary to make the diagnosis it does not prove definitively that the diagnosis is conversion disorder since stressful events can provoke any psychiatric disorder. Secondary gain is an essential element when making the diagnosis and the absence of any gain rules out this diagnosis. However, it must be remembered that gain may occur with physical illnesses also and so its presence does not prove the diagnosis. It is apparent that this is a diagnosis, which should be made only rarely and with extreme caution.

Management

Resolution of the symptoms usually occurs spontaneously although providing the patient with physiotherapy will enable the patient to 'save face' without having to acknowledge directly that the symptoms had a psychological basis. Thereafter psychotherapy can focus on the stressors and on their management as well as helping the patient achieve insight into the basis for the physical symptoms. It is unhelpful to tell the patient that the symptoms are imaginary and such an approach will compromise the doctor–patient relationship. Although used less frequently than in the past, abreaction with either hypnosis, amylobarbitone or diazepam also has a place, especially if symptoms are resistant to conservative approaches. This may also facilitate the identification of triggering events. The outcome is good for acute hysteria but once the symptoms have become entrenched the prognosis is poor and up to 50% remain symptomatic at 10 years.

Dissociative disorder

Dissociative disorder is a condition in which part of psychic function is separated from the whole. Thus memory for personal identity may be impaired while other aspects such as memory for skills remains intact. It is less common than conversion disorder. Dissociative amnesia is the most common symptom followed by fugues (wandering). While the psychoanalytic approach to dissociation emphasises repression and denial as the underlying defences provoking the disorder, the biological perspective emphasises that the problem lies in the underlying neuroanatomical and neurotransmitter systems. Although dissociative amnesia can occur spontaneously, this is rare and, more commonly, painful events associated with emotional conflict are described on history taking. Most patients are aware of the amnesia and are usually distressed. Amnesia may be localised, i.e. referring to a circumscribed period of time in the person's life, selective, in which there is amnesia for some but not all events during a specified period, and generalised, i.e. loss of memory for a whole lifetime. Localised amnesia is the most common. Some with dissociative amnesia may wander away from home and often present to casualty departments in a distressed state. However, when in a fugue state the patient may be unaware of the amnesia and a new identity may be adopted. As with conversion amnesia, fugues are associated with primary gain, e.g. a patient cannot recall the death of a parent thereby protecting herself from the emotional pain of this, and secondary gain, e.g. a soldier has amnesia and is removed from active duty. Dissociative amnesia must be distinguished from transient global amnesia and from dementia. Fugues and amnesia usually resolve spontaneously although on occasion abreaction using either hypnosis or intravenous barbiturates or benzodiazepines may be necessary. Recurrences are rare.

Other dissociative disorders

Hysterical pseudodementia gives the impression of severe generalised cognitive impairment and a variant, Ganser Syndrome, is associated with clouding of consciousness, approximate answers (e.g. Q. How many legs has a horse? A. 5) and hallucinations. These are rare conditions the symptoms of which were once thought to be knowingly fabricated, since they appeared to conform to a lay person's view of psychiatric disorder. It is now recognised that they may be indicative of schizophrenia or organic brain disease, unless the patient admits to or objective testing demonstrates that the symptoms are factitious.

Dissociative identity disorder, also known as multiple personality disorder, is a controversial diagnosis that is mainly made in the United States and rarely if ever in Europe. It is said to consist of two or more identities or personality states each with its own distinctive pattern of relating to others and self. These personalities are said to take control of the person's behaviour thereby depriving them of responsibility for this. Patients in whom this disorder is diagnosed are almost exclusively young women and studies vary between those that suggest it is extremely rare and is iatrogenic and those that believe it is grossly underdiagnosed.

FACTITIOUS DISORDER

This is a condition in which symptoms, usually physical but at times psychiatric, are intentionally produced with the objective of assuming the patient role. It is commonly referred to as Munchausen's syndrome after the fantastic tales of adventure described by that Baron. The patient's behaviour is directed to gaining admission to hospital or having multiple physical investigations. Sometimes urine or blood may be deliberately contaminated to achieve this end or sutures may be tampered with. Symptoms are often exotic, false names may be used and there may be a history of multiple operations. So convincing is the patient that preventing further investigations can be very difficult. The psychodynamic causes of factitious disorder are poorly understood since it is difficult to engage these patients in therapy. Anecdotal evidence is that many patients have a history of emotional deprivation, rejection or sexual abuse in childhood and of frequent hospitalisations at that time. The syndrome is believed to evolve from the perception of nurses, doctors, etc., rather than parents as carers and this is recapitulated in the sick role. A related but controversial diagnosis is Munchausen's syndrome by proxy (factitious disorder by proxy) in which a parent, usually a mother secretly harms her child in order to vicariously gain attention for herself. One of the problems with this diagnosis is that it is based on a subjective assessment of motivation by a third party. It is essential to explore all other possible causes for the child's signs and symptoms, even rare disorders, before making this diagnosis. Treatment of factitious disorder is very difficult since the sufferer has a specific treatment agenda and is usually unwilling to engage in further emotional exploration. Often the focus is containment and avoidance of admission by alerting hospitals and colleagues to the treatment seeking habits of these patients. There are no adequate studies of outcome in factitious disorders.

MALINGERING

Malingering is diagnosed when symptoms are feigned for the purpose of external gain. This differs from factitious disorder where the gain is internal or emotional. External gain includes compensation following road traffic accidents, repatriation from combat or avoidance of imprisonment for criminal offences. It can be a difficult diagnosis to make and the utmost care must be taken to obtain objective information concerning symptoms and functioning from doctors and other available sources before making this diagnosis. On the other hand it must also be considered as a possible diagnosis particularly where there is the likelihood of gain from the symptoms and where there is a discrepancy between dysfunction and symptoms.

While the symptoms are produced unconsciously in conversion and dissociative disorder (hysteria), they are feigned in both factitious disorder and malingering, although with very different motivations.

DEPERSONALISATION

This refers to an unpleasant state in which the patient feels detached and 'outside' themselves. A variant, derealisation, is the feeling that objects seem far away or unreal. These are not psychotic symptoms as is sometimes assumed. Depersonalisation and derealisation are usually secondary to some other condition, most commonly depressive illness or severe generalised anxiety and in these circumstances the treatment is of the primary disorder. These phenomena may occur in healthy people at times of tiredness, hunger or intense transient emotional states and they are then short-lived. Epidemiological studies have found that up to 70% of the general population describe these symptoms on an occassional basis and children may also experience them. Primary depersonalisation on the other hand is very rare and when it occurs seems to persist indefinitely. A brief trial of an anxiolytic may help in some. Otherwise there is no specific treatment except to support the patient.

SOMATOFORM DISORDERS

This group of disorders consists of conditions in which the focus is on the body – either physical symptoms, concerns about the possibility of physical illness or about the size/shape of certain parts of the body. Many involve the general practitioner at some point in their course although most patients with these disorders require referral for psychiatric opinion and intervention as they are very difficult to manage. They differ from malingerers and those with factitious disorder since the symptoms are not knowingly fabricated or exaggerated.

Somatization disorder

This disorder is characterised by the presence of numerous physical symptoms that cannot adequately be explained on the basis of physical investigations. A multiplicity of symptoms and of organs or systems is involved, with a propensity to be chronic and to begin before the age of 30. Occurring mainly in women, it was formerly called Briquet's syndrome. Although affecting less than 1% of the population, it causes significant distress and excessive medical help-seeking behaviour. It also causes frustration among doctors, patients and their families, as all seem to have different goals. The cause is unknown although a raft of psychodynamic explanations have been offered including social communication, emotional expression, repressed instinctual impulses, etc. A behavioural perspective emphasises the role of modelling, parental teaching and ethnic mores that somatise distress. Evidence for this comes from longitudinal studies demonstrating that children of parents who rate their general health as poor have more medically unexplained symptoms than controls (Hotopf *et al.*, 2000). Recurrent abdominal pain in childhood is a further risk factor although well-defined physical disease in childhood is not. Some studies described a neuropsychological basis for the unexplained symptoms due to a faulty perception and interpretation of incoming somatic stimuli. Patients often have very long, complicated histories and large case files. They often describe abuse, physical or sexual, and have impaired relationships in adulthood characterised by dependence. Treatment is difficult and is best managed by a single doctor. Regular appointments are necessary and investigations avoided unless absolutely clinically indicated. Psychotherapy, both individual or group, can be helpful in reducing treatment-seeking behaviour and the focus should be on coping with symptoms. The role of litigation is important in maintaining symptoms, such as chronic pain following traffic or other accidents due to the constant focus on and repetition of symptoms to medical personnel. This must be distinguished from malingering and factitious disorder.

Hypochondriasis

This term is used to describe the undue preoccupation with the possibility of serious disease. It differs from somatization disorder subtly in that in the latter there is excessive pre-occupation with multiple symptoms while in hypochondriasis the concern is with specific disorders. It results from the patient's unrealistic or inaccurate interpretations of bodily sensations. There is some evidence for a lower tolerance of physical discomfort; for example normal feelings of tension in the arms are experienced by the hypochondriacal person as pain and interpreted as evidence of illness. Theories of causation abound and include the desire to enter the sick role, a variant of depressive or anxiety disorders and psychoanalytic theories suggesting that the symptoms represent a transfer of angry feelings into physical complaints. Men and women are affected equally and up to 6% of medical out-patients suffer with hypochondriasis. Pain and gastrointestinal symptoms are the most common and the diagnosis should not be made when illness attribution is due to ignorance. For example the person getting chest pain during a panic attack may ascribe it to a possible myocardial infarct until the underlying cause is explained. Treatment is difficult as patients resist psychological explanations. However, interventions that focus on coping with symptoms and on explaining the physical basis for their symptoms, i.e. misinterpreting the normal physical signals to the brain, can keep them in contact with their therapist. Repeated investigations should only be carried out if clinically indicated and in this the general practitioner has a crucial role. Acknowledging that the patient is suffering rather than dismissing the symptoms as imaginary is the best approach. It is also helpful to request both patient and family to limit the amount of time during which the symptoms or supposed illness are discussed at home since the continuous preoccupation of the patient can alienate the family and reinforce the symptoms. Unfortunately the symptoms are often reinforced by herbalists, faith healers and well-meaning friends who encourage the patient to seek 'treatment' elsewhere. When the symptoms are symptomatic of some underlying disorder such as depression, panic disorder, etc., then the underlying condition must be treated.

In severe depression the hypochondriacal preoccupations may be of delusional intensity, e.g. when the person believes that cancer is present. Hypochondriacal delusions may also be part of a schizophrenic or monosymptomatic delusional state (see Chapter 16). The treatment is of the underlying disorder.

Body dysmorphic disorder

Formerly called dysmorphophobia, body dysmorphic disorder is a condition in which the person is preoccupied with some physical imperfection such as long legs, big ears, etc., in the absence of any objective evidence for this. In order to make the diagnosis it must be causing distress or impairment in personal, social or occupational life. Inevitably it leads to demands for corrective surgery. There is no information on its prevalence in the general population but in plastic surgery clinics it represents about 2% of patients. It also presents to dermatologists. More common in young women, the causes are unknown. Inevitably social learning theory has been offered as one possible cause resulting from society's preoccupation with physical perfection and stereotyped concepts of beauty. It is also associated with a higher than expected rate of mood disorders and obsessive–compulsive disorder in the family. As well as describing distress in association with the perceived flaw, many experience ideas of reference believing that others are looking at or talking about them, repeated mirror checking of the flaw and attempts to disguise it with make-up or clothing. Some patients become housebound as a result. Requests for cosmetic surgery should be resisted since the degree of deformity rarely warrants this. There is some evidence that treatment with clomipramine or the SSRIs is helpful in about 50% of cases. The long-term prognosis is unknown.

EATING DISORDERS

These are divided into three major types: anorexia nervosa, bulimia nervosa and obesity. Although they make good press and have attracted much media attention, they are difficult to treat and the role of the GP in their management is limited since most are referred for specialist help.

Anorexia nervosa

This condition was first described in 1868 and even then was recognised as being psychological in origin. It occurs most commonly in women and surprisingly the core symptom is not anorexia but a distorted attitude to shape, weight and food. The diagnostic features include loss of 25% of the standard body weight or a body mass index (BMI) less than 16 (BMI= weight kilos/height meters^2), an intense desire to be thin and amenorrhoea, often present before weight loss is obvious (in men loss of libido is present). The average age of onset is 16 and in boys is younger at 12. There is a marked socioeconomic gradient with the disorder being much more common in higher socioeconomic groups. It begins with dieting which is relentlessly pursued and as weight decreases body image becomes more abnormal. The pursuit of thinness may take the form of avoidance of certain foodstuffs, purging, vomiting or excessive exercising. A minority admit to stealing food and up to 50% have described regular binges when vast quantities of food are consumed, followed by excessive guilt, vomiting and purging (bulimia). There are also obsessional rituals around food and many will cook for the family on a regular basis while starving themselves. There are two broad categories of anorexia nervosa – the restricting and the binging/purging types. The latter have a poorer prognosis.

The lifetime prevalence of anorexia nervosa varies between 1.6 and 3.7% of the population depending on the definition, with an annual incidence of about 0.3%.

It is more common in certain groups such as fashion students and professional ballet dancers, both groups for whom bodily appearance and shape are of prime concern. Since many deny their symptoms and because milder forms may be undiagnosed it is likely that the prevalence is much higher and between 1 and 2% of university students in the United States may be affected by milder forms of the condition.

Causes

There is no evidence for a genetic contribution and the higher prevalence in siblings of those with an established eating disorder could be due to environmental factors. The importance of social attitudes to weight may be important since the condition is most prevalent in the middle and upper social classes and in certain professional groups. The name of Hilde Bruch is the one most associated with our understanding of the psychodynamics of anorexia nervosa. She suggests that the patient is attempting to gain control and autonomy and that control over food intake and weight is the symbolism of this. In particular those who come from a family which is preoccupied by food and which deprive the child of identity are most at risk. The significance of dieting in enabling the patient to escape from the turmoil of adolescence and regressing to childhood has been emphasised by others. Associated with these psychological understandings are the disturbed relationships which exist within the family and which have an important causative role in some.

Physical abnormalities

Hypothermia, bradycardia, lanugo, dependent oedema and hypotension are found on physical examination once the weight loss is apparent. ECG changes include flattening or inversion of the T waves, ST depression and lengthening of the QT interval. Hypokalaemic alkalosis is a further worrying complication.

Management

This is difficult since many patients project a veneer of normality both in their eating pattern and in the family relationships. Treatment has two aspects, one being weight gain to normal levels and the other relapse prevention. The first may require hospitalisation if weight loss is extreme. In general, medication is of little use and weight gain is achieved by a contractual agreement between the patient and therapist in which rewards to the patient are made contingent upon satisfactory weight gain. This objective can be achieved without much difficulty generally although it does require patience and encouragement from staff. More difficult is the task of preventing relapse and this requires on-going psychotherapy with the patient individually or if necessary in family sessions. The focus is upon the patient's difficulties and stresses as well as upon the problems within the family. The general practitioner is in a unique position in providing the therapist with information relevant to this task, especially in families who deny conflict. This information should not be used confrontationally but should provide direction to treatment. In addition other therapies such as social skills training may be required and if depression supervenes, as it sometimes does, antidepressants will be prescribed. Increasingly cognitive therapy is replacing the psychodynamic approaches to treatment with demonstrable success. Therapy will be required for months and sometimes even for years. Some patients will seek the advice of their general practitioner regarding self-help groups but, since there is no data available on their success or otherwise, caution must be exercised in view of the risks of reinforcement from meeting others with similar conflicts.

Outcome

Despite the therapeutic input, the outcome is gloomy and anorexia nervosa has a mortality of 5–18% depending on the study. Two-thirds return to normal weight and normal menses but relapses are common. Social and sexual functioning remains poor in the long term and up to two-thirds of patients remain preoccupied by food and weight while diet remains disorganised. Relationship difficulties lead to isolation and depression, anxiety, obsessional symptoms and sexual difficulties frequently supervene. Poor prognosis is associated with older age of onset, secondary bulimia, vomiting or purging, poor premorbid personality and male gender.

Bulimia nervosa

This is a disorder, first described in 1979, in which an intractable urge to overeat is associated with avoidance of the fattening effects of food by induced vomiting or purging and with a fear of becoming fat. Despite this, weight is usually within normal limits and amenorrhoea occurs in less than 50% of sufferers. During a binge there is a feeling of loss of control followed by depression, guilt and shame. It can thus be distinguished from anorexia nervosa although bulimia may sometimes be a symptom of this condition. It is more common in women than men and also has a later onset than anorexia nervosa, generally beginning in the late teens or early twenties. In view of the relative recency with which the condition was described there are some obvious gaps in relation to our knowledge of the aetiology, treatment and outcome. Its aetiology may be associated with the social pressures on young women to be shapely although why this should in some lead to anorexia nervosa and in others to bulimia nervosa is unknown. Biological factors such as the role of serotonin, noradrenaline and the endorphines have been suggested as mediators. The families of bulimics differ from those of anorectics in being more rejecting and many bulimics have a history of sexual abuse. The epidemiology is equally uncertain and depends on the definition chosen since up to 80% of female college students in the USA describe excessive eating, but only 4% admitted to self-induced vomiting. Clearly most who have occasional binges do not require treatment and it is only those meeting the criteria outlined above who need help, amounting to a prevalence of about 2% in women and 0.2% in men. Since sufferers perceive the loss of control over food as ego-dystonic, they are more likely to seek treatment than those with anorexia nervosa.

Physical problems secondary to purging and vomiting include dental caries, oesophagitis, salivary gland enlargement and electrolyte imbalance.

Diagnostically it may be confused with anorexia nervosa. Since many bulimics develop the capacity to vomit spontaneously it may resemble psychogenic vomiting but a careful history should clarify the diagnosis.

Treatment requires specialist help although there is uncertainty about the best approach. Many use a psychotherapeutic approach that combines support with exploration of the patient's background problems. In particular this may help those bingers who do so in response to personal difficulties. Providing structure in the patient's daily routine, especially when binging is related to boredom, and making the patient responsible for her food intake together with food diaries have also been advocated. The role of medication has received little attention until recently. However the SSRI fluoxetine has been found to have appetite stabilising properties and in doses of up to 80 mg per day is helpful in symptomatic control. It should always be combined with psychotherapy. In general, treatment is carried out on an out-patient basis and hospitalisation is required only when there are physical complications, such as potassium depletion or there is a risk of suicide. Little is known about the long-term outcome although it is probably a chronic condition that fluctuates. In general it has a better prognosis than anorexia nervosa. At three years less than one-third are completely well although symptoms do improve significantly in those who engage with treatment. About one-third have intractable symptoms.

Obesity

In most cases of obesity emotional factors do not seem to play an important aetiological role. However, in a small proportion excessive eating is related to such factors and psychiatric referral may be necessary. This group includes those who overeat to relieve boredom, anxiety or depression. By paying attention to these mood states and to the social reinforcers, which accompany them, the solace of food may be diminished and eating replaced by more appropriate behaviour. The use of positive rewards for weight loss and retraining of eating habits, e.g. eating more slowly, also aid management. Anorectic drugs have only short-term effects and the same is true for the more draconian method of jaw-wiring. In some grossly obese patients gastric reduction or jejuno-ileal bypass have been carried out with success.

SUMMARY

1. Obsessive–compulsive disorder is uncommon but debilitating. The main thrust of treatment is with behaviour therapy and anti-obsessional drugs, and referral to the specialist services is usual. The condition is associated with obsessional personality and the predominating symptoms are either rituals or ruminations. These symptoms can occur secondary to depressive or other illnesses.
2. The condition that was formerly hysteria has been subdivided into conversion and dissociative disorders. These disorders often resolve spontaneously although physiotherapy may assist in conversion disorder. Abreaction may be carried out if symptoms do not resolve. These conditions are most often secondary to depressive illness or organic states and then treatment is of the underlying disorder.
3. Somatoform disorders, including somatisation, hypochondriasis and body dysmorphic disorder are difficult to treat effectively and the focus is on support, recognition of the patient's distress and avoidance of repeated physical investigations.
4. The aetiology of anorexia and bulimia is related to social and personality factors. When weight is so low as to place the patient's life at risk admission to hospital may be required. Anorexia is best managed using cognitive therapy although some still advocate psychodynamic psychotherapy. Bulimia is also treated with cognitive therapy and fluoxetine is used as an adjunct.

CASE HISTORIES

Case 1

Miss X was a 25 year-old bank official referred with obsessional rituals. These had been present since the age of 15 and her decision to seek treatment was not because of any deterioration but because of her imminent engagement and marriage. The rituals included having to shower three times each day even though she would know she was not dirty. She insisted on putting her own clothes into the washing machine and removing them herself also. Each time she used the telephone or turned on the radio she had to wash her hands three times. There was no family history of psychiatric illness and her parents and boyfriend were supportive although they rarely saw her engaging in these rituals. At her first appointment she was asked to limit her showers to once each day and to monitor her level of anxiety after successfully resisting the urges. She was given instruction on replacing the thoughts of showering with thoughts about her wedding. She successfully overcame these rituals and her anxiety diary showed a slight increase in anxiety followed by a sustained drop. The next ritual which she chose to extinguish was that relating to washing her clothes. She was instructed to ask her mother to remove her clothes from the washing machine and she successfully overcame this ritual without any difficulty. Finally her hand-washing following using the radio or telephone was extinguished by a simple instruction not to do so. Her boyfriend then agreed to hold the telephone receiver and then request her to do so also. She experienced some initial anxiety at this and expressed fears of contamination but these disappeared following rehearsal over the following week. At the time of writing this girl is symptom-free.

Comment

This girl had a mild obsessive–compulsive disorder, a good premorbid personality and was highly motivated. She responded to very simple behavioural instruction. Had she responded less well it would have been necessary to treat her in her own home, more intensively and over a longer period of time.

Case 2

Miss X was a 17 year-old girl referred with a history of dieting since the age of 14. For about 1 year she had amenorrhoea and weighed 6.5 stone. Over the previous year she had returned to her normal weight of 8.5 stone without any specific treatment and was pleased about this but had then begun to binge eat. This occurred once every day and was associated with vomiting. She lived with her parents and was the eldest of four. Her relationship with her mother was good but she had not been close to her father and she resented him for being ambitious for the whole family and pushing them to excel in sports when they had little interest in this. At home she described him as overbearing and difficult and she avoided talking to him. She was irritated by the way in which he treated her mother, expecting her to do everything for him and especially by his eating habits, e.g. the noise he made, the way in which he held his cutlery, etc. When first seen this girl said she did not expect to benefit from therapy and had come at her mother's insistence. She was seen every week and therapy consisted of initially trying to build up a relationship of trust with this girl. Then her feelings about her father and herself were explored. Her self-image was negative but with encouragement and praise this improved. She was helped in this by doing simple tasks like writing down her positive attributes – prior to this she had seen nothing good in herself. She also started to draw again on the therapist's suggestion and felt pleased that she took this step. Her deep resentment of her father became more evident as therapy progressed and although her mother confirmed that his attitude to her had changed she made little effort to reciprocate. Requests to interview him were refused several times. Suggestions to her about reinforcing his change in attitude by simple greetings in the morning and at night were met with refusal. Despite this her binging became less frequent and she remains in therapy at the time of writing.

Comment

This girl had anorexia nervosa and a transition from this to bulimia is associated with a poor prognosis. Unless weight is very low it is important to shift the focus from diet to relationships and self-image. As this occurs in the patient the eating difficulty will improve also. Fortunately this girl admitted her interpersonal problems but many do not and insist that all is well. Therapy is usually long-term and this patient has already been seen for 6 months. Too prominent a concern with weight may distract from the cause of the problem and compromise dietary change.

Case 3

Mr X, a 35 year-old single man, was referred by a gastroenterologist with a 12–month history of unexplained abdominal pain and nausea. He had been experiencing increasing discomfort, weight loss and recent insomnia and in spite of extensive investigations by two other gastroenterologists, that included gastroscopy, ultrasound and barium studies, no physical abnormality was found. Mood and concentration was normal. He had a past history of aphonia several years earlier following the breakup of a relationship. He gave a history of major breakdown in his relationship with his sister because of his plan to sell the 50 year-old family business, in which she was a part shareholder. As a result they had not spoken to each other for 6 months, the period over which his physical symptoms had developed. The family was split on the decision he made and his relationship with some of them was also very poor. A diagnosis of somatoform disorder was made and a physical model by which distress can produce physical symptoms was offered by way of explanation. Symptomatic treatment with hypnotics and relaxation exercises was provided and advice on resolving the family conflict was also given. He was referred to a therapist who specialised in interpersonal therapy.

Comment

Care was taken not to dismiss this man's unexplained physical symptoms as 'in the mind' or 'psychological'. Instead an acceptable model involving explanation of the role of stress in causing autonomic symptoms was provided and accepted by the patient. All further physical investigations were stopped, as these would have reinforced his view of his symptoms as having an exclusively organic cause. Instead he was refocused on the real cause of his symptoms – the family dispute. He was treated symptomatically as well as being provided with professional help in resolving the interpersonal problems that were splitting the family. The differential diagnosis was of a depressive illness but as his mood was not low and his concentration was intact it was considered unlikely. His previous history of a conversion symptom (aphonia) indicates that this man expresses distress with physical symptoms.

REFERENCES

Chodoff, P. (1974). The diagnosis of hysteria: An overview. *American Journal of Psychiatry*, **131**, 1073–1078.
Hotopf, M., Wilson-Jones, C., Mayou, R., Wadsworth, M. and Wessley, S. (2000). Childhood predictors of adult medically unexplained hospitalisations. Results from the national birth cohort study. *British Journal of Psychiatry*, **176**, 273–280.
Kaplan, A. and Hollander, E. (1995). A review of pharmacologic treatments for obsessive compulsive disorder. *Psychiatric Services*, **54**, 1111–1118.

FURTHER READING

Fairburn, C.G. and Cooper, P.J. (1982). Self-induced vomiting and bulimia nervosa: an undetected problem. *British Medical Journal*, **284**, 1153–1155.
France, R. and Robson, M. (1986). *Behaviour Therapy in Primary Care. A Practical Guide.* Croom Helm, London.
Lazare, A. (1989). Current concepts in psychiatry. Conversion symptoms. *New England Journal of Medicine*, **305**, 745–748.
McCahill, M.E. (1995). Somatoform and related disorders: delivery of diagnosis at first step. *American Family Physician*, **52**, 193–204.
Reed, J.L. (1978). Compensation neurosis and Munchausen syndrome. *British Journal of Hospital Medicine*, **19**, 314–321.

SUGGESTED READING FOR PATIENTS

De Silva, P. and Rachman, S. (1999). *Obsessive–Compulsive Disorder. The Facts*. Oxford University Press, Oxford.
Fairburn, C. (1995). *Overcoming Binge Eating*. Guilford Press, London.
Palmer, R.L. (1980). *Anorexia Nervosa. A Guide for Sufferers and their Families.* Penguin Books, London.
Toates, F. (1990). *Obsessional Thoughts and Behaviour*. Thorsons, London.

USEFUL WEBSITES FOR PATIENTS

Anorexia and bulimia: www.rcpsych.ac.uk/info/help/anor/
Malingering: www.psychological.com/malingering.htm
Depersonalisation: www.benzo.org.uk

USEFUL CONTACTS

Eating Disorders Association
1st Floor, Wensum House
103 Prince of Wales Road
Norwich NR1 1DW
Tel: 01603 621 414
Website: www.edauk.com

Obsessive–Compulsive Foundation Inc
676 State Street
New Haven
CT 06511
USA
Tel: 203 401 2070
Email: info@ocfoundation.org

15

Psychiatric Aspects
of Physical Illness

For many years relations were strained between psychiatrists and physicians due in part to the grandiose claims of the psychosomatic school which believed that psychological factors caused physical illnesses. These were termed 'the psychosomatic illnesses' and included such conditions as hypertension, ulcerative colitis and cancer. In modern psychiatry this naïve claim has been abandoned and replaced by the view that psychological factors along with a number of genetic, environmental, and other unknown factors may interact in bringing about physical illness.

AETIOLOGICAL ROLE OF PSYCHOLOGICAL FACTORS IN PHYSICAL ILLNESS

Nowhere has the role of psychological factors been studied more closely than in relation to coronary artery disease. Numerous studies have found an association between what is termed type A behaviour and subsequent development of heart disease. Type A behaviour consists of hostility, competitiveness, high achievement and aggressiveness. Other factors such as hypertension, smoking and diabetes which are associated with coronary disease may provide the link between type A behaviour and this condition, although findings in this regard have been inconsistent. Intervention studies aimed at changing type A behaviour have shown a drop in the re-infarction rate when this behaviour altered (Friedman *et al.*, 1982).

Numerous data have been accumulated to support the view that major stress and bereavement are followed by an increased mortality in close relatives although the exact psychophysiological mechanism is not understood. An association between depression and cancer has been postulated but the evidence for this is conflicting as is the direction of the association. It has been suggested that depression alters the immune system thereby rendering the patient vulnerable to cancer. Any investigations of these links would need to be controlled for such intervening variables as smoking, drug taking and alcohol consumption which have a recognised association with personality and psychological disturbance and which may themselves be responsible for the development of a variety of physical ailments.

PSYCHOLOGICAL REACTIONS TO PHYSICAL ILLNESS

In all but the mildest of physical illnesses there are psychological symptoms occurring as a consequence of the symptoms and of the restriction placed upon the individual. These reactions may vary from transient distress, which improves as symptoms improve (or if the illness is chronic, the distress wanes as a new level of adaptation is reached) to depressive illness and even psychotic disturbances (see Chapters 5 and 6).

These disorders lie on a continuum, and identifying the point at which understandable unhappiness/distress ends and illness begins is extremely difficult and is bedevilled by the arbitrariness of what is understandable and what is not. As in any clinical situation the doctor attempting to distinguish one from the other will take account of such factors as the symptom cluster with which the patient presents, previous reaction to stress, past and family psychiatric history along with the degree of impairment occasioned by the psychological symptoms. In addition, the presence of an established psychiatric illness at the onset of the physical illness must also be taken into account. Overall, most studies on hospitalised patients with physical illness have confirmed that the dominant diagnoses are adjustment disorder, in which the psychological symptoms cause distress and impairment but resolve as the physical symptoms improve, and depressive illness (Smith *et al.*, 1998).

Adjustment disorders

Following myocardial infarction up to a quarter of patients develop significant psychological symptoms. In most patients these symptoms are transient and will have remitted within 3–4 months. When a diagnosis of carcinoma is made the symptoms are even more intense and are similar to those found in the acute phases of grief, with anger, denial, bargaining and depression being described. However these subside over the subsequent months and most patients, while remaining sad, do not require psychotropic medication but support and, at times, counselling. All serious physical conditions, including some that are not regarded as illnesses, such as termination of pregnancy and miscarriage, can induce these feelings and understanding and sympathy are the cornerstone of treatment.

Depressive illness

All physical illnesses can potentially cause depressive illness and where it is felt the patient has moved from the disorders classified as adjustment into depressive illness, antidepressant medication is required. There is however a group of medical conditions which are specifically associated with a tendency to develop depressive illness. These include:

- Painful musculoskeletal disorders, especially rheumatoid arthritis
- Hysterectomy

- Amputation
- Infectious mononucleosis
- Pregnancy, miscarriage and termination of pregnancy
- Carcinoma
- Cardiac by-pass

In some patients the depressive illness will antedate the physical disorder (see symptomatic depression) and those who were depressed prior to the onset of the condition have a poorer prognosis than those who become so subsequently.

SYMPTOMATIC DEPRESSION

Drugs

An increasing proportion of psychiatric disturbance, especially depression, is due to prescribed drugs. The affective disturbances cover the whole range from mild to severe depression. The weight of evidence suggests that those with drug-induced depression frequently have either a past or a family history of affective disorder. Antidepressants are not usually required since discontinuing the drug causes an improvement. If however symptoms persist then the treatment is as for any depressive illness. Antihypertensives are amongst the most commonly cited offenders in particular reserpine and methyldopa followed less often by the α- and β-receptor blockers. Most of the research on the relationship between depression and antihypertensives has been conducted on hospital populations. In a general practice setting the evidence for this relationship is much weaker.

Depression has been reported as a frequent complication of the use of oral contraceptives, especially those with a high oestrogen content, with a reported incidence of between 2 and 40% and it is the most common reason for discontinuation. Other disturbances such as anxiety and suicidal gestures have also been described. In general, attempts to clarify the association between this group of drugs and depression are fraught with methodological difficulties, not least being the possibility that many have a past or family history of depressive illness. The proposed mechanism is that high doses of oestrogen cause a deficiency of pyridoxine, which in turn impairs the metabolism of 5–hydroxytryptamine, the neurotransmitter believed to be responsible for depression. However, the addition of pyridoxine did not prove effective, when investigated in controlled studies.

Corticosteroids have frequently been reported as causing depression and less commonly hypomania or mania. One of the difficulties is that these drugs are widely used in medicine for conditions which themselves are associated with psychiatric complications. Non-steroidal anti-inflammatory agents have also been reportedly associated with depression although this may be associated with the conditions for which they are prescribed rather than the drugs themselves.

Major tranquillisers have long been considered a possible cause of depression and there have been many reports of suicide. Although depression is recognised as a common symptom in schizophrenia, it is only in recent years that the extent of this has been fully appreciated, and much of the depression, presumed due to treatment, may be part of the illness itself. A further confounding factor is the presence of insight into the nature of the illness together with the extrapyramidal side-effects which occur. Both of these may themselves contribute to changes in mood. Other drugs such as levodopa and cytotoxic agents especially the vinka alkaloids have a similar association with depression. The drug accutane isotretinoin, a retinoid receptor agonist, used in the treatment of acne has been widely reported as being associated with causing depression and even suicide in some users. Although the patient information sheets carry information cautioning its use in those with a history of mood disorder, it is still unclear if the drug actually causes depression. Among the problems with establishing a link is the relative frequency of depression among young people with a disfiguring condition and the failure to establish any putative mechanism (Hull and D'Arcy, 2003).

Symptomatic disorders

Many physical conditions are known to be associated with affective and other psychiatric disturbances. These are not just reactions to physical illness but are an inherent part of the disease process. The psychological symptoms may occur prior to the physical illness being diagnosed and this is especially true with carcinoma of the bronchus, of the pancreas and Hodgkin's disease. Manic and schizophrenic presentations are much less common than depression.

There is a strong link between neurological disorders and psychological disturbances, especially depression. Following a cerebrovascular accident, depression is frequently described. This is not due solely to the physical incapacity resulting from such disorders but is related also to the site of the lesion and right-sided infarcts in the posterior cortex are most likely to be associated with depression. Catastrophic reactions and dementia may occur also. Multiple sclerosis is associated with depression, mania and dementia and these are related to the degree of central nervous system involvement. Contrary to the belief that such disturbances do not respond to antidepressants, there is now convincing evidence that pharmacological intervention is indicated and can bring about a dramatic response. Parkinson's disease is also associated with a higher than expected occurrence of depression, as is Huntington's chorea and epilepsy. The treatment of depressive illness in Parkinson's disease is complicated by the effect the SSRIs may have in worsening some of the physical symptoms while tricyclics may worsen confusion. Lofepramine is probably the best choice, although there is no absolute contraindication to any antidepressant. On occasions temporal lobe epilepsy may be confused with schizophrenia especially when perceptual disturbances predominate. These normally subside when the epilepsy is brought under control.

Endocrine disorders such as hypoglycaemia may occasionally present with acute confusional states or with hypomania. Hyperthyroidism may be associated with anxiety, hypomania or depression and depression and paranoid illnesses are often found in hypothyroidism. Mood disturbances also occur in Cushing's syndrome.

Autoimmune disorders especially systemic lupus erythematosus are associated with a variety of psychological conditions when there is cerebral involvement. Of these depression is the most common.

SOMATIC PRESENTATION OF PSYCHIATRIC ILLNESS

It is well recognised that many people present to their general practitioner not with psychological symptoms but with their physical counterparts such as anorexia, fatigue, paraesthesia and palpitations. Chest pain is also a common presenting symptom to the casualty department and is frequently a manifestation of underlying anxiety. Abdominal discomfort due to anxiety or depression or urinary frequency may lead the patient to the gastroenterologist or urologist. More unusual presentations are with fits, vomiting and a feeling of a lump in the throat (referred to as globus hystericus). These so called hysterical symptoms are frequently part of an underlying depressive illness (see Chapter 14). Dentists frequently encounter facial or gum pain for which no physical cause has been found and there is convincing evidence that such patients benefit from tricyclic antidepressants. These symptoms are known as 'depressive equivalents'.

The hypochondriacal patient will often express the firm belief that he has cancer or some terminal illness and in some cases may commit suicide in order to avoid the 'diagnosis'. It is tempting to try to reassure such people by agreeing to numerous physical investigations. This however rarely achieves its objective, and once the doctor has satisfied himself that he has taken reasonable care to rule out an underlying organic cause, further investigations should be avoided. Failure to do so will reinforce the patient's beliefs of the physical rather than psychological basis of the symptoms. The management of such patients is to treat the underlying cause whether it be depression, anxiety or schizophrenia (see Chapters 6, 14 and 16).

A group of people, usually young women, who present with multiple physical symptoms for which no organic cause is responsible are said to have somatisation disorder (see Chapter 14). Other physical manifestations of psychiatric disorders such as malingering, factitious disorder and Munchausen's syndrome are discussed in Chapter 14.

Worries of a physical deformity, frequently focusing on the nose or ears, are referred to as dysmorphophobia or body dysmorphic disorder (see Chapter 14). In more severe cases the patient may be deluded and suffering from a monosymptomatic psychosis, now called persistent delusional disorder (see Chapter 16). The former group generally requires help with their own self-esteem and with inter-personal relations since such individuals are frequently shy and isolated. Surgical intervention rarely resolves their difficulties and symptom substitution may occur or the focus of concern may shift to some other part of the body. Monosymptomatic psychosis requires pharmacological treatment and pimozide is believed to have a specific effect on this disorder.

CHRONIC FATIGUE SYNDROME

Chronic fatigue syndrome (CFS) defies classification and three aetiological views have been expressed depending on whether the syndrome is regarded as either psychiatric, physical or straddling both. The condition has attracted unprecedented interest and even the name has caused controversy with the term myalgic encephalomyelitis (ME) implying a strong organic basis for the symptoms. Although the term is seldom used, the syndrome does bear more than passing resemblance to what was in the past termed neurasthenia.

Aetiology

The most common belief among sufferers is that the origin of the fatigue arises from a viral illness, and retroviruses, enteroviruses (Coxsackie virus) or the Epstein–Barr virus (EBV) have all had their adherents. The prominence of fatigue and myalgia has led some to suggest that CFS is a disorder of neuromuscular function. EMG studies have confirmed abnormalities of muscle structure but function is not impaired suggesting that the abnormalities are consequent upon disuse, a common result of the symptoms.

The possibility that this is an immunological disorder has been mooted by American researchers since the swollen glands, allergies and sore throats that preceed the onset mimic some disorders of immune function. Abnormalities of T-lymphocytes have been suggested as underlying CFS although such abnormalities have also been described in depressive illness and there are similar findings among controls.

The suggestion that CFS is primarily a psychiatric disorder evokes negative reactions from some doctors and the majority of patients, although up to two-thirds of patients with CFS meet the diagnostic criteria for major depression, anxiety disorder and somatisation disorder, in that order. It is likely that there is overlap in the diagnostic criteria, making the finding of a high prevalence for psychiatric disorder an artefact. Alternatively CFS may be a form of 'masked' depression but antidepressants fail to make an impact on the symptoms in many patients. Thus the aetiology is still uncertain.

Prevalence and classification

Up to 2.5% of attenders in primary care may suffer with CFS. However, this may be an over-estimate since three distinct groups exist in the primary care population. First, there are those who, as part of a depressive illness, complain of fatigue and myalgia. The second includes those who develop the symptoms over several months and become increasingly concerned at its impact on their lives. As a result they are eager for help. A third group, the most difficult to treat, cling assiduously to the belief that their symptoms are due to CFS, often reinforced by family, friends, the Internet and a local support group. Unfortunately, this latter group through their reading will have come to regard rest as an essential component of management based on the 'energy-bank' model. This says that each person has a limited supply of energy, which if used too quickly causes a deficit (overdraft) requiring rest to replenish it. This theory is validated for them by the fact that they suffer fatigue even after simple exercise. These patients are therefore likely to oppose any efforts to reintroduce a graded exercise programme and are often reluctant to attend their doctor for that reason. They also subscribe to theories that allergies, yeast infections and vitamin deficiencies contribute to it. Infections may or may not have preceeded the fatigue. Over half of all cases of CFS are female and it is most common in young adults.

Features

CFS is diagnosed when the patient describes fatigue for more than 6 months that interferes with everyday activity by 50% or more. Generalised muscle pains, post-exertional fatigue and mental fatigue, such as poor concentration and difficulty thinking and focusing are also prominent. Sleep, although normal in quantity is not refreshing and headaches, painful glands and a feverish sensation (but no actual rise in temperature) are also described. Depressed mood and anxiety is often secondary to the incapacity.

Investigations

A careful history with particular focus on the sequence of symptom development will assist in out-ruling depressive illness. Physical examination is important since physical causes must be excluded but also this helps build up trust between the patient and doctor as patients with CFS often feel their symptoms are not believed. There are no investigations specific to this condition or definitive in making the diagnosis. Routine tests such as Hb, FBC, ESR, LFTs, U and Es, urinalysis and thyroid function tests are probably all that are required in the presence of a normal physical examination and typical history. Other investigations should be determined by the history and physical abnormalities since these may reinforce the patient's belief that CFS is a disease process that further tests will eventually identify.

Natural history and prognosis

Poor prognosis is associated with long duration of symptoms and with physical attribution of the syndrome. Belonging to a patient support group is also a negative indicator as these generally subscribe to the medical or viral theory of causation. Children and adolescents have a better prognosis while continuing medical investigations or granting early retirement worsens the outcome also. Without treatment the outcome is poor with between 13% and 18% improving after one year and only 6% becoming symptom-free.

Treatment

The relationship between doctor and patient is especially important in the disorder due to the anger and mistrust which these patients evoke. Reassurance that the symptoms are taken seriously and not just regarded as 'all in the mind' has to be balanced against colluding with the patient's belief that the symptoms are purely of organic origin. It is important to explain that while the onset may be viral other factors are prolonging the condition especially inactivity.

The cornerstone of treatment is graded activity. Many will have been cautioned against activity and will describe worsening myalgia and fatigue following exercise. Activity must be gradual and balanced and 'boom and bust' exercise, a common feature of sufferers, must be avoided, as must total inactivity. Patients must also be informed that myalgia will increase temporarily after activity begins but coupled with suitable rest periods is not damaging and is part of recovery. Antidepressants can be used when depressive illness accompanies the disorder.

Analgesics have little effect on myalgia and there is no evidence that vitamins, nutritional supplements or specific dietary exclusions are helpful. At presentation many patients will be taking herbal or other medicines and these need not be stopped unless there is evidence of harm or cost becomes a factor. However, reliance on medicines, even those that are complementary, may undermine the rehabilitative core treatment. An excellent review of treatment is provided by Wessely (1995).

CANCER

As described above, emotional disturbances may at times herald an occult carcinoma or the distress may be a direct result of the threatened loss of life. There are a number of factors which predispose patients with cancer to becoming clinically depressed and these are enumerated below:

(i)   Impending disability or death
(ii) Pain

(iii) Isolation and stigma
(iv) Pre-existing depression
(v)   Spiritual difficulties
(vi) Treatment for cancer especially radical surgery or chemotherapy
(vii) Cerebral metastases.

Much of the early research supported the view that the patient's reaction to his illness affected the prognosis in early cancer. This was widely studied in relation to breast cancer where those with short-lived distress and those who express and resolve their emotional distress either by developing a 'fighting spirit' or by denial, were thought to have a more favourable outcome than those who lapsed into apathy and hopelessness. However recent studies have failed to replicate these findings although the belief that the patient's attitude to illness can affect the outcome remains a popular one.

Management of depression in the terminally ill

When the diagnosis of cancer is first made many people will need their own time and space to adjust. Distress, suicidal ideation and completed suicide are highest in the period immediately following diagnosis. Most people reach a state of equilibrium and a new level of adjustment with passage of time. Those who fail to do so however may require additional help along psychotherapeutic lines. In particular this may involve the family discussing the condition with the patient, or the patient working through their inevitable grief. Failure to reach a state of equilibrium may be indicative of a depressive illness which needs pharmacological treatment.

Caution must be exercised in affixing diagnostic labels in these circumstances. The seriously ill patient who is diagnossed as clinically depressed and treated as such may in fact be denied the right to feel emotionally upset about the future. The feelings of sadness which will be exhibited may be dismissed as due to depressive illness and relatives may unwittingly use this to avoid their own sadness. On the other hand, the person wrongly diagnosed as going through an understandable reaction to the circumstances may be deprived of a potentially powerful tool for alleviating depressive symptomatology and improving the quality of life during their last months in this world. The distinction between adjustment disorder and depressive illness is therefore of more than intellectual importance and the doctor will look to any family and past history of psychiatric disturbance, together with the current symptom pattern in making the diagnosis. However, many of the symptoms found in depressive illness are not useful in those on chemotherapy or who are in the late stages of illness since they are part of the physical illness itself. These include anorexia, tiredness, insomnia and lassitude. Symptoms such as persisting tearfulness, diurnal mood swing and panic attacks may be helpful in making the diagnosis. In practice, the distinction is extremely difficult to make.

The appropriate treatment of depressive illness is a humanitarian exercise that will improve quality of life, reducing the suicide potential and possibly lessen the intensity of physical symptoms especially pain.

PREMENSTRUAL SYNDROME

Originally called premenstrual tension by Frank in his original description of the syndrome, it is now termed premenstrual dysphoric disorder (PMDD). However, most clinicians are in agreement that irritability is often more distressing and disabling than low mood, as noted in the early description of the condition.

Prevalence

Accurate estimates are difficult to come by since 20–40% of all women seek medical help at some time for incapacitating premenstrual symptoms and over 80% of women report significant physical or psychological changes during the premenstrual phase of their cycle but these are usually not disabling. Among those keeping diaries and evaluated prospectively, 3.5% of women meet criteria for PMDD that is associated with multiple symptoms and impaired social, occupational or family functioning. However up to 10% of women retrospectively report such features although some also wrongly ascribe psychological and physical symptoms to premenstrual syndrome due to the menstrual exacerbation observed in many psychiatric conditions.

Aetiology

Twin studies strongly support a genetic contribution to PMDD. The relationship to hormonal change has not been substantiated and neither ovarian function nor changes in gonadal steroids distinguish those with or without the disorder.

Some studies have explored the role of gaba-amino-butyric acid, of β-endorphins and of allopregnanolone (a metabolite of progesterone) and identified some abnormalities although these findings have taken second place to serotonin, which has been found to be low in blood and platelets as well as showing decreased uptake during the luteal phase of the cycle. Coupled with the effects of serotonin deprivation on aggression in animal studies these findings suggest that underactivity in this system is a contributor to the psychological symptoms of PMDD especially irritability.

Diagnostic features

The clinical features are a mixture of psychological and physical symptoms that occur in the premenstrual phase of most cycles and remit in the week post-menstruation. These consist of depression, hopelessness, anxiety, tension, lability of mood, irritability or anger, decreased interest in usual activities, tiredness, increased or decreased appetite, hyper-somnia or insomnia, weight gain, feeling bloated, breast discomfort and feelings of being overwhelmed or out of control resulting in impairment in occupational and interpersonal functioning. Irritability is one of the most common symptoms in the condition and one that probably has most impact on family and colleagues. Many of these symptoms can be found in association with menstrual exacerbation of other psychiatric disorders and when this occurs the diagnosis and treatment is of the underlying disorder.

Menstrual diaries can help in deciding whether there is follicular phase remission since this is crucial in making the diagnosis and the impact on family members should be confirmed by collateral interview.

Treatment

Non-pharmacological

Many of these are of unproven efficacy but remain popular for mild symptoms and in those who do not wish to take pharmacological agents. These include aerobic exercise, reduction in caffeine intake, relaxation exercises, high fibre or low salt diets, the latter being useful only when symptoms due to fluid retention are prominent.

One of the treatments that has been shown to be effective is cognitive behaviour therapy. However, this requires access to specialist services and may be impractical for many family doctors. PMDD support groups have also been shown to be effective but many women may be reluctant to discuss such a personal matter in this setting.

If the family response to PMDD is abnormal then the exacerbation of interpersonal problems may require referral to a specialist family therapy centre.

Pharmacological

Oral contraceptives remain the most commonly prescribed pharmacological treatment for PMDD yet there is no evidence that psychological symptoms improve and they may even become more severe although some physical symptoms do respond. The SSRIs are the most effective treatment (Dimmock *et al.*, 2000) and there appears to be no difference between individual products although the slight difference in side effect profile suggests that citalopram and fluoxetine have fewer sexual side effects. Unlike the antidepressant response, the response in PMDD occurs very rapidly and in light of this the intermittent use of SSRIs during the luteal phase only is a possibility. Several studies have successfully used this regime. Clomipramine, a tricyclic antidepressant, in doses of 10–50 mg, has also been found to be effective and trials of venlafaxine and nefazadone are currently underway.

Antidepressants should be discontinued after about 1 year to evaluate symptom recurrence.

Other pharmacological agents including buspirone and alprazolam are supported by some empirical evidence and diuretics are of use if cyclical weight gain is evident although their efficacy in other symptoms is uncertain. Pyridoxine (vitamin B6) and calcium supplements may be effective but well designed studies are required and similar caveats apply to L-tryptophan and evening primrose oil. There is no evidence for the benefits of herbal remedies in spite of their popularity.

SUMMARY

1. The association between physical illness and psychological problems is well recognised.
2. Physical illness may have an *aetiological* role in causing psychological disturbance along with other factors. The emotional symptoms may be a direct result of physical pain or of the incapacity and threatened loss. They correspond with the categories known as adjustment reaction and depressive illness.
3. Some disorders are *symptomatic* of physical illness including certain cancers, some endocrine abnormalities and strokes. The role of drugs in causing depressive symptomatology is also recognised.
4. Chronic fatigue syndrome is a difficult to treat condition and graded exercise is the best treatment.
5. Cancer is associated with depressive symptoms for a number of reasons and both counselling and, at times, medication are necessary.
6. Premenstrual tension is of uncertain aetiology and SSRIs are the most effective treatment although oral contraceptives are most commonly prescribed.

CASE HISTORIES

Case 1

Mrs X was a 65 year-old woman who had suffered a stroke 6 months earlier. She made a good recovery but had some residual left-sided weakness and walked with a limp. She always used her husband as a physical support by holding his hand although she was deemed to be capable of walking alone and unaided. Within a few days of hospitalisation following the stroke she complained of feeling sad and upset at what had happened. She had some appetite disturbance and initial insomnia. It was felt initially that these symptoms were the result of mild incapacity in a previously active woman who had been involved in local community work. Her family of three daughters and her husband were all supportive and there were no major problems in the family. She was referred to the psychiatric out-patient clinic 6 months after her stroke because of her feelings of sadness, her insomnia and poor appetite, but above all because of the discrepancy between her residual physical symptoms and her level of functioning after rehabilitation. A diagnosis of depressive illness was made and she improved both emotionally and functionally following a course of antidepressant treatment.

Comments

This lady's depressive illness was mistaken for an adjustment reaction. The discrepancy between physical symptoms and functioning was important in helping make the diagnosis since both should improve simultaneously in a patient of normal personality successfully undergoing physical rehabilitation. There is now much evidence to support the use of antidepressants in post-stroke patients suffering from depressive illness.

Case 2

Mrs X was a 36 year-old married woman with metastatic carcinoma of the cervix. She was being nursed in a hospice but was largely uncommunicative with the staff and rarely looked directly at any of them when speaking. When the doctors came to see her on their ward rounds she would look at a magazine although it was felt she was not reading it. Her carcinoma had been diagnosed one year earlier and she was fully aware of the diagnosis. Her husband was also aware of the diagnosis but he was a heavy drinker and unsupportive. She had two children, a daughter, 17, born before marriage from another relationship and a son, 10, from her marriage. They were aware of the illness and its consequences in general terms only. The family visited her regularly but little was ever said during the visits. She was by nature a reserved, aloof woman and had never discussed problems with anybody. Mrs X was referred for assessment because of her behaviour as outlined above. When seen at interview she made no eye contact and fiddled with her book throughout. She was monosyllabic initially but as the interview progressed she became more forthcoming telling me of her fear of dying. She especially feared suffocating as she had experience of nearly suffocating as a child. She was angry with her husband because of his poor understanding of her now or in the past. She also spoke of her children and her worries for their future although she had asked her sister to care for them after her death and she was agreeable to do this. She said she had never discussed her illness with anybody and the nursing team who had treated her at home prior to admission verified this – she would never sit and was frequently absent when they visited, even by appointment. It was felt that this woman had never resolved her feelings about her illness and her death. Within two days of the first interview she had become more communicative with the nurses and had put aside her books and magazines when seeing the doctors. It was decided that a nurse, whom she already knew on the ward, should be involved in encouraging this patient to talk and express her grief whenever she wished to do so. She responded to this approach and at the time of writing the patient had returned home and was coping emotionally.

Comments

By her behaviour this lady was keeping those who could talk to her at a distance and they therefore did not broach the subject. Her husband's attitude also did not facilitate communication and her personality was such she always kept her problems to herself. Before embarking on discussing her illness and its consequences the interviewer had to ascertain what she was willing to admit about her illness. In fact she was very knowledgeable about it and had no obvious denial. It was therefore appropriate to proceed further to discussing more openly her fear and her feelings about the future. Had she denied knowing about her illness it would be unwise to proceed in this way without first getting to know the patient better and even then it may be inadvisable. This woman's behaviour was a manifestation of her distress, and once she was allowed to acknowledge this openly, her behaviour improved, allowing intervention to continue from the counsellor. This approach worked for this patient. It is not to be used for every patient who is terminally ill since intervention, if it is required, has to be individually tailored. It must be remembered that some patients resolve their grief themselves without any outside help or with the minimum and forcing counsellors or psychiatrists upon them is unnecessary and clumsy.

Case 3

Mr X was a 37 year-old man with a 3 year history of dyspepsia and occasional vomiting. He had been referred sequentially to a gastroenterologist, a surgeon and a physician for assessment. No physical cause was found and he was referred to the psychiatric services for assessment. He described feeling depressed and apathetic because of the dyspepsia. He was free from dyspepsia when on holiday but immediately he returned to work the symptoms recurred. His appetite was reduced, he had little interest in reading although he had been a keen reader prior to his symptoms. He admitted that he was in debt and this caused friction with his wife. The hospitalisations also put a strain on the relationship and she was angry that no cause for his symptoms had been found. He slept for 6–7 hours each night but never woke refreshed and had nightmares over the past year. He worked at senior management level and his work was suffering because of his absences. Also he did not enjoy the personnel aspects of his work for which he felt himself ill-trained. A tentative diagnosis of depressive illness was made and he was commenced on antidepressants. His physical as well as his psychological symptoms resolved completely. At the time of writing he was off all medication, had been given advice on dealing with his work-related difficulties but had refused an offer of marital therapy.

Comments

The physical symptoms were of anxiety, which was secondary to depressive illness. The differential diagnosis was of somatoform disorder. The history that his dyspepsia improved when on holiday helped in making the diagnosis along with the presence of other background problems in his life prior to the onset of his illness. Although this man attributed his depression to his physical symptoms, this explanation is often the result of rationalisation rather than insight.

REFERENCES

Campion, P.D., Lynch, S.P.D. and Blenkiron, P. (1999). Chronic fatigue syndrome: UK primary care perspective. *Primary Care Psychiatry*, **5**, 31–36.

Dimmock, P.W., Wyatt, K.M, Jones, P.W. and O'Brien, P.M. (2000). Efficacy of selective serotonin-reuptake inhibitors in premenstrual syndrome: a systematic review. *Lancet*, **356**, 1131–1136.

Friedman, M., Thoresen, C.E., Gill, J.E. *et al.* (1982). Feasibility of altering type A behaviour pattern after myocardial infarction. Recurrent coronary prevention project study: methods, baseline results and preliminary findings. *Circulation*, **66**, 83–92.

Hull, P.R. and D'Arcy, C. (2003). Isotretinoin use and subsequent depression and suicide: presenting the evidence. *American Journal of Clinical Dermatology*, **4**, 493–505.

Smith, G.C., Clarke, D.M., Handrinos, D. and Dunsis, A. (1998). Consultation-liaison psychiatrists management of depression. *Psychosomatics*, **39**, 244–252.

Wessely, S. (1995). Chronic fatigue syndrome – the current position: 2. Assessment and treatment. *Primary Care Psychiatry*, **1**, 87–98.

FURTHER READING

Condon, J.T. (2001). Premenstrual syndrome in primary care: an update. *Primary Care Psychiatry*, **7**, 85–90.

Creed, F. and Pfeffer, J. M. (Eds) (1982). *Medicine and Psychiatry*. Pitman, London.

Parkes, C.M. (1979). Terminal care: Evaluation of in-patient services at St Christopher's Hospice. *Postgraduate Medical Journal*, **55**, 517–522.

Robertson, M. and Katona, C. (1996). *Depression and Physical Illness*, Wiley, Chichester.

Wyatt, K.M., Dimmock, P.W. and O'Brien, P.M.S. (2004). Selective serotonin re-uptake inhibitors for pre-menstrual syndrome. *Cochrane Library*. Issue 1, Wiley, Chichester.

USEFUL WEBSITES FOR PATIENTS

Cancer: www.nimh.nih.gov/publicat/depcancer.cfm
Premenstrual tension: www.pms.org.uk

16

The Psychoses

SCHIZOPHRENIA

Kraepelin and Bleuler are the founding fathers of the concept of schizophrenia and Bleuler described the core symptoms, known colloquially as the four As: ambivalence, altered associations, autism and blunted affect. Many of the symptoms described by them, such as delusions and hallucinations, were known to occur in other conditions and the core symptoms were sufficiently ill-defined and subjective to make validation of the condition unsatisfactory. Schneider identified and described the first rank symptoms and advanced the process of refining the diagnosis and validating the condition.

Prevalence

The lifetime risk for developing schizophrenia is about 1% while the annual prevalence lies around 2–4/1000. The number of new cases each year lies between 0.2 and 0.5/1000. There is a slight excess of men over women and the age of onset is earlier in men, with a peak age of onset between 15 and 25 and a decade later in women. It is very rare before the age of 10.

Aetiology

Genetic

The importance of a genetic contribution to this illness has been apparent since the early part of the last century although it is clearly identifiable in only a minority of cases. The magnitude and type of this contribution is still a matter for debate. A number of genetic mechanisms have been investigated with ambiguous results and these include both monogenic and polygenic modes as well as genetic heterogeneity. Moreover, the view that what is inherited is not a certainty of developing the illness but an increased vulnerability is now gaining credibility. Almost half of all chromosomes have at some point been thought to be linked with schizophrenia and the most common associations are with the long arms of chromosomes

5,11 and 18 and the short arm of chromosome 19 and the X chromosome. The risk where both parents have the condition is about 35%, where one parent is affected 12% and a second degree relative 2.5%. For monozygotic twins the concordance lies between 35 and 60% and for dizygotic twins between 9 and 26%, while for a non-twin sibling the risk is about 8%. Genetic studies into the traditional subtypes (hebephrenic, catatonic and paranoid) have found no evidence that they breed true although there may be a slightly lower risk of schizophrenia in the relatives of those with the paranoid type.

Family

Older theories of schizophrenia and also of the antipsychiatry school focused on the role of family psychopathology in the genesis of the condition. The most popular theory, dubbed the 'double bind', suggested that the dissonance between the verbal and non-verbal cues which the child faced in his day-to-day life made schizophrenia the inevitable and indeed the only 'sane' response. This view with its legacy of blame and guilt has happily never been scientifically proven and has been abandoned. An equally judgmental view, referred to as 'schism' and 'skew' described the balance of dominance within the family and this was thought to be a risk for producing schizophrenic members. This theory has also been relegated to the archives. The importance of the family however has not been ignored and there is now a convincing body of opinion, backed up by research, that the ultimate prognosis is determined, in part, by family attitudes known as 'Expressed Emotion' (EE) (see under Social Management).

Personality

The existence of an association between schizoid pre-morbid personality and schizophrenia is a commonly held belief. Recent evidence has questioned this and suggests that many schizophrenics who show evidence of schizoid personality may in fact have incipient schizophrenia. Also, only a minority of those with this type of personality disorder develop schizophrenia. Further problems arise with regard to schizotypal personality disorder which is regarded in the DSM classification system as a personality disorder (see page 153, Chapter 11) while the European classification (ICD) includes this as a variant of schizophrenia.

Environment

The recognition that many sufferers with this illness belong to the lower social classes suggested that there may be some risk factor in these socioeconomic groups which predisposed to this disorder. Closer scrutiny of their family background clarified that this was the effect of the illness with the associated social drift downward, rather than any inherent pathogen in the social environment *per se*.

As with depressive illness many schizophrenic episodes follow upon major psychological trauma although the type of event has been shown to be non-specific. Those episodes which have a definite precipitant have a better prognosis than those which arise spontaneously. However, such events would not act as a trigger unless there was a prior vulnerability to the illness.

Another approach to environmental causes has focused on the observation that significantly more schizophrenics are born in the winter months than at other times of the year thus raising the possibility that some pathogen such as a virus may be the basis for this disorder. The influenza virus has received considerable attention as a possible candidate. The role of birth trauma and temporal lobe dysfunction has been suggested also. Other authorities suggest that it may be a reflection of a wider neurodevelopmental disorder since is has been found in some studies to be associated with 'soft' neurological signs.

Biological theories

There has been considerable interest in the specific areas of the brain that may be the primary site of pathology in schizophrenia. These include the basal ganglia, the frontal cortex and the limbic system. Several post-mortem studies have found a decrease in size of this area including the amygdala, hippocampus and the parahippocampal gyrus and these replicate the findings of MRI studies in living patients. Studies focusing on the basal ganglia, while finding an increase in D_2 receptors in certain parts have failed to establish if this is the result of medication or the underlying neuropathology of the condition. As the basal ganglia are connected to the frontal cortex this area has also become a focus for investigation.

The theory that abnormalities in dopamine turnover or in dopaminergic receptors are responsible has been proposed for more than 25 years. The simplest theory is that schizophrenia results from too much dopaminergic activity. In particular D_2 receptors have been linked to the positive symptoms and D_1 with negative symptoms. Other receptors such as D_5 being related to D_1, and D_3 and D_4 to D_2 amplify this picture as increases in D_4 receptors have been found in post-mortem samples from schizophrenia patients.

Other receptors have also been the subject of major investigation. Serotonin turnover, especially that linked to $5HT_2$ receptors, has been implicated in the negative symptoms. A decrease in function in the prefrontal cortex, the area with the highest density of $5HT_2$ receptors, and an increase in size of the lateral ventricles may be associated with negative symptoms. Recent imaging studies have shown a decrease in the size of the temporal and limbic areas of the brain, changes that may play a part in the positive symptoms of schizophrenia. Norepinephrine, glutamate and GABA have also been investigated.

Brain imaging

The earliest imaging studies, i.e. CT studies, showed enlargement of the lateral and third ventricles and a reduction in cortical volume. Other studies have shown cerebral asymmetry, altered brain density and reduced cerebellar volume. However, these abnormalities have also been reported in a variety of psychiatric and organic brain disorders. Attempts to clarify whether the brain changes are static or progressive are inconclusive. Overall, what these investigations have demonstrated is that schizophrenia is an illness associated with structural abnormalities. However, the magnitude of these changes is small and so CT scanning is unhelpful in making the diagnosis in clinical practice.

MRI studies have amplified the findings from CT studies in identifying a reduction in volume in the hippocampal-amygdala complex and the parahippocampal gyrus. Some have also found differences between the right and left hemispheres although others have not. The greater sophistication of positron emission tomography (PET) and magnetic resonance spectroscopy (MRS) is also now being used to further our knowledge of the neurobiological aetiology of schizophrenia but as yet without any definitive conclusion.

Symptoms

The acute phase

In the absence of biological markers, the most common approach in clinical practice is to base the diagnosis of schizophrenia on the presenting symptoms. These include auditory hallucinations, commonly in the third person, delusions of persecution or reference, delusions of control (also called passivity), delusional mood, occasionally olfactory, gustatory, tactile or somatic hallucinations, perplexity of mood and disorders of the form of thought. Depression may occur concomitantly and if persistent requires treatment in its own right. Many of these symptoms may occur in other conditions, so making the diagnosis difficult.

In an attempt to overcome this difficulty, Schneider proposed a set of symptoms, known as symptoms of the first rank (Table 16.1), which he believed to be pathognomonic of schizophrenia, in the absence of any organic cause (Mellor, 1970). This has considerably improved the reliability with which the diagnosis is made although the occurrence of some of these symptoms in mania makes them less than perfect. Nevertheless, they have gained widespread acceptance in clinical practice.

The residual (chronic) phase

The striking feature is the personality change which afflicts those with the chronic syndrome. Volition is reduced, interest in social encounters is diminished and personal hygiene is often poor. It is these symptoms which relatives find most difficult to understand and often attribute them to laziness. Behaviour may be stilted

Table 16.1. First rank symptoms of schizophrenia.

- Thought insertion
- Thought withdrawal
- Thought broadcasting
- Primary delusions
- Passivity of thoughts, actions or impulses
- Echoe de la pensée
- Third person auditory hallucinations discussing the patient or commenting on his actions
- Somatic hallucinations

---

with mannerisms and/or stereotypes. Hallucinations and delusions may occur, as in the acute syndrome, but the latter are often fixed and systematised. Affect is blunted making rapport difficult and formal thought disorder is often gross. An unexpected but common finding is age disorientation, and some patients display intellectual deficits when tested psychometrically.

Syndromes of schizophrenia

The older classification of schizophrenia into the *simple, paranoid, hebephrenic* and *catatonic* subtypes has largely fallen into disuse due in part to the overlap between them when presenting clinically. Also the picture may vary between episodes and they do not breed true. Apart from the paranoid type, with its better prognosis and the lower risk to relatives, these classifications are of doubtful validity. In particular, caution should be exercised when making a diagnosis of simple schizophrenia since it is based on the absence of features rather than on positive symptoms and some sources recommend its abandonment.

It is apparent that not all those who have an episode of schizophrenia progress to the chronic residual state. This led to the use of the term *schizophreniform* to describe those patients whose illness had a precipitant, an acute onset, prominent depressive features and clouding of consciousness. Prognosis is also believed to be better.

Schizoaffective psychosis is a controversial label being interposed between schizophrenia and manic depressive illness and describing a condition in which typical schizophrenic and depressive or manic episodes succeed each other, or occur concurrently. The prognosis is good and its proponents suggest lithium as the preferred maintenance treatment. Many believe that as depression or excitement are commonly part of schizophrenia their presence does not warrant a specific label and that this additional term confuses rather than clarifies.

Management

Acutely disturbed behaviour

The general practitioner plays a crucial role in managing acutely disturbed and sometimes violent behaviour, either when a patient has relapsed or during a new and untreated episode of illness. The use of intramuscular, intravenous or oral haloperidol and lorazepam in combination is the most effective method of achieving rapid tranquillisation.

Zuclopenthixol acetate (Clopixol Acuphase) may be used after repeated attempts at tranquillisation have failed although it is not useful when an immediate response is required since its onset takes up to 2 hours. It should not be given until a period of 15 minutes has elapsed since the last IV injection and 60 minutes since the last IM medication. It is given in an IM dose of 50–150 mg spaced at least 24 hours apart up to a maximum of 400 mg over 2 weeks. Zuclopenthixol use is almost always in a hospital setting since the maximum dose is set at a low threshold.

First episode schizophrenia

While in hospital the mainstay of treatment is with major tranquillisers which are instituted immediately the diagnosis is made. There is little to choose between the phenothiazines or butyrophenones in terms of efficacy but the spectrum of side effects may influence this decision. In particular, the butyrophenones such as haloperidol are more likely to cause extrapyramidal symptoms but are less sedative than the phenothiazines. Doses of up to 2000 mg of chlorpromazine orally, or its equivalent, may be required initially and anticholinergic agents should not be given unless side effects develop as these lower blood levels. During this period, the patient is best managed in a tranquil environment since over-stimulation may provoke a recrudescence of disturbance.

The older first generation antipsychotic agents have been replaced by the newer second generation (atypical) medications as the first line treatment for schizophrenia. These have fewer extrapyramidal side effects lessening the necessity for antiparkinsonian medications. The agents available at present include risperidone, olanzapine, quetiapine, amisulpiride, aripiprazole and ziprasidone and while all of these reduce positive symptoms the evidence for their effect on negative symptoms is uncertain with the most robust data supporting amisulpiride.

Although neurological side effects are less common with the newer medication, other problems are to the fore. There is concern about weight gain with agents such as olanzapine while QT prolongation is of concern in some at risk patients taking ziprasidone. The risks and benefits have to be carefully considered in each patient individually. A further issue of relevance is whether the second generation antipsychotics are all equally efficacious. A recent meta-analysis concluded that there were differences and that olanzapine, risperidone and amisulpiride should be considered as first-line treatments in view of the greater efficacy and side effect profile when compared with other antipsychotic agents (Davis *et al.*, 2003). If there is a likelihood of non-compliance, depot preparations may be necessary (see below).

Following discharge, medication is continued for two years following a first episode. Where there have been prior episodes, treatment is generally for life. Antidepressant and at times ECT may be required if depressive symptomatology

Table 16.2. Commonly used depot neuroleptics.

Drug	Duration of therapeutic activity[a]	Dose range[a]
Flupenthixol decanoate	2–4 weeks	20–400 mg
Fluphenazine decanoate	2–4 weeks	12.5–100 mg
Clopenthixol decanoate	2–4 weeks	200–600 mg
Pipothiazine decanoate	4 weeks	25–200 mg
Haloperidol decanoate	4 weeks	2–20 mg
Risperidone	2 weeks	25–50mg

[a]There may be individual variation and, if in doubt, consult the relevant manufacturer.

supervenes and persists. This is now believed to be an inherent part of the illness and not due to medication or to insight into the illness as was formerly suggested.

Resistant and residual (chronic) schizophrenia

Many patients require long-term medication and there is no therapeutic benefit in using depot in preference to oral preparations except to reduce non-compliance (Table 16.2). As a general rule, the risks of tardive dyskinesia are higher with depot than with oral preparations and this should be borne in mind when considering long-term treatment. The recent availability of risperidone in a depot format is a great advantage in this regard.

Clozapine is a newly available dibenzodiazepine with an affinity for a host of receptors. It is finding use in the treatment of negative symptoms and in the treatment of those with resistant positive symptoms, estimated to occur in 5–25% of those receiving standard antipsychotic medication. Although it has the serious side effect of agranulocytosis, reported in up to 13/100,000 patients, it now has a significant part to play in the treatment of this difficult group and it is estimated that 30–50% of patients unresponsive to other treatments show a positive outcome with this drug. A period of up to 6 months is required to achieve improvement. It must be administered in hospital initially and until a dose of 300 mg per day has been reached. Thereafter monitoring can take place as an out-patient, consisting of weekly white cell counts for the first 18 weeks, then every 2 weeks for the remainder of the first year and then every 4 weeks thereafter, as the risk of agranulocytosis is greatest in the first 18 weeks of treatment and after one year has the same risk as with standard antipsychotics. Other side effects include nocturnal enuresis, sialorrhea, seizures, hypertension and vomiting.

Management of neurological side effects

Anticholinergic agents should only be given when parkinsonism develops and the commonly used preparations are biperiden or procyclidine. For acute dystonic reactions these will be required intramuscularly. Thereafter, they should be continued regularly. Akathisia or 'restless legs' can be difficult to distinguish from agitation but in the former the patient is unable to control the movement. The treatment of choice is with diazepam, unless the offending drug can be reduced. Tardive dyskinesia is more serious than the other side effects because it may be irreversible. It is preventable by using the minimum required dose of drug and by avoiding antiparkinsonian agents. The effectiveness of 'drug holidays' in prevention is in dispute. When the condition is diagnosed, a reduction in medication may temporarily lead to a worsening of symptoms. Thereafter a number of drugs may be tried although none is universally successful. These include pimozide and tetrabenazine. Unfortunately many patients remain chronically symptomatic.

Social therapy

An important aspect of long-term treatment is the environment in which the patient lives. Understimulation will worsen the negative symptoms while overstimulation may precipitate relapse. Thus, a moderately stimulating milieu which includes occupational therapy is superior, on the one hand, to an unstructured timetable devoid of activities and, on the other, to more intense treatments such as psychodynamic psychotherapy, which may provoke relapse.

Family work has an important role for some in reducing the risk of relapse. Several studies have found that families who are hostile, critical or over-involved, known as high EE (expressed emotion) families, contribute to relapse even when prior protection is given with medication but low EE families are not associated with such a risk. Psycho-education along with family therapy to improve the emotional tone of the family have been shown to reduce EE and subsequent relapse rates.

Differential diagnosis

Mania

Acute schizophrenia with its attendant excitement and delusions may be difficult to distinguish from mania. The presence of first rank symptoms is helpful, although manic patients sometimes have these symptoms also. The content of the delusions is not helpful in making the diagnosis. It may only be possible to make a definitive diagnosis in retrospect, having considered the course of the illness.

Drug-induced psychoses

Drug-induced psychoses present with schizophrenic-like symptoms and a drug screen should be carried out in every young schizophrenic having their first episode. Nevertheless, even those episodes that are drug-induced may exhibit the same course as schizophrenia with relapses and remissions, or with negative features. The risk is particularly high in those abusing cannabis (Arseneault, 2004), amphetamines and ecstasy.

Acute and transient psychotic disorder

Brief psychotic disorders can occur in response to major emotional stressors and are of sudden onset. Consciousness may be clouded and although psychotic symptoms are present the full range of schizophrenic symptoms is lacking. Clinically these are very difficult to distinguish from those with a schizophrenic illness of acute onset. Treatment is with antipsychotic agents and hospitalisation is usually required. There is a risk of depressive symptoms in the immediate post-psychotic phase. Treatment is required until symptomatic recovery is complete and close monitoring in the follow-up period is required for indications of relapse or for the emergence of a typical schizophrenic illness, an occurrence in an unknown percentage of such patients.

Depressive illness

The apathetic and withdrawn state of the chronically ill patient may resemble that of severe depressive illness. A detailed history of the previous episodes and, especially, of the level of functioning between these should clarify the diagnosis. It is recognized that depressive illness may occur following a schizophrenic episode and it should be treated with antidepressants.

Outcome

A number of factors influence outcome. Onset during teenage years, insidious presentation, negative symptoms and poor premorbid personality augur badly for the future as do low IQ and a family history of schizophrenia. The features which are associated with favourable outcome are acute onset, precipitating stress, affective symptoms and late onset. Women have a slightly better prognosis than men. The adverse effect of belonging to a high EE family has been outlined above.

The prognosis of schizophrenia has improved over the last 30 years, although it is still recognised as the most serious psychiatric disorder and a high proportion require long term medication. Follow-up studies of patients discharged from hospital after acute episodes suggest that 25–33% make a complete symptomatic and social recovery while up to 25% remain psychotic, if followed up for 2 years. The remainder has an intermediate prognosis. The concomitant abuse of illicit drugs has an adverse effect on outcome since they have a destabilising effect and result in frequent relapses and re-admissions.

Rehabilitation

Those patients with negative symptoms who are being rehabilitated need help with the basic skills of everyday life including self-care, household management and social skills. This necessitates adequate occupational and re-socialisation therapy, usually provided by occupational therapists. Basic social skills training can be provided by nurses, social workers or psychologists. To encourage the patient in better hygiene, or in more appropriate social behaviours, a token economy system of rewards for acceptable behaviour can be devised by a psychologist. Retraining for work may be feasible for those whose illness is under control and who have satisfactory social and personal skills.

Long-term care is needed only for the most incapacitated, and hostels, group homes and individual flats are better suited to the less disabled (see Chapter 19). Most patients with schizophrenia live independently or with their family.

A key worker in the area of rehabilitation is the community psychiatric nurse who is often the person most frequently in contact with the patient following in-patient discharge. He/she is the link between the hospital and the community-based services and in addition to giving continuous support, also deals with issues such as default from treatment, depot clinic appointments and may be the person to administer depot injections to those who cannot or will not attend the hospital for these. A part of the multidisciplinary team, the community nurse has a crucial role in supporting the family and in assisting with rehabilitation options.

PERSISTENT DELUSIONAL DISORDER (PARANOID AND OTHER PSYCHOSES)

A group of disorders that previously had such names as paranoid psychosis, monosymptomatic delusional psychosis, delusional jealousy, etc., have been grouped together in the modern classifications under the rubric 'persistent delusional disorder' since they share the common features of delusions, in the absence of hallucinations or other psychotic symptoms, and, unlike schizophrenia, are characterised by good preservation of personality.

Paranoid psychosis

The relationship between paranoid psychosis and both schizophrenia and paranoid personality is a matter of debate. Paranoid psychosis and its variants differ from schizophrenia in arising without the hallucinations or thought disorder that characterise the condition. It usually has an insidious onset, the delusions are often systematized and even with treatment they often persist. Because personality is intact the patient is frequently able to continue to work and perform socially with the symptoms impinging only upon those who are close to the patient.

Delusional jealousy

A variant of paranoid psychosis is delusional jealousy (Othello syndrome). This may sometimes be associated with alcohol abuse. The patient constantly asks for 'proof' of his partner's fidelity, who may initially accede to these and other requests. This should be discouraged since it will offer only temporary respite from the doubts and queries and may reinforce the delusions. If the delusions fail to respond to treatment the couple may be advised to separate especially if threats of violence are being made by the patient.

Other delusional states

Delusions of love or erotomania (De Clerambault's syndrome) are also difficult to treat and the person to whom they are directed may be frequently harassed by the patient. Other monosymptomatic delusional states are associated with delusions that *bodily appearance is abnormal* (dysmorphic delusions), e.g. the ears are misshapen or that the body emits smells or harbours some serious illness or infection. This latter state must be distinguished from severe depressive illness, which may be associated with similar delusions. At times of stress those with paranoid personality disorder may *decompensate* into a psychosis and immigrants are also vulnerable to short-lived psychotic episodes.

The treatment of all the above disorders is with antipsychotic medication although forming a therapeutic relationship is often difficult since the recommendation that medication should be taken is often perceived as an indication that the doctor is colluding with those who disbelieve the patient or are his persecutors. Some authorities recommend pimozide in those with persistent delusional disorder, especially of the somatic and dysmorphic types. When agitation is severe, as may occur during periods of decompensation, then intramuscular sedation may be required.

ORGANIC PSYCHOSES

These may be divided into two groups: the acute and the chronic states. The latter are referred to as the dementias.

Acute organic syndrome

This is commonly associated with physical illness and is found in up to 15% of patients in medical and surgical wards but may be higher in intensive care units. The most common symptoms are confusion and disorientation, which vary in intensity throughout the day, being usually worse at night. Perplexity may lead to agitation, noisiness and restlessness. Concentration is impaired and psychotic

Table 16.3. Common causes of acute organic syndrome.

- Infections; systemic or intracranial
- Cerebral tumours
- Major organ failure
- Hypoglycaemia, hypothyroidism
- Surgery, especially open heart and cataract operations
- Withdrawal from alcohol or certain drugs
- Poisoning, e.g. anticholinergic, anticonvulsants, lithium, industrial poisons, etc.
- Dehydration or water intoxication
- Electrolyte imbalance
- Nutritional deficiency
- Epilepsy

symptoms such as hallucinations, especially visual, and delusions may occur. Plucking movements with the hands may also be noticed. The common causes of acute confusional states are listed in Table 16.3.

A detailed physical examination, including neurological assessment is mandatory. Initial haematological and biochemical tests should include ESR, liver, thyroid and renal function, as well as fasting blood sugar. A focus of infection, including syphilis, should be ruled out. Skull X-ray, EEG and CAT scan may occasionally be necessary as well as lumbar puncture. The treatment is of the underlying cause. The patient must be nursed in a single, quiet room, which is well-lit by day and which can also be lit by night. Major tranquillisers that do not have anticholinergic properties such as haloperidol are the first choice when agitation control is required and they may be used intramuscularly or orally. Short acting benzodiazepine may be required additionally to reduce insomnia. If delirium tremens is diagnosed then long-acting benzodiazepines are the medication of choice along with high doses of thiamine in order to reduce the risk of fits and of Korsakoff's psychosis.

Chronic organic disorders

A number of causes have been identified and these are listed in Table 16.4.

Alzheimer's disease

The most common of the chronic organic disorders is senile dementia, or more accurately Alzheimer's disease, as it is called in those under 65. The pathology is similar in both. In both pre-senile as well as senile type Alzheimer's disease women are over-represented. The course is progressive and death occurs usually within 7 years from the onset of symptoms.

Aetiology. There is a definite genetic component to this condition although the magnitude is unknown. Neither is the mode of inheritance understood.

Table 16.4. Common causes of chronic organic disorders.

Primary degenerative
- Alzheimer's disease/senile dementia
- Atherosclerotic dementia
- Multiple sclerosis
- Normal pressure hydrocephalus
- Parkinson's disease
- Pick's disease
- Jacob–Creutzfeldt disease
- Huntington's chorea
- Lewy body dementia

Symptomatic
- Cerebral tumours, subdural haematoma
- Cerebral infections, e.g. encephalitis
- Collagen diseases. e.g. SLE
- Anoxia
- Poisoning from alcohol, lead or other metals
- Vitamin deficiency especially B_{12}, thiamine
- Endocrine disorders. e.g. hypothyroidism, hypoglycaemia
- Head injury

Nevertheless, there is an increased risk in the relatives of probands and this is highest when the onset is before the age of 65. There have been suggestions that an excess of aluminium may be the cause of Alzheimer's disease but the evidence is conflicting.

Pathology and neurochemistry. The pathological changes in the brains of Alzheimer's patients are no different from those of normal ageing although their frequency is much greater. Macroscopically there is shrinkage of the brain with enlarged ventricles and widened sulci. There is cell loss on histological examination and neurofibrillary tangles and senile plaques abound. There is a possibility that the degree of cognitive impairment is related to the density of plaque formation. Acetylcholinesterase and choline acetyl transferase are reduced, suggesting that the selective loss of acetylcholine may be responsible for some of the cognitive symptoms.

Symptoms. The early symptoms consist of forgetfulness which progresses insidiously. This may lead to frustration and catastrophic responses when under pressure. Mood may be depressed and in the early stages of the disease, delusions, usually paranoid in content, and hallucinations may be found. As the disease progresses personality changes, agitation may increase and focal parietal lobe signs such as dysphasia may occur. Acute confusional states may at times be superimposed. Weight loss is noticeable and in the terminal stages of the illness the patient is bed-bound.

Treatment. There is as yet no treatment for Alzheimer's dementia. Major tranquillisers may be necessary to reduce agitation and thioridazine or promazine, beginning in doses of 25 mg orally as required, are preferred to other phenothiazines since they have fewer anticholinergic and or extrapyramidal side effects. The atypical antipsychotics such as olanzapine can also be used. Antidepressants may also be needed to relieve any associated depressive symptomatology.

There are some treatments that improve memory although there is no known cure as yet. Donepezil, rivastigmine and galantamine, all acetylcholinesterase inhibitors, act on acetylcholinesterase to prevent it metabolising acetylcholine, the neurotransmitter thought to be deficient in Alzheimer's disease. However, they are only of benefit in mild to moderate disease. The action of memantine differs from these as its effects are on glutamate release and it is of benefit in the middle to late stages of Alzheimer's disease. There is a suggestion that it may slow the disease process itself. None of these drugs are addicitve and the most common side effects with donepezil, rivastigmine and galantamine are gastrointestinal while hallucinations, tiredness and confusion can occur with memantine. It is unclear if these drugs help other forms of dementia although they are sometimes prescribed for Lewy body disease. Memantine may be helpful in vascular dementia although not yet licensed for this.

Most patients should be cared for at home, if possible, and support provided by the day hospital and by relief admissions to allow for holidays, etc. The relatives of sufferers need help initially in coming to terms with the disease and in grieving about this. The daughter who has cared for her mother all her life, and who is no longer recognised by her, will have as profound a grief reaction as if her mother had actually died. Many relatives do not grieve at the time of death since they have already done so during the course of the disease.

Lewy body disease

This is a form of dementia that has features of both Alzheimer's disease and Parkinson's disease although it is often misdiagnosed as the former with the true diagnosis only becoming apparent at post-mortem. It may form up to 15% of all cases of dementia. Lewy bodies are protein deposits that are found in the cerebral nerve cells although the reason for their development there is unknown. It is characterised by memory impairment that fluctuates on a daily basis, symptoms of Parkinson's disease, faints and falls and daytime drowsiness. In addition there may be complex visual hallucinations, often of animals.

Although the diagnosis is difficult to make it is important to attempt to distinguish it from other forms of dementia since those with Lewy body disease are particularly sensitive to neuroleptics. As well as worsening the Parkinsonian symptoms they can cause sudden death. When neuroleptics are prescribed to control agitation or hallucinations they should be used with great caution and very closely monitored. Antiparkinsonian drugs help in reducing these symptoms but may worsen memory and hallucinations. The medications used to treat Alzheminer's disease may help in Lewy body disease although they are as yet not licensed for this.

Multi-infarct dementia

This condition is associated with multiple infarcts in various sites. It is slightly more common in men than women and generally affects the elderly. There is atrophy which in the early stages is localised, but later becomes generalised. Areas of infarction are present and can be seen on scan.

Initially the symptoms may follow a cerebrovascular accident, but this is not invariable. Mood is labile and the memory impairment fluctuates. The progression is step-wise and there is often a seemingly total recovery from the initial episodes. Death is from vascular disease elsewhere, or from cerebral infarction.

There is no permanent treatment although vasodilators are used by some and the evidence for benefit is conflicting. Treatment of associated hypertension may slow the progress of the disorder.

Rare dementias

Other rarer cause of dementia include *Pick's disease, Huntington's chorea* and *Jacob–Creutzfeldt disease.* These belong to the presenile group of dementias while *normal pressure hydrocephalus* is most common in the elderly. The latter may be treatable and is therefore important to diagnose.

Pick's disease is characterised in the early stages by changes in social behaviour, rather than memory impairment, although in most patients there is nothing to distinguish it from Alzheimer's disease and the diagnosis is usually made at post-mortem. Jacob–Creutzfeldt disease is associated with neurological signs, including cerebellar ataxia and extrapyramidal symptoms. This is a rapidly progressive condition and is believed to be caused by infection with a slow virus. Huntington's chorea is inherited by autosomal dominant transmission. Usually the neurological signs precede the dementia but occasionally the reverse can occur. Depression is a frequent accompaniment, even in the absence of knowledge about the disease. A schizophrenia-like picture has also been found in some patients. Suicide is a common cause of death not only in Huntington's chorea sufferers but also in relatives unaware of the diagnosis. The dementia is slowly progressive and death may not occur for up to 15 years following diagnosis. Normal pressure hydro-cephalus is associated with slowness and memory impairment and may resemble depressive illness. There is no treatment for any of these conditions except normal pressure hydrocephalus, where a shunt may improve the symptoms.

Assessment

This involves a number of haematological and neurological investigations to rule out treatable causes of dementia especially vitamin B_{12} deficiency, hypothyroidism and cerebral tumours. CAT scan is required to exclude tumours or dementia although in the early stages of the dementing process the scan may be normal. A normal scan should also raise the possibility of another cause of the condition, especially depressive illness. In the early stages of dementia a neurocognitive assessment is likely to be more sensitive in identifying the disease than a CAT scan. The most commonly used test is the Weschler Adult Intelligence Test (WAIS) where discrepancies between the verbal and performance IQ are indicative of possible brain damage. Other tests are also available to detect generalised or localised abnormalities. Clinical testing for agnosia and apraxia are helpful in localising parietal lobe lesions. An EEG may be useful since both senile and pre-senile dementias are associated with slowing of the α-rhythm and the appearance of diffuse delta activity. In pre-senile dementia the activity may disappear totally. Vascular dementias show a similar pattern but may also exhibit focal abnormalities. Huntington's chorea and Jacob–Creutzfeldt disease also have characteristic patterns. However, a normal EEG may sometimes occur even with advanced dementia and this is indicative of the limitations of this investigation.

The Mini Mental State (Folstein *et al.*, 1975) is a practical and clinically useful test in screening for dementia. Out of a possible score of 30, a score of less than 25 suggests impairment and of less than 20 indicates definite impairment.

Differential diagnosis

The distinction from depressive illness may seem easy in theory. In practice it may be difficult, especially in the elderly, where confusion may be attributed to dementia. Those with depressive illness often exhibit confusion and disorientation as part of their illness, i.e. pseudodementia (Raskind, 1998). A careful history is essential, paying special attention to the recency of the confusion and its relation to other symptoms of depression. In addition, the failure to find any haematological, biochemical, CAT scan or EEG abnormalities should suggest a depressive illness. Cognitive assessment is generally unhelpful in making the distinction. The difficulties in distinguishing one from the other have been confirmed in many studies and up to a third of patients in whom a diagnosis of senile dementia is made with confidence are later reclassified, usually, as having depressive illness.

SUMMARY

1. Schizophrenia has a prevalence of between 2–4/1000 with a slight excess among men.
2. The cause is unknown, although there is a genetic component in some, and the concordance is higher among monozygotic than among dizygotic twins. The mode of inheritance is unknown.

3. Causes originating in the family or relating to social class have been disproven.
4. The distinction from mania may be difficult during an acute episode.
5. Following a first episode, treatment is continued for two years. If relapse occurs, then it will be required for life.
6. The family environment and the milieu in which the patient lives are important in preventing relapse.
7. The prognosis has improved over the past 30 years.
8. Those who develop negative symptoms show some abnormalities on CAT scan.
9. The dementias have many causes but few are treatable. The most common are the senile and atherosclerotic types.
10. Depressive illness may be easily mistaken for dementia and the distinction is vital, since the former can be treated.

CASE HISTORIES

Case I

Miss X was a 22 year-old girl in her third year at university. During her last year she had become anxious and even agitated at times and felt she could not cope. She felt inordinate pressure was being put on her by her tutors and that she was not liked by them. One day she threw a chair at one of them and was referred for counselling. She became increasingly distressed and finally decided to return home the month prior to her exams. When seen by her local general practitioner she was agitated, claiming that people were sending messages to each other about her by telepathy and that there was a plot going on to prevent her getting her degree. She believed she heard people laughing at her through the wall of her bedroom and felt one of these was the tutor. Her general practitioner made a diagnosis of schizophrenia having also obtained a urine sample immediately she returned from university which was negative for opiate metabolites or amphetamines. He treated her with trifluoperazine 5 mg b.d. and when her symptoms settled after a few days referred her to the psychiatric services for confirmation of the diagnosis and for on-going treatment. Because she had Parkinsonism even with antiparkinsonian drugs she was changed to thioridazine and at the time of writing was symptom-free, functioning normally and had returned to university.

Comment

This girl's increasing disturbance was heralding a schizophrenic illness. Had this been diagnosed earlier counselling would have been contraindicated because of the risk of provoking an acute reaction. Her family were reluctant to have her treated as an in-patient but assured the general practitioner that if she did not begin to respond within 2 days of commencing treatment they would then not object to admission. She responded rapidly, and although suffering from side effects, these went when her phenothiazine was changed. Because of the acute onset the prognosis is good. Depot injections are not necessary since this girl complies with treatment. She will be continued on medication for 2 years from the date at which she showed symptomatic improvement.

Case 2

Mrs X, a 72 year-old lady, was referred with a 2-year history of increasing memory impairment and episodic agitation. Her recall for recent events was the most affected and she had to make notes of day-to-day needs in the house. Her agitation was especially bad in the morning and when her husband tried to go out to play golf. She could not date the onset of her problems but her husband felt they had followed an operation for cataracts 2 years earlier. She also complained of hyperacusis such that even the clinking of cups distressed her. She felt very sad, got no enjoyment from life and slept badly. She woke at 5 a.m. and could not return to sleep. Both she and her husband felt that her memory problem and her dependence on him were the worst aspects of her illness. A tentative diagnosis of depressive illness was made in view of the biological symptoms, the loss of confidence as evidenced by her increasing dependence on her husband and the fact that the symptoms had followed a surgical procedure with a known relationship to depressive illness. A differential diagnosis of early dementia was made, she was commenced on a trial of antidepressants to which she had a dramatic response. CAT scan was normal.

Comment

This lady's presenting problem may be considered to be more suggestive of an organic than a depressive illness. However the degree of memory impairment bears little relationship to the diagnosis and even those with depressive illness may have marked difficulties. Her memory disturbance is best described as a pseudo-dementia.

Case 3

Mr X had been treated at home by his general practitioner since he became depressed following an unsuccessful operation for congenital talipes equinovarus. In fact, he was less well able to walk and had to use a zimmer frame, where before he used a stick. He had never been depressed before. Prior to admission, his general practitioner felt that he was worsening and two days prior to admission became acutely confused necessitating his admission. As he was receiving tricyclic antide- pressants these were discontinued but without effect. An MSU, chest X-ray, full blood count, electrolytes and ESR were normal. CAT scan was normal as were thyroid and liver function. A neurological opinion was sought but failed to find evidence of neurological disease. A lumbar puncture was also normal. During this period, lasting about one month, Mr X became bed-bound and doubly incontinent. He said little, did not recognise his family and gazed vacantly into space. In view of the history of depressive illness of increasing severity prior to his admission and the failure to find any organic cause for his deterioration a (reluctant) diagnosis of depressive stupor was made and he was commenced on ECT as well as restarting antidepressants. He responded dramatically to ECT and after three treatments was speaking, continent and recognising family although still disorientated for time and place. As treatment continued, his confusion improved, he became mobile to his post-operative level and his depression lifted. He was discharged home and at follow-up arrangements had been made for a further orthopaedic opinion. He has maintained his improvement.

Comment

This case is unusual and the general practitioner is unlikely to have to deal with many such patients. He does illustrate the difficulty of distinguishing depressive illness from organic disorders. The decision to administer ECT was made on the basis of negative physical and biochemical investigations and on the prior history of depressive illness. The author is not recommending this treatment for acute confusional states but only where this is indicative of profound depressive illness. Such patients require full physical, radiological and biochemical investigations to rule out any organic cause for the confusion or the depression.

REFERENCES

Arseneault, L., Connon, M., Witton, J. and Murray, R.M. (2004). causal association between cannabis and psychosis: examination of the evidence. *British Journal of Psychiatry*, **184**, 110–117.

Davis, J.M., Chen, N. and Glick, I. (2003). A meta-analysis of the efficacy of second genera- tion antipsychotics. *Archives of General Psychiatry*, **60**, 553–564.

Folstein, M.F., Folstein, S. and McHugh, P.R. (1975). Mini-mental state: A practical method for grading the cognitive state of patients for the clinician. *Journal of Psychiatric Research*, **12**, 1189–1198.

Mellor, C.S. (1970). First rank symptoms of schizophrenia. *British Journal of Psychiatry*, **117**, 15–23.

Raskind, M.A. (1998). The clinical interface of depression and dementia. *Journal of Clinical Psychiatry*, **59** (Suppl. 8), 9–12.

FURTHER READING

Guirguis, W.R. (1981). Schizophrenia: the problem of definition. *British Journal of Hospital Medicine*, 236–247.

McKeith, I., Mintzer, J., Aarsland, D. *et al.* (2004). Dementia with Lewy Body. *Lancet*, **3**, 19–28.

Nott, P.N. and Fleminger, J.J. (1975). Presenile dementia: the difficulties of early diagnosis. *Acta Psychiatrica Scandinavica*, **51**, 210–217.

Ruhrmann, S., Schultze-Lutter, F. and Klosterkotter, J. (2003). Early detection and intervention in the initial prodromal phase of schizophrenia. *Pharmacopsychiatry*, **36** (Suppl. 3), 162–167.

SUGGESTED READING FOR PATIENTS

Fuller Torre, E. (1995). *Surviving Schizophrenia – A Family Manual, 3rd edn.* Harper Collins, London.

Howe, G. and Kingsley, J. (1997). *Getting into the System – Living with Serious Mental Illness 1.* Rethink, London.

Howe, G. and Kingsley, J. (1998). *Mental Health Assessments – Living with Serious Mental Illness 2 .* Rethink, London.

Martyn, C. and Gale, C.   (1995).*Understanding Forgetfulness & Dementia.* Family Doctor Series, British Medical Association, London.

Reveley, A. (1998). *Does Severe Mental Illness Run In Families?* National Schizophrenia Fellowship (free of charge).

Svantesson, I. (1990). *Mind Mapping & Memory: Powerful Techniques to Help You Make Better Use of Your Brain.* Kogan Page, London.

USEFUL WEBSITES FOR PATIENTS

Alzheimer's Society: www.alzheimers.org.uk
Royal College of Psychiatrists' information on dementia: www.rcpsych.ac.uk/info/help/memory/
Royal College of Psychiatrists' information on schizophrenia: www.rcpsych.ac.uk/info/help/schiz/

USEFUL CONTACTS

The Schizophrenia Association of Ireland
4 Fitzwilliam Place
Dublin 2
Ireland

Rethink (formerly The National Schizophrenia Fellowship),
30 Tabernacle St
London
EC2A 4DD
Tel: 020 7330 9100.
Email: info@rethink.org

The Alzheimer's Society of Ireland
43 Northumberland Avenue
Dunlaoighre
Co. Dublin
Ireland
Tel: 00 353 1 2846616.

Alzheimer's Society
Gordon House
10 Greencoat Place
London SW1P 1PH
Tel: 020 7306 0606
Email: info@alzheimers.org.uk
Website: www.alzheimers.org.uk

17

Counselling

Those who are familiar with the literature on counselling will realise that the term is used loosely to describe those therapies which do not utilise drugs. For some writers it encompasses behavioural psychotherapy as well as some of the common psychotherapies. This includes such theoretical approaches as transactional analysis, Gestalt therapy, client-centred therapy and a host of others. The present chapter focuses principally on the client-centred, *non-directive* approach of Carl Rogers, since this is one of the more accessible techniques and is also the most commonly used. Behaviour and cognitive therapy are not included in this chapter but are referred to elsewhere (see Chapters 8 and 12).

Every family doctor spends a large portion of his working life listening to and in dialogue with patients. This may be nothing more than the doctor advising his patient about the proper taking of medicines. Frequently, however, the interaction is of a more personal nature concerning relationships and emotional problems. It is in this context that the term counselling is used. It is often assumed that every interview which addresses emotional issues is itself a counselling session – this is naïve and does an injustice to the special skills and training necessary for good counselling. It is also a gross oversimplification of the aims and aspirations of Carl Rogers, the man who fathered 'client-centred therapy', in the 1940s and 50s.

PSYCHOTHERAPY v. COUNSELLING

Many will question the differences between psychotherapy and counselling, and at times there may be very few. Indeed counselling and supportive psychotherapy are terms which are often used interchangeably. There are marked differences between in-depth psychotherapy and counselling. In the former, problem solving is eschewed and the aim of the therapist is to help the patient achieve insight by interpreting his behaviour in terms of past experiences and by understanding the transference. To be receptive to such an approach, which may be lengthy, strict patient selection is essential. By contrast a counselling approach is applicable to a wider range of patient problems and selection criteria are less stringent. A further difference is that the time span over which therapy is carried out is invariably much shorter. Interpretation of transference does not occur in counselling and the sessions home in on current emotional issues rather than on childhood or past experiences.

The distinction from supportive psychotherapy is less obvious but pertinent nevertheless. This form of treatment has limited aims, these being generally to provide a listening ear and to help at times of crisis. There is no specific focus for therapy, whereas in counselling a particular area of difficulty is being remedied and in the process the individual grows. The latter is conducted regularly while supportive psychotherapy is offered as and when the need arises. Thus a counsellor will see a client every two or three weeks for a session while the person receiving supportive psychotherapy will be seen at times of renewal of prescriptions or times of special need. In supportive therapy little attention will be paid to such issues as unexpressed feeling, the recognition of the patient's own feelings or insight, while such principles are germane to counselling.

REQUIREMENTS IN THE PATIENT

1. The person must have a capacity to express himself emotionally and have a basic acceptance of the role of psychological and emotional issues in his life – commonly referred to as psychological mindedness.
2. The absence of any gross instabilities such as schizophrenia or major personality difficulties is essential since relapse or decompensation may occur in these patients during therapy.
3. A desire for help at the outset is an advantage but not essential since this may crystallise during the sessions. For example a client may not wish to have marital therapy but after a few meetings with the therapist become more positive. Resistance may derive from ignorance or fear and reassurance is the keynote to overcoming these difficulties. However if the client continues to resist there is little point in continuing although the family or friends of the client may put considerable pressure on the therapist. It is thus important to obtain permission from the client to commence counselling, since an insistence on pursuing this therapy against the client's wishes will compromise the therapeutic relationship.
4. The patient must be relatively independent emotionally and of average intelligence. Those who have a tendency to dependence may transfer this to the counsellor and frustrate attempts at establishing mature behaviour.
5. The patient must be mature enough to cope independently with life and yet be flexible enough to have some capacity for change. It is thus difficult to be chronologically rigid about this since there is great individual variation, but the emotional age of the patient is the principal concern.

REQUIREMENTS IN THE THERAPIST

1. The counsellor must be empathetic towards the patient. If he finds it difficult to sympathise with the problem or indeed for some reason dislikes the patient (and this does happen) then a therapeutic relationship will be impossible. It is important to recognise that resentment of, or lack of regard and respect for the patient are not the basis for a psychotherapeutic liaison. The counsellor must possess 'unconditional positive regard' for his patient and attempt to instil this sense of self-worth in him. The doctor who feels he dislikes the patient should not blame himself, unless of course it is a regular occurrence where it may reflect a particular problem in the doctor himself, but should have the wisdom to refer the patient to a colleague who will be in a position to help.
2. The therapist who is cold or aloof will be unable to form the necessary bond with his patients or will certainly not win the care or respect of his clientele.
3. By contrast the counsellor must not become over-involved with his clients either, and the capacity to detach himself from his work when at home is mandatory. A therapist who becomes over-involved may be unable to step back and form an objective view of his patient and his needs, and will also have grave problems in coping with an unsuccessful outcome. It is for this reason that doctors, irrespective of their counselling skills, are advised to avoid working with their own friends or family. This is known as therapeutic distance and it is ignored at peril.
4. An essential feature in the therapist is psychological mindedness. The doctor who views emotional problems in simple physical terms or whose approach is a 'black and white' one should be mature enough to admit his unsuitability for this type of work. The person who prefers giving advice to listening and understanding is also unsuitable. Many neophyte counsellors do not realise that counselling is not about giving advice or giving the client 'a good talking to', but about helping the client make his or her own choices.
5. It is now accepted that the competent therapist must be free from serious psychological disturbance. The presence of unresolved emotional conflict may lead to over-identification with some clients and inability to handle others. While there is no requirement for psychological perfection (if it exists!) an ability to deal effectively with problems in one's own life is necessary.

CAVEATS IN COUNSELLING

1. Do not apportion blame. Many patients will express a feeling of guilt at their own behaviour. The counsellor's role is to help adjust to this and not further accentuate the self-blame. Statements like 'You should feel guilty about this' are unhelpful and unprofessional.

2. In general avoid asking 'why' questions. The patient is attending for help in understanding his feelings, and queries about the likely cause serve only to undermine the client's confidence in the therapist. Also the explanations offered to the therapist may be incorrect.
3. Avoid personal disclosures like 'That happened to me and I also felt as you do'. Occasionally, personal revelations may be helpful but they are generally best avoided. The sessions are not about the therapist's feelings but about the patient's emotional state.
4. Never undermine the clients feelings by saying 'No, you're not feeling angry at all'. The feelings of the client are real to him and although they may be inappropriate to the circumstances or difficult to understand, they are a source of pain and deserve to be acknowledged.
5. There is a common belief that counselling is a catch-all therapy which can be of benefit in almost any situation. This is incorrect and while supportive psychotherapy is indeed of universal benefit, there are risks attached to the inappropriate use of non-directive counselling. These relate to both the therapist and the client. These include the risk of precipitating psychosis in those who are so predisposed. The possibility that counselling may be recommended where another approach, e.g. behaviour therapy or drug treatments, may be more appropriate is also a serious consideration. In the author's experience the inappropriate prescription of counselling is the most common difficulty. Other problems with counselling are the inappropriate use of interpretations or summaries which may lead the patient to a false view of his problems. The general practitioner must also have suitable training in this technique if he is to deal with such issues as the patient's feelings for him, overtalkativeness, manipulation, etc. Training consists of seeing patients under supervision, reading background theoretical material and learning the appropriate interviewing skills.

BEGINNING THERAPY

Counselling is not a non-specific treatment, but a method of dealing with *problems*. Inevitably therefore, it is mandatory to *clarify* them from the outset. In many patients the source of difficulty may be vague and uncertain or the problems may continually shift. This pattern is a contraindication to counselling since at best the therapist will flounder and in so doing alienate the patient. The failure to identify the specific areas of difficulty will not only waste the therapist's time but also that of the patient.

A further prerequisite is *setting the goals and aims of treatment.* If this is neglected, therapy may become interminable with all the problems of dependence that this entails. These goals must be identified with the patient and if they are unrealistic the therapist should hesitate before beginning and a more realistic aim outlined. Allied to this is the *time limit* that is set. There is a tendency to give open-ended counselling but this may delay change in the patient's behaviour and the experienced counsellor is well aware of the benefits of setting a limit on the number of sessions over which treatment will be available. There are of course exceptions to this, such as the bereaved, but as a starting principle it is useful. In particular in marriage counselling this form of contract may stimulate the couple to work on their difficulties where otherwise they may stall.

ACTIVE THERAPY

The components of counselling may be divided into two parts – listening and intervening.

Listening

This is the largest part of counselling and often the most difficult to sustain since speech is central to our interactions with others. Some believe that listening is a passive state, but this is incorrect and it is best described as 'active inactivity'. The therapist is attentive to his client and is not distracted by peripheral stimuli. Attention is paid to the actual content of what the client says but also to the hidden agenda. Aspects of *language* to which attention must be paid include speed, volume and hesitations. This may throw light upon embarrassments, sources of tension and conflicts. The words, phrases and metaphors used must also be noted for their idiosyncratic use or non-use may reveal areas of difficulty. For example the terminally ill patient who never uses the word cancer but refers to the illness as 'it' may be having problems accepting the diagnosis, or may be avoiding the word because of fears about the family's reaction to the illness. *Non-verbal cues* are as important as the spoken word and the body language of the client often discloses much about their personality and problems. The person who sits with drooping shoulders and head cast downward creates a sense of being passive while the person who fidgets when certain topics are raised may have difficulties in that area. Observing this may be the only clue to the cause of the distress especially if problems are strongly denied by the client.

It is clear that listening is an active and sometimes draining part of the counselling process. The doctor who is talkative by nature will thus be unsuited to counselling unless he has the insight and commitment to change.

Intervening

This refers to the more obvious aspect of the client/counsellor interchange and can be divided into the verbal interchanges that facilitate and stimulate the client to talk and those that are therapeutic in themselves.

Facilitating

The patient's flow of speech may be hesitant in the early stages of counselling. *Open questions* like 'Tell me about your problem' are more likely to provoke spontaneous disclosures than are closed, interrogative questions. The habit of asking many questions and of being verbally active during sessions, known as floorholding, serves only to stifle spontaneity and results in the common complaint of 'I couldn't talk to him'. It is essential even at the first interview to establish the style and flow of the interaction since changing at a later phase in therapy may be strange and difficult for the client. The other extreme from the interrogative interview is the totally free-floating interchange.This is best avoided also since the diffuseness it generates may suggest to the client that the therapist is aloof or disinterested and that nothing is being achieved.

Echoing either parts or the whole of the client's last sentence also encourages continuity. If used too often, it can be irritating to the client and caricature the counsellor. More general statements like, 'Tell me more about that' or 'How did that feel?' are useful also as a stimulus to further dialogue.

Offering empathetic comments, e.g. 'That must have been terrible for you' is essential if trust and confidence in the therapist are to be built up. They suggest that the therapist has understood the problem and has entered the client's world.

Summarising is a useful technique when a lot of material has been divulged quickly or indeed when the therapist is uncertain if he has understood fully what has been said. Not only will it demonstrate the therapist's intention to grasp the problem, but it may give meaning to confused emotions. For example the client may say, 'Everything is dreadful at home, I'm in debt, my mother lives with us and she's a handful and work is awful', and this could be clarified and packaged by saying, 'So you're saying you've got problems at home and at work'. This focuses the problems and the session can then proceed to discuss the individual difficulties in each of these areas.

Closed questions are necessary to clarify difficulties or to elicit specific symptoms that may not have been mentioned. Their use should be restricted to the closing stages of the interview. *Confrontational questions* such as, 'Do you still love your husband?' are useful at times but should not be used early in therapy as they may appear insensitive and alienate the client.

The charge that doctors often lose sight of the *therapeutic* nature of their work is as pertinent to counselling as to any other method of treatment. While the process is important in itself, its purpose is to bring about change in the patient's state. A large component of counselling is concerned with exploring and allowing the *expression of feelings* and thereby effecting change. The most common of these are anger, guilt and grief. Most commonly they have been suppressed and the therapist's role is to encourage their expression since failure to do so may lead to clinical depression, physical symptoms of anxiety or on-going anger and guilt. The effect of these on the personal, emotional and spiritual life of the sufferer is immeasurable. The therapist at times has to give permission to the client to be angry, sad or guilty. This *permission giving* component is important for those who are ashamed to express their true feelings. Equally important is the terminating of the anger or guilt or sadness. The widow may feel guilty because she is beginning to enjoy life again without her husband. One of the dangers of counselling, or indeed any form of psychological treatment, is that emotions are churned up and vented but there is often no facility for healing these. Thus, discussing death with a seriously ill patient may be unhelpful if the therapist is not available to facilitate resolution of the emotion that has been generated. There are times when the therapist may have to decide that further discussion of the problem is unhelpful and that continuing to do so may provoke rather than resolve unwanted emotions. The belief that expression of emotion is the only ingredient in good counselling is erroneous and harmful. Permission therefore extends to encouraging resolution of emotions as well as their initial expression.

The exploration of feelings may be relatively easy where the patient is in touch with their emotions. On the other hand the well-defended patient may deny any emotions at all even where they would ordinarily be expected, e.g. losing a spouse. A few simple techniques can be used to provoke emotion including the description of emotional scenes, e.g. the wedding day or the funeral. The 'empty chair' technique is also useful in these circumstances. The client is asked to imagine the person to whom the emotion refers sitting on the empty chair (it is important to actually place an empty chair beside the client as this brings the setting to life) and to direct their conversation to this. For example the client who feels angry with her son for leaving home will be advised to imagine him sitting on the chair and to articulate her resentment. This is a form of abreaction and, as with any emotional expression, may be associated with a dramatic catharsis. The therapist who feels unable to deal with this should avoid further counselling until he has become more skilled, since emotional outpourings are commonplace especially in the bereaved or in those who have been sexually abused.

During therapy clients must be encouraged to use the *correct terms* for the situations or events they are describing. Thus, the bereaved person who describes her loved one as having 'passed on' may be fearful of the word 'dead'. Similarly, the girl who has been sexually abused may speak of 'it' or 'you know' when she means penis or penetration. Euphemisms have a particular purpose, i.e. to modify the emotional content of the words to which they refer. In the initial stages of therapy they may be allowed but as it progresses the therapist may have to intervene actively to replace them with the correct word. This can be done by saying, 'Tell me what happened, and I want you to use to proper words', or if the client hesitates, 'I know what you mean but it is important that you learn to use the correct words no matter how painful'.

Explaining the reasons for an abnormal piece of behaviour may be helpful at times. For example the housewife who constantly shouts at her children may in fact be angry with her spouse and 'taking it out' on her family. The client who understands this may then be able to deal with her feelings more appropriately. This is known as interpretation and should be used with extreme caution and even with reluctance. It may give the therapist a spurious sense of knowledge, but used inexpertly can also make him seem just silly. A common misinterpretation is the belief that those with panic attacks are using their symptoms to control their spouses. This may be true for some but in many cases the control is the result rather than the cause of the symptoms.

A further tool is the *summary*, which has been mentioned above in the context of facilitating dialogue. It is also a powerful therapeutic force when used to clarify what is being said or to make explicit what has, until then, been implicit. As with interpretation, if summarising occurs too frequently it makes the therapist seem uncertain and hinders emotional progress.

Confrontation may be necessary but must never be a verbal assault on the patient. The therapist must at all times remain calm and professional and also maintain the warmth which is central to all aspects of counselling. The woman who says she does not wish her daughter to leave home may need to be confronted with the likelihood that it is her own loneliness she fears. The danger of inappropriate confrontation is obvious and more than anything else may fracture the therapist–client relationship if done awkwardly.

ENDING THERAPY

For general practitioners this section may be considered unnecessary since the end of counselling may not, and indeed usually does not, mark the end of contact. Nevertheless, it is important to at least make explicit the end of this particular aspect of treatment for the sake of clarity. Of course for the patient who consults infrequently this may indeed mark an end to consultations for a long time.

Terminating treatment should not come as a surprise to the client since a time limit will have been contracted at the outset. Inevitably, however, therapist and client get close and due warning has to be given of the plans to terminate treatment. This should be mentioned in passing at some time during the last three or four sessions to allow disengagement to occur. The client may often produce new problems at this point in the hope of prolonging therapy. Assurance must be given that further therapy will be forthcoming at a later date should the need arise. In general those who have difficulties with separation are also likely to find separation from the therapist difficult. The skilled and sensitive counsellor is keenly aware of this and facilitates separation, which should occur without misgivings or anxieties. In the author's experience the patient frequently fails to attend for the final appointment.

COMMON DEFENCE MECHANISMS

These are the techniques used by the psyche to protect itself from stress and their presence may explain some of the response patterns observed in patients. It is seldom worth interpreting these to the client since they may appear glib and create a feeling of 'being analysed' in the patient's mind. Furthermore, they are not entities in themselves, but explanations derived originally from psychoanalysis to explain behaviour. They are thus no more or less than hypotheses but, despite their limitations, do provide an understanding for at least some behaviours. The list below is not exhaustive but describes those that may be of use in the general practice setting.

Denial is of relevance to general practice, especially to those with serious physical illnesses, where the patient denies being told of the presence of any illness in themselves or their loved ones. It may persist despite constant reiteration of the facts. It is defined as the denial of painful thoughts and as it is unconscious must be distinguished from the knowing avoidance of a painful thought.

Repression is characterised by the unconscious forgetting of painful ideas or impulses in order to protect the psyche. It overlaps with denial.

Identification with the aggressor is observed where the victim begins to assume the qualities or faults of the opponent. This may show itself as the battered wife believing she deserves to be beaten and justifying her husband's aggression to her.

Altruism describes the mechanism of satisfying one's own needs through the lives of others. The man who wished he had become a doctor may 'push' his family into this career and blame himself if they do not fulfil his expectations.

Displacement is the process by which interest is shifted from one object onto another so that the latter replaces the former. Thus the person who loses a child in a road accident and thereafter devotes herself tirelessly to campaigning against dangerous driving is exhibiting this defence. The child is replaced by the ideals of the campaign!

Finally, *projection* is the defence against unpalatable anxieties, impulses, etc. in one's own psyche and these are attributed as being external in origin. The person who attributes indecision to others may be projecting his own indecisiveness.

TRANSFERENCE AND COUNTER TRANSFERENCE

Transference derives from classical Freudian psychoanalysis and refers to the patient who behaves towards the therapist as if he was somebody from a much earlier period in development, e.g. mother, father, etc. He has the same emotions, expectations and needs of the therapist as of his parent. In psychoanalysis, interpretation of the transference is considered the key to therapy. More loosely, the term transference is used to describe the patient's emotional attitude to the therapist. Its use in counselling is that it may provide a clue about the client's behaviour with family and friends. Thus the client who expects the therapist to make all the decisions for him may behave in this fashion with his spouse, thereby leading to marital problems. It is appropriate to reflect this to the client as it may provide an important insight into why the interpersonal problems exist. As with all interpretations it must be done sensitively and appropriately. Implicit in transference and its usefulness in giving insight to the patient is that the therapist has an emotional reaction upon which to base his observations and interpretations. This reaction is known as counter transference.

COUNSELLING IN SPECIFIC SITUATIONS

Terminal illness

The reaction to a diagnosis of serious terminal illness in oneself is analogous to that of a bereavement. However the patient may deny the illness or refuse to discuss it. Denial may have a protective effect on the physical as well as the emotional status of the patient since 'deniers' have been shown to have better prognoses than those who emotionally accept their illness. The denial may need to be dealt with where the patient is not fully successful in the denial and where pockets of insight are known to exist. It is best to begin by probing gently about the patient's fears for the future, for the family and especially for their children. Many patients fear the dying moments and especially the fear of pain or of suffocating may be foremost. These are groundless fears with modern pain relieving techniques and this needs to be explained. Once a relationship has been established and the grieving process is under way the illness will need to be discussed gently and openly, avoiding euphemisms while still retaining some hope and a positive attitude. The response of the family is often a cause of distress to the patient and such comments as, 'Every time I try to talk to my husband he says that I'll be all right and I know I won't' are commonplace. Involving the family in counselling is therefore essential. To the frequent question, 'Should the patient be told?' the response must be, 'It depends'. The personality, intelligence and previous coping capacity of the patient must all be taken into account. It must also be borne in mind that many say they would like to know the truth but in fact do so only wanting to be told of a negative diagnosis. The true meaning of the patient's wishes are very much a matter of clinical judgement.

Sexual abuse

In this more than in any other area, the inexperienced or uncertain therapist should be cautious about commencing therapy. Those who have been the victims of sexual abuse often have repressed their pain, and provoking an emotional reaction can be difficult and frightening both for the client and therapist. There may be some for whom such exploration is not advisable. In particular intense guilt, panic and depression with behavioural decompensation, such as parasuicide or violence, may occur.

The counsellor should be aware of the reluctance of the abused person to use sexually explicit language. This avoidance should be discouraged once a relationship has been built up. Once the client begins to use appropriate and explicit words openly and without distress it is obvious that most of the emotional work has been done. During therapy feelings of anger, dirtiness, depression and panic occur frequently. Allowing the client space to ventilate these feelings either verbally or initially in writing is to be encouraged. There is often some initial difficulty in expressing anger and the client must be given permission to express this, even to the extent of using vitriolic language. It is worth remembering that many who have been abused sexually present with or develop depressive symptomatology. Antidepressant therapy may be required and it is naïve and ethically unsound to suggest to clients that therapy will only be offered if drugs are avoided. The concomitant use of antidepressants is no contraindication to counselling the sexually abused.

Marital disharmony

The function of marriage counselling is to encourage the emotionally distanced couple to begin communicating verbally again. This is based on the assumption that communication has broken down. It is useful to ask the couple to identify their problem areas and to deal with these in turn. The therapist does not give advice but his intervention allows the couple to explore the areas of conflict in a safe environment. Suggestions or possible solutions may be presented to the couple but it is they who decide on the course of action. For marriage counselling even to begin it is necessary for the counsellor to prescribe specific time for the couple to be alone together so that communication can proceed. In general, marriage counselling is much less directive than the behavioural approach of marital contract therapy (see Chapter 12).

For bereavement counselling see Chapter 5, pages 45–47.

PASTORAL COUNSELLING

This is an approach to counselling used by ministers of religion. It encompasses the principles mentioned above but also includes a religious dimension for those who have religious beliefs. The essence of pastoral counselling however is no different from that used in a secular setting.

ARE THERE DANGERS IN COUNSELLING?

As with any therapy, counselling too has its dangers. One of these is excessive dependence on the therapist leading to difficulties in terminating the treatment. An experienced therapist will identify this if it is developing but will also prevent its occurrence by setting firm boundaries during therapy. For this reason appropriate training is imperative. Another difficulty that arises is the release of painful memories that the person may have actively dismissed from day-to-day recall. Thus, speaking about a bereavement may trigger overwhelming feelings of sadness and sorrow and if the event was traumatic may at times provoke suicidal ideation.

However, a problem identified in the past few years is the role of counselling in triggering new memories of sexual abuse in childhood, i.e. memories that have heretofore been absent but surface during therapy (see Chapter 13). These are termed recovered memories although others dispute their reality and have called the phenomenon 'False Memory Syndrome'. The theory underlying recovered memories is that during abuse the person dissociates and represses the memory leading to amnesia for the events. It is believed that during therapy these are unlocked and resurface. However, they are believed by some to arise as a result of suggestion in vulnerable individuals by a powerful therapist. Among psychiatrists there is a strong, although not universal view, that such memories cannot be totally forgotten since they are too painful and extensive to cause total amnesia (Brandon *et al.*, 1998) and that what appears to be repression is in fact deliberate 'putting to the back of the mind'. It is crucial when memories of abuse do arise *de novo* during therapy that the person is not led during their assessment. A free narrative should be allowed with as few questions as possible. Corroborative evidence should also be sought with the patient's permission. Ultimately, there is no way of determining the factual truth or falsity of a recovered memory except through external confirmation.

THE EVIDENCE BASE

Numerous studies show that patients have a preference for counselling over medication in the treatment of emotional problems and this in part may be linked to the proliferation of counsellors in general practice in Britain, although not, as yet, in Ireland. Not surprisingly this has been studied most in relation to the treatments for depression. In spite of this preference not all studies have found a relationship between treatment choice and outcome (Thornett, 2001) although other studies have recommended giving patients the choice of counselling or antidepressants for mild to moderate depression (Chilvers *et al.*, 2001).

In an economic analysis antidepressants were found to be superior to generic counselling in a randomised trial of antidepressant therapy in those with mild–moderate depression (Miller *et al.*, 2003). In a study comparing general practitioner 'treatment as usual' against counselling for those with chronic depression there was some evidence of limited superiority in those referred for counseling but there was an attendant increase in treatment costs (Simpson *et al.*, 2003). However, a recent meta-analysis of seven studies confirmed the superior clinical effectiveness of counselling compared with 'treatment as usual' in the short term but not the long term (Bower *et al.*, 2003). Clearly more studies are required, in order to resolve these conflicting findings. It is important that the exact nature of what is being treated be clarified since 'depression' is a broad term that, in the context of general practice, might describe a range of emotions and/or disorders including unhappiness, adjustment disorder or depressive episode, states that may resolve without intervention. It also remains to be confirmed that optimum antidepressant treatment, as distinct from 'treatment as usual', is superior to counselling in the management of depressive illness.

Other psychosocial approaches have also been explored for treating a variety of emotional problems in primary care and problem solving has emerged as the most positive for depressive disorders (Dowrick *et al.*, 2001; Huibers *et al.*, 2003), while cognitive therapy, behaviour therapy and counselling for disorders that include smoking cessation, alcohol reduction and somatisation are of limited value or have shown conflicting results (Huibers *et al.*, 2003). Again further information on the non-pharmacological interventions that have the best effect await further trials.

SUMMARY

1. Counselling is a specific therapy which is useful for some problems. It is not a 'catch all' or inactive treatment.
2. Successful counselling depends upon the attributes of the patient and also those of the counsellor.
3. Counselling is based upon the principle that exploration of conflicts and expression of emotion bring about resolution of the symptoms.
4. The beginning of therapy should be confined to defining the problem and organising details of the sessions.
5. The middle stage of therapy is when most emotional work is done. Techniques such as summarising, confronting, facilitating and interpreting are but some of the approaches available to the therapist.
6. The end of therapy should not come as a surprise to the patient.
7. The common defence mechanisms are denial, displacement, projection, altruism, etc. These are methods by which the psyche defends itself from overwhelming emotion.
8. There are dangers associated with counselling and it is important to be alert to these.
9. Evidence for the benefits and/or superiority of counselling over antidepressant treatment is uncertain.

REFERENCES

Bower, P., Rowland, N. and Hardy, R. (2003). The clincial effectiveness of counselling in primary care: a systematic review and meta-analysis. *Psychological Medicine*, **33**, 203–215.

Brandon, S., Boakes, D., Glaser, D. and Green, R. (1998). Recovered memories of childhood sexual abuse: Implications for clincial practice. *British Journal of Psychiatry*, **172**, 296–307.

Chilvers, C., Dewey, M., Fielding, K. *et al.* (2001). Antidepressant drugs and generic counselling for treatment of major depression in primary care: randomissed trial with patient preference arms. *British Medical Journal*, **332**, 772–775.

Dowrick, C., Dunn, G., Ayuso-Mateos, J.L. *et al.* (2001). Problem solving and group psycho-education for depression: multicentre randomised controlled trial. Outcomes of Depression International Network (ODIN). *British Medical Journal*, **321**, 1450–1454.

Huibers, M.J., Beurskens, A.J., Bleijenberg, G. and van Schayck, C.P. (2003). The effectiveness of psychosocial interventions delivered by general pratitioners. *Cochrane Database of Systematic Reviews*, **2**, CD003494.

Miller, P., Chilvers, C., Dewey, M. *et al.* (2003). Counselling versus antidepressant therapy for the treatment of mild to moderate depression in primary care: economic analysis. *International Journal of Technology Assessment in Health Care*, **19**, 80–90.

Simpson, S., Corney, R., Fitzgerald, P. and Beecham, J. (2003). *Psychological Medicine*, **33**, 229–239.

Thornett, A. (2001). Assessing the effect of patient and prescriber preference in trials of trreatment of depression in general practice. *Medical Science Monitor*, **7**, 1086–1091.

FURTHER READING

Berne, E. (1964). *Games People Play*. Penguin, Harmondsworth.

Brandon, S., Boakes, D., Glaser, D. and Green, R. (1998). Recovered memories of childhood sexual abuse: Implications for clincial practice. *British Journal of Psychiatry*, **172**, 296–307.

Burnard, P. (1989). *Counselling Skills for Health Professionals*. Chapman and Hall, London.

Frankl, V. (1975). *The Unconscious God*. Simon and Schuster, New York.

Hinton, J. (1972). *Dying*. Penguin, Harmondsworth.

O'Byrne, S. (1979). *Fundamentals of Counselling*. Fredrick Press, Dublin.

Rogers, C.R. (1951). *Client-Centred Therapy*. Constable, London.

SUGGESTED READING FOR PATIENTS

Bates, T. (1999). *Depression. The Common Sense Approach*. New Leaf, Dublin.

Lake, T. (1984). *Living with Grief*. Sheldon Press, London.

Weeks, C. (1983). *Self-Help for Your Nerves*. Angus Robertson.

USEFUL TELEPHONE NUMBERS

Please fill in the following telephone numbers of your local organisations:

CRUSE (Britain) ....
Widows Association (Ireland) ....
LIFE (UK) ....
LIFE (Ireland) ....
Sudden Infant Death Association ....

18

The General Practitioner and the Law

DRUG ABUSE

Britain

The law relating to drug abuse is contained within the Misuse of Drugs Act, 1971 and the Misuse of Drugs Regulations, 1973.

The areas within the Act of relevance to general practitioners are those dealing with controlled drugs and their classification. Drugs are grouped into three classes: Class A includes all natural and most synthetic opiates, cocaine, LSD, injectable amphetamines and cannabinol (the active ingredient in cannabis). Class B includes oral amphetamines, codeine and its derivatives, as well as some barbiturates, and Class C includes methaqualone, cannabis and its resin, some amphetamine-like drugs and benzodiazepines. Class A attracts the most severe penalties and there is a difference in penalties for possession and for trafficking. The doctor who prescribes irresponsibly could be disciplined under this Act.

Under the Regulations it was mandatory for doctors to notify the Home Office of any patient whom they believe to be addicted to opium or its derivatives or to cocaine but this regulation has ceased to apply since 1997. Doctors are prohibited from prescribing heroin, dipipanone or cocaine to addicts unless licensed by the Home Office to do so, although prescribing these drugs for the treatment of organic conditions is allowed. Failure to act within these Regulations could lead to disciplinary proceedings.

Under the new Mental Health Act 1983 dependence upon drugs or alcohol has been excluded as grounds for compulsory treatment unless there is evidence of concomitant mental illness.

Ireland

The law relating to illicit drugs is contained within the Misuse of Drugs Act, 1977 (amended 1984) and has three classes of drugs as in Britain but cannabis remains a class B drug. Unlike the law in Britain there has never been a requirement to notify the Department of Justice of known opiate or cocaine abusers. Under the

Act the prescribing of methadone and buprenorphine is governed by The Misuse of Drugs Regulations (1988). These specify that patients can receive these drugs in community pharmacies or from drug treatment centres with dispensaries attached. For the former a treatment card specifying the name of the treating doctor, the name of the designated pharmacy and the patient's name and photograph must be provided. The Regulations also specify that GPs may treat drug addicts and different levels of training are recognised. For example, a 'level 1' doctor will have received some training in substance misuse and can only treat those addicts who are stable. Each practice is capped at 15 in order to disperse treatment and expertise across practices. A 'level 2' doctor has greater expertise in treating addicts by virtue of training and links to specialist drug treatment centres and these can take on the care of less stable patients.

COMPULSORY ADMISSION

England and Wales

The Mental Treatment Act, 1983 protects and regulates the care of the mentally ill. It also provides for the compulsory admission and treatment of psychiatric patients and of mentally abnormal offenders. The act states that nobody should be deemed to suffer from a mental disorder, within the terms of the act, by reason of alcohol or drug abuse, promiscuity or other immoral conduct.

Assessment Orders

Section 4 allows for the emergency detention of patients for assessment for up to 72 hours. This should only be used when there is insufficient time to obtain the opinion of an approved doctor who could complete Section 2 (see below). Section 4 requires an application to be made by the nearest relative or an approved social worker. A medical recommendation must also be made by one doctor who has examined the patient within the previous 24 hours. This Section is usually completed in the patient's home by the family doctor but may occasionally be also used in the Casualty Department. It is recommended that Section 4 be converted to a Section 2 order as soon as possible. The patient can be discharged by the responsible medical officer.

Section 2 orders allow for assessment of patients for up to 28 days or for their assessment and treatment. Certain treatments such as ECT, hormone implants and psychosurgery are excluded from this. Application must be made by the nearest relative or by an approved social worker who has seen the patient within the previous 14 days. The medical recommendation requires the approval of two doctors one of whom must be approved under Section 12 as having special experience in the diagnosis and treatment of mental illness. They must not be on the staff of the same hospital. The responsible medical officer, the hospital managers, the nearest relative or the Mental Health Review Tribunal can discharge the patient.

Section 5 orders allow for the emergency detention for up to 72 hours of patients who are already in hospital as voluntary patients but request to leave. It applies to patients in any hospital and not just in psychiatric units. It requires the recommendation of one doctor who is in charge of the patient or of a doctor on the staff of the hospital who has been nominated by the doctor in charge. If a doctor is not available a 6 hour holding order may be implemented by a registered mental nurse. The responsible medical officer has the power to discharge the patient.

Two other sections allow for the removal of a mentally disordered person to a place of safety by the police (Section 136) or for a social worker to obtain a warrant to search and remove a patient unable to care for himself to a place of safety (Section 135).

Specifications of Section 2, 4 and 5. The patient must be suffering from a mental disorder, which need not be specified and admission must be in the interests of the patient's health and safety or the safety of others.

Treatment orders

Section 3 is used where treatment is required in the longer term and this section is valid for up to 6 months, with the option of renweal. The involvement of the GP will be as in Section 2 in making the medical recommendation along with a doctor approved in the diagnosis and treatment of mental illness. The grounds for making the recommendation must be stated and these include mental illness, severe mental impairment or psychopathic disorder. In relation to psychopathic disorder or mental impairment such treatment must be deemed likely to prevent or alleviate deterioration in the patient's condition and such treatment is necessary for his safety and wellbeing or for the safety of others. The application is made as in Section 2.

Sections 7 and 8 allow for the treatment of patients living in the community. The application, recommendation, duration and renewal of the orders are as in Section 3.

Consent to treatment

A detained patient may be competent to give informed consent to treatment. Where such a patient is incapable of giving consent, withdraws consent or refuses to give consent, treatment may be imposed in certain circumstances and provided certain requirements are met.

Emergency treatment may be given without consent or a second opinion if it is necessary to save the patient's life or is necessary to prevent serious deterioration in the patient's condition or to prevent the patient from being an immediate danger to himself or others.

Consent or a second opinion is required to administer ECT and medication (other than in an emergency), if it has not been given for the previous three months of the detention. The second opinion must be provided by a doctor who consults with two people, one a nurse, the other neither a nurse nor a doctor, in relation to the patient's state.

Consent and a second opinion are required for irreversible treatments such as leucotomy or hormone implants.

Mentally abnormal offenders

These include Section 37, which commits an offender to hospital as in Section 3 above, Section 47 allowing for transfer from prison to hospital and Section 41 which places a restriction on the patient's discharge from hospital. Since these sections do not involve the general practitioner they will not be considered further.

Further developments

It is proposed that those with 'dangerous and severe personality disorder' (DSPD) shall be detained even when no crime has been committed if such people might potentially be a danger to the safety of others. Detention will take place in specialist units dedicated to the treatment of such disorders. Not surprisingly there is much resistance to this proposal from psychiatrists, human rights groups and advocacy networks and the necessary legislation is yet to be enacted.

Scotland

The law operating in Scotland was enacted in the 1984 Mental Health Act. This is less complex than its counterpart in England and Wales. A new act, the Mental Health (Care and Treatment) (Scotland) Act, 2003 has been enacted but will not become operational until late 2004. The following headings relate to the 1984 Act.

Emergency admission

Section 24 allows for the emergency admission of a patient deemed to be suffering from mental disorder (mental illness or handicap) or mental impairment. Those who are dependent upon drugs or alcohol, promiscuous or exhibiting sexual deviance are excluded under the Act. The recommendation is made by a registered medical practitioner, usually the general practitioner, provided that he has seen the patient on that day. There is no application but if practicable the nearest relative must be notified and consent obtained. The sheriff's approval is not required. The hospital to which the patient is being admitted need not be named nor the form of mental disorder specified. Admission must be urgently required for the protection of the patient or of others and use of the full procedure (Section 18) would involve undue delay. If the patient is not admitted within 3 days of the date of recommendation, the order becomes invalid.

This section may be used in an emergency when an informal patient wishes to discharge himself and when so doing would place him or others at risk. It also allows for certain nurses to detain a patient for a maximum of 2 hours until a doctor arrives to examine the patient.

Section 18 allows for the admission of a patient for 6 months in the first instance. Application is made by the nearest relative or a mental health officer. The recommendation is made by two medical practitioners, one of whom is recognised under the Act as having special experience in the diagnosis or treatment of mental disorder and the hospital to which the patient is being admitted must be named. The form of mental disorder must be specified and the sheriff's approval for detention sought. He must take into account the objections that are raised by the nearest relative or mental health officer. Admission must follow within seven days of his approval and the order is valid for up to 6 months from the date of admission.

Section 26 allows for the detention of a patient already detained under Section 24 (see above) for a further 28 days provided that a medical recommendation is made by an approved doctor and with the consent, if practicable, of the nearest relative or a mental health officer. If the latter is not available a written explanation must be furnished. If continuing detention becomes necessary only Section 18 can be used.

Patients may appeal against their detention to the Mental Welfare Commission.

Consent to treatment

Drug treatments may be given under the above sections for up to 3 months. Thereafter it becomes necessary to implement *Section 98* and this involves obtaining the opinion of a doctor appointed by the Mental Welfare Commission. If an involuntary patient requires ECT at any time following compulsory admission, this section is also utilised. Those patients who become involuntary during their hospitalisation and who are capable of giving informed consent are treated as voluntary patients for the puspose of ECT or long-term drug treatments.

Section 97 applies to treatments such as psychosurgery and hormone implants. These may be given only with the consent of the patient and a favourable opinion from a doctor appointed by the Mental Welfare Commission.

Within the terms of the Act patients so detained must be informed of their rights both orally and in writing although there is no specification on how this should be done and it is left to individual hospitals to decide. Other sections allow for policemen to remove from a public place to a place of safety for 72 hours a person deemed to be in need of psychiatric care (*Section 118*). A mentally disordered person who is being ill-treated may be removed to a place of safety for 72 hours by a policeman or a mental health officer. This section (*Section 117*) also allows for a warrant to be obtained in order to see such a person if entry is refused.

Mentally abnormal offenders

Sections 174 and 375 allow for the detention in 'State Hospitals' of convicted offenders before passing final sentence.

2003 Act

This new Act has not yet been implemented. For the purposes of the 2003 Act, mental disorder includes learning disability, personality disorder and mental health problems. The greatest change in this act is that relatives are no longer required to consent to detention although they can object and have a right to be heard by the tribunal.

Emergency detention. This allows for the detention in hospital of somebody for up to 72 hours where such assessment is required. It must be recommended by a doctor and if possible the agreement of a social worker specially trained in mental health (mental health officer) should be obtained.

Short-term detention. This allows detention in hospital for up to 28 days on the agreement of a mental health officer and a psychiatrist. It is not necessary to have been on a prior emergency order.

Compulsory treatment order (CTO). This order has to be approved by a Tribunal. A mental health officer applies to the tribunal with two medical recommendations and a careplan for the patient. The patient, his/her primary carer and the patient's named person (see safeguards) are entitled to have objections heard by the Tribunal. There is also an entitlement to free legal representation. A CTO is valid for 6 months but can be extended. This order allows for treatment in hospital or in the community.

Other provisions. If a person is receiving voluntary treatment in hospital and decides to leave, an appropriately qualified nurse can hold the patient for up to 2 hours to allow for a medical assessment. This can be extended by another hour once the doctor arrives.

The police may also remove a person to a place of safety if he/she appears to have a mental disorder and to be in need of treatment. The person can be kept there for up to 24 hours to allow assessment and arrangements for the patient's care to be made.

Safeguards. A Mental Health Tribunal, comprising a lawyer, doctor and one other person, will replace the Sherriff's Court as the forum for reviewing compulsory treatment orders. A patient will be able to choose somebody to support him/her and protect their interests in tribunal procedings under the Act. If there is no named person, then the primary carer or nearest relative will fulfil that role. Under the new act all service users, even those not being detained compulsorily, have the right of access to independent advocacy and a duty is placed on Health Boards to ensure that these are available.

Advance statements can also be set out detailing how a patient would wish to be treated at some point in the future and these would have to be taken into account by treating doctors. In addition, there are now safeguards for those receiving ECT or psychosurgery.

In terms of service provision, Health Boards will have to provide mother and baby units to allow for the joint admission of mothers with their babies when being treated for puerperal disorders.

SUPERVISED DISCHARGE

The Mental Health (Patients in the Community) Act 1995 came into effect in April 1996. This allows for the insertion of new sections in the 1983 Mental Health Act in England and Wales and in the 1994 Mental Health (Scotland) Act introducing supervised discharge, referred to as 'aftercare under supervision' in the legislation. The principal element is that each patient, detained under section 3, 37 or 41, will have a treatment plan negotiated with them and their carers prior to discharge and a requirement to attend for treatment. A nominated key worker, usually a community psychiatric nurse, will ensure the discharge of the agreed treatment and will have the power to convey a patient to a place 'for medical treatment, occupation, education or training'. However the legislation does not allow for compulsory treatment in the community and should a patient refuse to be 'conveyed' the only sanction is an obligation on the clinical team to review whether the patient should be detained in hospital under the Mental Health Act (1983). Although now law, the bill was opposed by the Royal College of Psychiatrists as being antitherapeutic and clinically and medicolegally flawed.

Ireland

The Mental Treatment Act of 1945 is now outdated and, although new legislation has been enacted, it is not yet operational and doctors still work under the 1945 act which is largely concerned with administrative issues containing very few protections for the patient. Patients' rights however are protected under the constitution (bodily integrity and habeus corpus). A patient may also seek a judicial review where unlawful detention in hospital is believed to have occurred. The specific circumstances under which compulsory admission is requested are not specified in the Act but are determined by Common Law. Therefore the protection of the patient or of other people are the usual grounds.

Under the Act patients are either voluntary or involuntary. Even the former must put in writing their agreement to hospitalisation, hence the term 'signing in' and they are required to give 72 hours notice of their intention to self-discharge. Non-voluntary patients are further divided into 2 groups – 'temporary' patients who are likely to recover within 6 months and 'persons of unsound mind' who require more than 6 months for recovery.

To bring about a compulsory admission the next of kin, defined under the Act, or if there is none, a welfare officer, make an application. The recommendation is made by a doctor within 24 hours of examining the patient. The doctor is ordinarily the general practitioner but need not necessarily be so. The patient has the right to request a second medical examination before being taken to hospital. The hospital to which the patient is being admitted must be specified. The psychiatrist then accepts or rejects the request. Admission in these circumstances is valid in the first instance for 6 months, when the procedure must be repeated if compulsory detention is still necessary. The patient may request a judicial review. There is no provision for compulsory treatment following discharge and consent to treatment is not addressed in the Act. In practice a patient who refuses treatment is first detained under the Act and permission sought from the next of kin.

New Legislation

The Mental Health Act, 2001 allows for the compulsory admission to hospital of somebody suffering from a mental disorder but specifically excludes personality disorder, addiction to alcohol or drugs or socially deviant behaviour although it does include severe dementia and significant learning disability. Moreover there must be a serious likelihood that the person may cause immediate and serious harm to himself/herself or others or there must be an impairment of judgement such that failure to treat the person would lead to a deterioration in his/her condition. Finally, there must be the likelihood of benefit from such treatment.

An application for admission may be made by a spouse, relative, garda, authorised health board officer or any other person (over the age of 18). Members of the governing body or staff of the approved centre or anybody with an interest in the payments made to the centre may not apply. A medical assessment is carried out within 24 hours of making the application and a recommendation for compulsory detention is made if this is deemed appropriate. The admission must take place within 7 days.

On arrival at the psychiatric centre the person must be examined within 24 hours by a consultant psychiatrist on the staff and if compulsory admission is felt to be justified an order for involuntary admission is made. This is valid for 21 days. Renewal orders may be made after this time for periods of two months. In situations where a patient is already in hospital as a voluntary patient and it becomes necessary to change this to a compulsory order then it must happen within 24 hours of the decision.

All patients must be informed that they are being compulsorily detained and a general description of the treatment provided also. Information concerning the legal right to appeal must also be included. This is also forwarded to the Mental Health Commission who will refer it to an appointed tribunal consisting of a lawyer as chairman, a consultant psychiatrist and a person who is not a lawyer or doctor. Its role is to review the detention of the patient within 21 days and a designated psychiatrist must examine the patient. It also has to ensure that proper procedures were followed. The tribunal has similar powers to a high court and it can compel witnesses and the production of documents. Where a patient is unhappy with the decision of the tribunal he/she may appeal to the Circuit Court.

Electroconvulsive treatment can only be given with the patient's agreement or when it is authorised by the patient's psychiatrist and another consultant psychiatrist. Psychosurgery can only be used with the consent of the patient or is authorised by a tribunal.

FURTHER READING

Anon (1945). *Mental Treatment Acts.* Stationery Office, Dublin.

Anon (1983). *The Mental Health Act, 1983. Summary of the Main Provisions.* Royal College of Psychiatrists, London.

Anon (1983). *The Mental Health Act.* Her Majesty's Stationery Office, London.

Hamilton, J.R. (1983). The Mental Health Act. *British Medical Journal,* **286**, 1720–1725.

USEFUL WEBSITES

Summary of The Mental Health (Care and Treatment) (Scotland) Act 2003:
www.mwcscot.org.uk/act.htm

Summary of the Mental Health Act 2001 for Ireland:
oasis.gov.ie/health/mental_health_act_2001.html

USEFUL CONTACTS

The Medical Defence Union
3 Devonshire Place
London W1N 2EA
Tel: 020 7202 1500
Email: mdu@the-mdu.com
Website: www.the-mdu.com

Medical Protection Society
33 Cavendish Square
London W1G 0PS
Tel: 020 7399 1300
Email: info@mps.org.uk
Website: www.medicalprotection.org

UK Advocacy Network (UKAN)
14–18 West Bank Green
Sheffield, S1 2DH
UK.
Tel: 0114 2728171
Website: www.u-kan.co.uk

Irish Advocacy Network
Tel: 047 38918

19

The General Practitioner and the Psychiatric Services

The view of psychiatrists as the dustmen of medicine is outmoded and the most exciting development in modern psychiatry has been the recognition that psychiatry treats and helps patients on a par with any other branch of medicine. Patients are no longer consigned to 'bins' and psychiatrists now work alongside paediatricians, obstetricians and all the other acute medical specialties in general hospitals.

FACILITIES

Traditionally treatment was concentrated in mental hospitals throughout Britain and Ireland. These were established before there were any scientifically recognised treatments for psychiatric disorders and consequently became the enclaves of people with a variety of problems ranging from chronic schizophrenia to the those who were unwanted because of some perceived disgrace, such as illegitimacy. Clearly many did not need lifelong hospitalisation and the growth of libertarianism in the 1960s led to the 'open door' policy. This coincided with the development of more efficient treatments for psychiatric disorders, so whether the philosophical or the scientific insights led to this change is debatable.

In-patient services

In-patient facilities are essential to the good practice of psychiatry. Unfortunately the move to 'community' psychiatry has led the naïve to assume that this inevitably meant the closing down of the available facilities and the total care of the patient in his or her own environment. This was a travesty of the truth and has been shown to be unrealistic. Far from weakening the acute facilities it should re-emphasise the necessity for acute admission units with full back-up facilities and staff to deal with acute psychiatric disorders.

Recent years have seen the growth of acute psychiatric units in general hospitals so that psychiatrists now work alongside their medical and surgical colleagues. Also there is an interchange of patients from medical to psychiatric wards and vice versa as is deemed appropriate. This has led somewhat to the demystification of psychiatry and psychiatrists although some stigma continues. The added advantages of modern buildings and location in the geographic area that they serve has also made the specialty more acceptable.

Previous government documents both in Ireland and Britain have recommended that areas should be served by units in general hospitals and 0.5 acute adult beds per 1000 population should be the target. However there have been no such specific recommendations in recent years due to the difficulty of making these calculations taking into account patient mobility and demographic changes.

The goal of in-patient units is short-term treatment, perhaps for 2–3 weeks followed by out-patient follow-up as in any of the acute specialties. While there has been a shortfall in the provision of acute beds in some areas and over-provision in others, the target of short hospitalisation has been achieved and psychiatry is now becoming aligned with its sister specialties, at least in terms of admission policies and aftercare.

As well as serving the acutely ill, the humanitarian care of the long-term ill and the provision of asylum must not be forgotten. While the 'new long-stay' are few in number, the responsibility for their care falls to the health services especially when they are unable or unwilling to live at home. The Utopian ideal of community care may be advocated, but where the family are elderly or poor, or where the burden of care is too great, then alternatives must be sought. Some patients drift away from their families, and the State, by default, becomes responsible. The choice in these circumstances is between long- or medium-stay units in the patient's locality, designated high support hostels, or less commonly admission to old-style psychiatric hospitals. The location and title of the facility are less important than the core ingredient, i.e. the ambience. These should provide day-time activities as well as recreation compatible with the patient's level of functioning. Regular reviews by the responsible medical staff are necessary to identify those who are capable of moving on to rehabilitation or to more independent living. Care in these units is not an end in itself but constitutes one aspect of the treatment and rehabilitation of those with severe psychiatric illness. Facilities of this kind are still necessary for the compassionate treatment of a small and voiceless but challenging group of patients. Unfortunately, it has been the plight of many, that discharge to inadequate facilities resulted in destitution and homelessness and the insistance on discharge to the community, at all costs, has been criticised by many (World Health Organisation, 1980).

Home care

First promoted in the early 1980s, home care of the acutely ill represented a natural extension of the philosophy of community care. It stems from the belief that it is possible to manage all but the most suicidal or psychotic of patients at home, provided there is adequate nursing and medical support. Home care involves multiple visits from the team each day until symptoms settle and treatment can be transferred to day-hospitals or other venues. A further argument in its favour is that patients and carers alike prefer this and that outcome is not adversely affected. However, there are disadvantages, among them the unsuitability of some patients for treatment at home such as those who are suicidal or aggressive. This points to the necessity for a very thorough initial assessment in order to out-rule these. In addition the ability of some carers to cope with an acutely ill patient in a home setting must also be considered and where diagnosis is uncertain the benefit of constant observation by mental health professionals is lost. For those who live in inner cities and who may be isolated with inadequate support or living alone the problems with home care are obvious. Carers and patients remain more satisfied with treatment at home although the treatment teams have been found in a recent study to be low in morale. A recent meta-analysis of the benefits on home-care was inconclusive (Catty *et al.*, 2002).

The day hospital

The first day hospital was set up in 1945 by Joshua Bierer in London and since that time the provision of day care has been recognised as essential to the psychiatric services. Day hospitals vary greatly in the type of patient they accept and in the range of treatments provided. Some will only accept those with schizophrenia, others deal exclusively with those not ill enough to require in-patient care, and some take a mixed group including those with alcohol problems, psychotic illnesses and personality disorders. There is as yet no information on the patient groups who are most likely to derive maximum benefit from treatment in this setting or indeed what proportion of those who are acutely ill can be successfully managed as day-patients. The overall aim is therapy and the policy is against long-term attendance. A range of treatments is provided including behavioural, psychological and pharmacological in groups as well as individually. Day hospitals may be located near the psychiatric unit or in some other location. Many sectors now have their own day hospital serving that geographical area exclusively. The staff of the modern day hospital should consist not only of psychiatrists but also nurse therapists, psychologists and occupational therapists and the recommended norm for Great Britain is 0.3 places per 1000 adults. An equivalent figure for Ireland is 0.75 places per 1000 but this also includes day centre places.

Day centres

Day centres have a different philosophy and more limited goals. The main aim is to provide an outlet, company and activity for those who need it. In particular those with long-term mental illness, the old and lonely and those with physical or mental handicap benefit from this approach. Unlike the day hospital many patients are long-term attenders. They are usually run by the Local Authority and in Britain 0.6 places per 1000 adults is recommended.

Hostels

The first hostels were established in the 1950s and since then have become an integral part of modern psychiatric rehabilitation. Three types exist – low support or short-stay hostels which provide acommodation for those who move on rapidly through the rehabilitation services to independent living; medium support for those whose progress is less rapid; and high support for the patients, now resident in psychiatric institutions, who will continue to need indefinite supervision and nursing care as well as the small group described as the 'new long-stay'. Hostels are staffed by nurses although the patient:nurse ratio depends on the type, with more nurses inevitably being employed in high support units. The psychiatrist and the multidisciplinary team have regular patient reviews so that any change in the patient's condition, for better or worse, will result in further input either behaviourally for rehabilitation, or with medication to control recrudescent symptoms.

Group homes

These houses are the closest that many patients will have to a home and although they are owned by health boards the occupants function independently of the medical services. Thus patients live with others of similar capacity and care for themselves with the minimum of supervision usually from the community nurse. Some may eventually move on to independent accommodation.

PERSONNEL

The psychiatrist

The development of community psychiatry has ushered in the transfer of patient management from the hospital to settings in many different environments. These include health centres, day hospitals situated in the locality, hostels and in some areas even total home management. These new developments are not without their critics. A radical approach, which is rarely included in discussions of 'community psychiatry' has been the move into the realms of general practice psychiatry. As the prognosis for the major mental illnesses improved it became increasingly apparent that many conditions designated as 'neurotic' and by implication less serious in nature, were in fact incapacitating and a challenge to the profession. These have generally been managed with varying success by the general practitioner but the increasing use of modern therapies such as behaviour therapy and cognitive psychotherapy has resulted in the frontiers of psychiatry being extended into this domain.

Since the late 1970s the interface between general practice and psychiatry has become more diffuse. Up to 50% of psychiatrists in Britain now have clinics in general practitioner's surgeries. While greeted with cynicism and charges of treating the 'worried well' initially, it has become increasingly apparent that psychiatrists have an important role to play in dealing with those patients who would not normally be referrred to the hospital-based psychiatric services. Several approaches to this model of liaison are available.

The replacement model

The replacement model operates where the psychiatrist sees his out-patients in their local practitioner's surgery. This is likely to lead to greater compliance on the part of patients and less stigma at having psychiatric treatment. Inevitably the numbers referred to such an accessible service are likely to increase and the demands made of psychiatrists that this would entail would be excessive. There are cogent arguments for discouraging any dramatic increase in referrals to the psychiatric services and for strengthening the role of the general practitioner in competently managing the majority of his patients with psychological difficulties.

The educative model

The educative model aims to carry out this important task. For many this model is perceived as a threat since its goal is to equip the family doctor to recognise and adequately treat most of those in the community with emotional problems without recourse to the psychiatric services. Harnessing the GP's skills for the good of the patient is central to this philosophy. The work of Balint, dealing with the psychotherapeutic aspects of the patient and the consultation, was seminal to this model although it is now recognised that a much broader approach is required if this model is to achieve its aim of therapeutic success coupled with holism.

The liaison model

In this model education combines with consultation and, while not diminishing the role of the family doctor, provides practical support and help for GPs and their patients. Central to the operation of this scheme is the development of close working relationships between the psychiatrist and one or two family practitioners. Regular visits to the surgery by the psychiatrist and discussion or assessment of selected patients results in an increase in knowledge by the GP along with the opportunity to manage the patient without relinquishing responsibility. Should difficulties arise then referral to the psychiatric services would occur in the usual way. This model has the advantage of fully utilising the GP's knowledge of the patient's background and personality and has been shown to be an effective and relevant model for over a quarter of patients seen in primary care with emotional disturbances, provided both psychiatrist and general practitioner show a willingness to initiate face to face contact (Darling and Tyrer, 1990).

Whichever model is chosen the aim is to help the general practitioner recognise psychiatric disorder at an early stage, provide effective treatment and institute preventive measures where this potential exists.

Cost-effectiveness

One of the spurs to provide treatment to patients in locations that are accessible to them is the desire to make financial savings, stemming from the earlier referral of patients to such a service, thereby avoiding hospital admission. There is some evidence that admissions among those with depressive illness are reduced with primary care based community services although no such reduction has generally been shown for schizophrenia. However, duration of stay is shorter. Among those with depressive illness, clinical and social outcomes are similar for community based and mental hospital based services. However, the failure to reduce the number of admissions among those with schizophrenia as well as the greatly increased number of referrals to the primary care based service mean that there is no overall cost saving to the Health Service. This has implications for fund-holding general practices in Britain (Goldberg *et al.*, 1996).

The community nurse

The role of the community nurse was once confined to dealing with recently discharged patients, assisting in depot clinics and providing an extension of the hospital services into the patient's environment. These roles are still essential but as the diagnoses seen in the out-patient clinic have beceome more diverse, the nature of the task performed by the community nurse is also changing. In addition, the involvement of the psychiatrist in general practice has necessitated this change in function.

In recent years community nurses have gained additional qualifications especially in behaviour therapy and have an important therapeutic role often specialising in behaviour and cognitive therapy. The involvement of nurses in prescribing certain medications is also presently being piloted. A number of studies have now examined patient satisfaction with nurse therapists and the results generally have been positive. Until recently, nurses worked in close liaison with the psychiatrist but their links with general practice have now been intensified with concerns being expressed that this will encourage the fragmentation of the psychiatric services. The counter argument that the links to general practice may have a preventive function is plausible but as yet unproven. Thus the modern community nurse has, in the eyes of many, a therapeutic role but an uncertain accountability.

This issue has yet to be clarified and the debate about direct referral to psychiatric nurse therapists has only just begun. What has been established is that community nurses are invaluable as supports and as 'keyworkers' for those with long-term difficulties. They have a recognised therapeutic potential although the limitations, answerability and autonomy need to be examined in depth.

The psychologist

The clinical psychologist's role is as uncertain as that of the community nurse. They too have been establishing close links with general practitioners and in many instances accept direct referral independent of the psychiatrist. Again the issue of clinical responsibility, e.g. in the event of suicide, has to be worked out. Not only are clinical psychologists accused of usurping the psychiatrist's role, but psychologists in turn feel that nurse therapists are intruding upon their area of practice. In many centres, especially in Britain, psychologists have been replaced by behaviourally trained nurse therapists who now undertake all the marital, cognitive and general behaviour therapy for the team. Inevitably, psychologists feel that their therapeutic role is being eroded.

The occupational therapist

The role of the occupational therapist (OT) is largely to evaluate the functional capacity of the patient. Assessments of the person's ability to shop, manage money, cook and maintain self-care and care of others such as children can be carried out either on the ward or at home, the latter by the community based OT. This evaluation is especially helpful when arranging discharge following lengthy hospitalisation or following an episode of severe psychiatric illness. Indeed, functional capacity is arguably a more relevant target for assessment than is symptom evaluation since it is impairment in functioning that is often the trigger for psychiatric referral and admission. Moreover functioning usually improves more slowly than do symptoms and understanding this time frame is pertinent when deciding on changes to treatment. Those areas where there is a deficit can also be targetted for specific interventions aimed at enhancing practical activities that are part of the daily routine.

The social worker

The social worker has many functions in dealing with the psychiatrically ill. These range from the practicalities of sorting out social welfare payments to the more 'glamorous' work of family and marital therapy. They may also have a role in preventing psychiatric problems especially at times of crisis in the lives of those who are vulnerable. These include the elderly, the isolated, the bereaved or those with few supports. GPs have been shown to be especially welcoming of the social worker's involvement, often due to the new light which is shed upon the patient's background but also due to the opportunity they provide to share the emotional burden of treating problem patients. The face to face contact and the lack of formality makes them easy working partners. As with community nurses and psychologists their boundaries and accountability as therapists have yet to be clarified particularly within the multidisciplinary approach, where non-medics may make decisions concerning the appropriate therapist to provide treatment.

APPROACHES TO COMMUNITY CARE

The Care Programme Approach

The Care Programme Approach (CPA) has been called the cornerstone of the British Government's mental health policy since 1991. It forms the basis for the care of all those with serious mental illness treated outside hospital and is the approach used for those with schizophrenia and severe mood disorders. In many cases, the CPA comes into play while someone is receiving in-patient treatment (not necessarily detained under the Mental Health Act), and creates the framework for discharge planning and aftercare. It is multidisciplinary in approach and for each patient a key worker is identified who takes the lead in the individual patient tracking, monitoring and care delivery. Both patients and carers are involved and it must be flexible so as to adapt to the patient's changing needs. It is proactive and so identifies early relapse and initiates appropriate action.

There are four stages to the CPA and these are:

1. A systematic *assessment* of the person's healthcare and social care needs.
2. The development of a *care plan* agreed by all involved, including the person herself/himself and any informal carers, as far as this is possible, and addressing the assessed needs.
3. Identifying a *key worker* to be the main point of contact with the person concerned and to monitor the delivery of the care plan.
4. Regular *review* of the person's progress and the care plan, with agreed changes to the plan as appropriate.

Not everyone who is a patient of specialist psychiatric services will require an equally full or complex CPA approach. In practice, three levels of the CPA exist. Minimal CPA is appropriate for those with few health care needs, those who have high levels of social support and are likely to remain stable. A higher level will be needed for those requiring more social support and whose illness is more severe and are less likely to remain well. Full multidisciplinary CPA will be necessary for those with poor social function and poor support, those who may be unstable or volatile or present a risk to themselves or others. In these circumstances the care plan is likely to be detailed with special attention paid to communication between the professionals so that the patient does not 'slip through the net'.

Supervision Registers

If it is judged that the person poses a significant risk to themselves or others, then they may be placed on a Supervision Register. Established in 1994 the British Government required all mental health providers to establish such registers with the aim of flagging those patients with severe mental illness who are at risk to themselves, by suicide or neglect, or to others, by violence and ensuring that they receive appropriate care in the community. Both the Royal College of Psychiatrists and MIND have expressed doubts about their usefulness and their utilisation varies from one Trust to another, and indeed between consultants also. Gradually however their implementation has extended from England to Scotland and Wales although not yet to Northern Ireland. Before placing a patient on the Register the patient must be informed, evidence must be presented to the multidisciplinary team meeting that this is necessary and regular contact with the patient must be ensured. The register list is not distributed to other agencies such as the police. Even though there is no legislation underpinning the Supervision Register, failure to place an 'at risk' patient on the register could lead to severe criticism of the responsible consultant and/or Trust in the event of an adverse incident involving the patient.

Assertive outreach

Traditionally mental health services are delivered in clinics, hospitals or health centres. However, a proportion of patients do not engage with this and as a result default and eventually relapse. Assertive outreach is the term used to describe a way of working with those who disengage partially or fully from the usual psychiatric services. Instead a key worker will review them, in their own environment, be it their home, a café or where ever the patient is most accessible and comfortable. Many sectors in Britain have dedicated assertive outreach teams while others are part of the generic team. However they are constituted, assertive outreach workers expect to review their patients several times per week. With such intensive and flexible follow-up the case-worker/patient ratio is low. Recent studies have shown that although enhanced community management may reduce admission among heavy users of the services, there was no additional clinical benefit and the savings resulting from reduced in-patient admissions were offset by the cost of intensive community follow-up when compared with treatment as usual (Harrison-Read *et al.*, 2002).

Early intervention services

As far back as 1990 it was suggested that the optimum treatment for non-affective psychosis was intervention in the prodrome or in the early stages of illness.

Impetus was given to this view by the findings that the shorter the duration of untreated psychosis the better the prognosis and although the evidence is not definitive it is robust enough to warrant development of early intervention facilities linked to studies of outcome.

There are two elements to such services – one is the ready availability of assessment and early treatment where appropriate. This means assessment within 1 to 2 days and the acceptance of referrals from a variety of sources other than the general practitioner alone, as has traditionally applied. These diverse referral agents include schools, family members, friends, community workers, self-referral, etc. Some centres have a dedicated early detection team.. The second element is the educative one. People at risk of these disorders will not be referred if the public has little knowledge, or only misinformation about schizophrenia and related disorders. Thus education about attitudes to mental illness that use multiple points including schools, cinemas, etc., and with a variety of media, e.g. newspaper advertisements, radio discussions, etc., are central to achieving this. A recent study found that such a multi-faceted approach reduced the duration of untreated psychosis from 114 weeks to 26 weeks (Johannessen *et al.*, 2001). It remains to be seen if such a proactive approach improves prognosis.

SELF-HELP

Patients frequently seek advice about self-help and the advice given will very much depend on the quality of the local groups. Self-help groups have several goals. *First*, they have a supportive role and many patients feel that meeting others with the same problem is not only comforting but helpful in dealing with the difficulty. *Secondly*, they have an educative function and they disseminate information about particular disorders. This is obviously beneficial but has an especially helpful effect in relation to psychiatric disorders where knowledge will reduce stigma. *Thirdly*, self-help has the aim of prevention and groups such as the widows' association, infertility groups and a host of others provide vital supports to those who are isolated, lonely and vulnerable. *Finally*, they aim to treat emotional disorders and groups such as Alcoholics Anonymous have been particularly successful in achieving this. In addition to these laudable aims, self-help harnesses the resources within the sufferer and also draws on the experience of those who have suffered to bring about change.

Having enumerated the advantages of self-help groups it is important to be aware of their limitations. In particular those who constitute the group may not in fact be suffering from the condition at all. Since they are run by lay people for lay people there is no way of ensuring the homogeneity of the group. Thus a group for depressives may also have those who are primarily unhappy or even those with personality disturbance. A further difficulty lies in the fact that all its members are, in principle, experiencing the same difficulty. This may be a problem with chronic sufferers who instead of motivating may adversely affect the newer members and convey a feeling of hopelessness rather than optimism. A third problem lies in the motivation of some self-help members who come to depend upon the group rather than use it as a stepping-stone to well-being. Finally, but uncommonly, self-help may be antithetic to medicine and may be part of the 'no drug' culture erroneously advising its members to 'do it themselves'. In psychiatry this can be detrimental but is fortunately a rare occurrence and in the author's experience self-help groups generally work in liaison with doctors rather than the converse.

SUMMARY

1. Care in the community is now the norm and this has extended in many areas to treating the acutely mentally ill at home.
2. A number of recent developments include the provision of supervision registers for those who pose a special risk.
3. Assertive outreach represents a flexible approach to follow-up in the community.
4. Early intervention in the prodrome or early symptom phase of schizophrenia is now being developed, by targeted education and flexible rapid assessment for those believed to be at risk.

REFERENCES

Catty, J., Burns, T., Knapp, M., Watt, H., Wright, C. (2002). Home treatment for mental health problems: a systematic review. *Psychological Medicine*, **32**, 383–401.

Darling, C. and Tyrer, P. (1990). Brief encounters in general practice: liaison in general practice psychiatry clinics. *Psychiatric Bulletin*, **14**, 592–594.

Harrison-Read, P., Lucas, B., Tyrer, P. *et al.* (2002). Heavy users of acute psychiatric beds: randomised controlled trial of enhanced community management in an outer London borough. *Psychological Medicine*, **32**, 403–416.

Goldberg, D., Jackson, G., Gater, R., Campbell, M. and Jennett, N. (1996). The treatment of common mental disorders by a community team based in primary care: a cost-effectiveness study. *Psychological Medicine*, **26**, 487–492.

Johannessen, J.O., McGlashan, T.H., Larsen, T.K. *et al.* (2001). Early detection strategies for untreated first-episode psychosis. *Schizophrenia Research*, **51**, 39–46.

World Health Organisation. (1980). *Changing Patterns in Mental Health Care. Euro Reports and Studies 25.* WHO, Copenhagen.

FURTHER READING

Corney, R.H. (1980). Factors affecting the operation and success of social work attachment schemes to general practice. *Journal of the Royal College of General Practitioners*, **30**, 149–157.

Department of Health and Social Security. (1975). *Better Services for the Mentally Ill*. Her Majesty's Stationery Office, London.

Department of Health, Ireland (1984). *The Psychiatric Services. Planning for the Future*. Government Publications, Dublin 2.

Mazhindu, D. and Brownsell, M. (2003). Piecemeal policy may stop nurse prescribers fulfilling their potential. *British Journal of Community Nursing*, **6**, 253–255.

Skidmore, D. and Friend, W. (1984). Community psychiatric nursing: Specialism or escapism? *Community Outlook*, June, 203–205.

SUGGESTED READING FOR PATIENTS

Drew, T. and King, M. (1995). *The Mental Health Handbook*. Piatkus, London.

USEFUL CONTACT

Inspector of Mental Hospitals
Department of Health
Hawkins House
Dublin 2
Ireland

20

Stress in Doctors

Studies of psychiatric morbidity in doctors have focused on the 'minor' disorders using screening questionnaires such as the General Health Questionnaire and, using this approach, possible, rather than definite, 'cases' are identified. Very few have gone to the next stage of conducting face-to-face structured diagnostic interviews to assess major psychiatric illness.

In general, health professionals have higher rates of psychiatric morbidity than their equivalents in other sectors and anxiety, depression and substance abuse are the main diagnoses. Some studies have examined suicide rates among doctors and these have been found to be higher than in other professions as are sickness absences and staff turnover. In addition, marital problems and divorce are also more common in doctors than other professionals.

PREVALENCE

A prevalence of up to 27% for minor psychiatric disorders has been found in a large sample of NHS staff when compared with non-health service staff and female doctors and managers were particularly at risk (Wall *et al.*, 1997). Using self-report measures to identify vulnerable doctors (Caplan, 1994), 55% of general practitioners were possible cases of anxiety and 27% possible cases of depressive illness. The figures were somewhat lower for consultants and although this was a screening study without a diagnostic interview the results point to a very high potential prevalence of stress-related disorders among doctors. Although other health service professionals have been studied less intensively, studies point also to a higher rate of psychiatric morbidity in nurses.

Broadly speaking psychiatric disorders in doctors can be classified into three categories. First, that which is profession related. Secondly, that which is independent, including major mental illness such as severe depression and psychotic disorders. The third overlapping category represents those episodes that, although triggered by work-related problems, subsequently recur independently. Irrespective of the aetiology of the disorder, work is likely to be impaired if it persists.

RISK FACTORS

A number of factors are thought to be associated with the development of work-related emotional disorders in doctors. In particular doctors have the invidious task of being warm and caring to patients while at the same time being expected to remain detached and calm even in the face of terrible suffering. These conflicting but professional requirements may make us more defensive of admitting emotional difficulties when we experience them ourselves and also inhibit us from seeking help. This is borne out by a study that found us to be reluctant patients, avoiding the sick role by self-diagnosis and self-prescribing (Forsythe *et al.*, 1999).

Work-related factors found to be associated with abnormal stress among doctors include work overload and its effect on home life, poor management and resources, excessive managerial responsibilities and dealing with patients' suffering. Similarly, variables which contribute to job satisfaction and protect against work-related stress include good relationship with patients and staff, professional status and esteem, intellectual stimulation, autonomy and good management and resources (Ramirez *et al.*, 1996). Certain specialties are also associated with a greater risk of psychiatric morbidity than others especially those that deal with high levels of trauma or mortality such as accident and emergency departments, intensive care units and neonatal units. Those working in areas where there is a risk of personal assault such as psychiatric units and accident departments as well as those who feel isolated in their work, e.g. doctors working in the community, have also been shown to be vulnerable.

Stressors unrelated to work may also cause symptoms which impinge upon the doctor's working life. These include marital and family related difficulties, financial and health related (in self or family) problems and bereavement. However, a recent study of depressive and anxiety disorders among hospital staff found that while stress outside work and prior vulnerability due to a past history contributed to these disorders, work-related problems also contributed independently as did the absence of a confidant and feelings of poor support from management (Weinberg and Creed, 2000).

Psychodynamic explanations have also been offered to explain the high rate of emotional disturbance among doctors and these include the suggestion that choosing a career in medicine may be a defence against feelings of abandonment resulting from childhood loss due to illness or death. Some have described the choice of a career in medicine as an attempt to remedy earlier emotional neglect by the compulsive giving of care to others to compensate for what was absent from the doctor's childhood. This has been termed the 'helping professional syndrome'. Psychodynamic theory suggests that such professionals perceive others' needs as demands which they try to satisfy. If they are unsuccessful they render themselves vulnerable to depression. These theories are still speculative and require much more empirical exploration.

Doctors will also carry the vulnerability factors that are relevant to major mental illness in any person irrespective of their work and these include family history, past history of abuse, separation from parents in childhood and inadequate social supports.

BURN-OUT

This is a vague but fashionable concept. Doctors and others who are reluctant to speak of their emotional distress are attracted by the destigmatising nature of the term. In consequence we hear people speak of burn-out who would otherwise be unwilling to admit emotional problems. The term itself entered the mental health lexicon in 1974 as a description of work-related symptoms that include physical depletion, helplessness and hopelessness, the development of a negative attitude to work and patients, and cynicism with regard to all aspects of life, in a previously idealistic person. There is often a fear of work and the doctor may become less caring of patients and more protective of himself. Thus burn-out is an end-point rather than an event and it represents the accumulation of multiple stressors over time over which he has little control and to which he responds in a maladaptive manner. Although a lot has been written about burn-out there is little that is scientific and much that is anecdotal and advice ridden.

VIOLENCE

The risk of violence to doctors is not a new phenomenon although the fatal stabbing of a general practitioner in Scotland in 1994 highlighted the seriousness of the risk. One in 20 NHS staff has been threatened with a weapon and 73% of all staff on medical premises suffer verbal abuse and threats. Among general practitioners, 63% experienced violence or abuse during the previous 12 months, 3% sustained minor injury and 0.5% serious injury (Hobbs, 1991). Violence is perceived by general practitioners to be increasing particularly in the inner city.

Not surprisingly the presence of a threat of violence will affect the approach of doctors to their work leading to fear of house calls, the abandonment of home visits especially at night, increasing use of the deputising service, increased prescribing, increased referral of threatening patients to secondary care services and removing patients from their lists. In such a climate it is not surprising that doctors' psychological wellbeing will be adversely affected leading to a host of symptoms including anxiety, insomnia, depression and irritability.

Strategies for reducing the risk of violence

1. Assume each patient is potentially threatening unless the patient is well known.
2. Place the desk and chair near an exit with the patient furthest from the exit.

3. If possible ensure that the surgery has a feeling of space and has natural light.
4. Be aware of your instinctive reaction to the patient's demeanour.
5. Keep your distance. Imagine there are four 'bubbles' around the patient. These spatial subdivisions are termed 'proxemics'. The first lies about 18 inches from the patient and is the *intimate zone*. The second or *personal space*, lies between 18 inches and 4 feet and is the area for touching and close non-intimate contact. The third subdivision, termed *social space*, lies from 4 to 12 feet and is the area for communicating with friends while not allowing physical contact. The fourth or *public space* extends from 12 feet outwards. It is best to remain in social space or outside it when initially dealing with an unknown patient. If a gesture of friendship or concern such as touching the shoulder is made, this will necessitate a move into personal space and should be avoided until the patient has been fully assessed. Not only will the patient not feel confronted or overwhelmed by remaining in social space but the distance is too great to allow for serious physical contact in the event of a violent incident.
6. Avoid confrontation about such matters as smoking rules on the premises, etc., until the patient has been fully assessed.
7. Install a panic button.

SUICIDE

The British Medical Association in 1993 paid special attention to the problem of suicide among doctors and a large number of papers, of variable quality, have addressed this problem. A comprehensive review, using only studies that met specific inclusion criteria based on both method and quality, confirmed the view that doctors are at increased risk of suicide compared with the general population or other academic occupational groups (Lindeman *et al.*,1996) and most of the increased risk is accounted for by women doctors who have three times the rate of suicide as their counterparts in the general population. A recent study of doctors in Britain found a suicide rate among male and female doctors to be 19.2 and 18.8/100,000 respectively confirming that the rate among males was lower than in the general population while among female doctors it was higher although the overall rate was similar in both sexes. This study also found differences between specialties, with anaesthetists, community health doctors, general practitioners and psychiatrists being most at risk (Hawton *et al.*, 2001).

Possible risk factors include the pre-morbid personalities of doctors whose supposedly obsessional tendencies make them more prone to depression and hence to suicide. Others have cited the knowledge of drugs and their lethality as a factor while the higher prevalence of drug and alcohol abuse among doctors when compared with other professions might also contribute. Finally, the demands of family and the dissatisfaction with medicine as a career have been identified, particularly in relation to female suicides (Anon, 1994). However these theories are still speculative and require further study.

Suicidal thoughts are also present in many doctors and, when compared with hospital consultants, general practitioners have a significantly higher incidence of such ideation (5% and 14%, respectively). Even among medical students and recently qualified doctors suicidal ideation was present in 14% of those interviewed at some point in the previous year and while the proportion who planned suicide was high at 8%, only 1.4% made an attempt, a figure that is lower than in the general population (Tyssen *et al.*, 2001). However, other studies have found much lower rates for suicidal thoughts at 3% in ICU doctors, a group considered at high risk of suicide (Coomber *et al.*, 2002).

HELPING SICK DOCTORS

Doctors are often reluctant to advise their colleagues to seek help although it is obvious that such assistance is necessary and such reticence is detailed clearly in the work of psychiatrist Professor Kay Redfield-Jamison (1995) who describes her colleagues' reluctance to address her increasingly obvious bipolar disorder. Ideally, when a doctor becomes worried that a colleague is unwell, he should be approached and advised to contact the Occupational Health Department (OHD) of the hospital/Trust or visit the general practitioner. Many doctors may be worried that contact with the OHD may lead to the involvement of management and decline this although doctors in these departments are bound by the same rules of confidentiality as any other doctor. Furthermore, many doctors do not have a general practitioner and a recommendation should be made to visit the appropraiate specialist/consultant for treatment. If these informal approaches are rejected, more formal procedures may be required, especially if patient care is jeopardised.

In British hospitals, doctors known as the 'Three Wise Men' are elected by the local medical community and provide advice and support for those with emotional or other problems which are impacting on their work. For general practitioners the local Medical Committee has the same role. Both of these bodies have legal obligations to report to the employer any doctor whose problem is placing patients at risk. For this reason their advice is often met with resentment from the practitioner who refuses to acknowledge that help is needed. They may then have to arrange the suspension of the sick doctor by Management or report the doctor to the General Medical Council (GMC) at that point.

The National Counselling Service for Sick Doctors offers confidential advice in a non-threatening manner and has no links with employing authorities nor any responsibility to it. This service was initiated by the GMC and the British Medical Association (BMA) working in concert. However, due to its strict adherence to confidentiality it does not publish reports and there is no information on its uptake or effectiveness. Finally, the GMC's Health Committee, during the screening stage of assessing complaints, may direct a practitioner to helping agencies thereby avoiding a full enquiry.

In Ireland the Sick Doctors' Scheme, a helping agency initiated by the Irish Medical Organisation, offers support and advice to doctors with alcohol and drug-related problems. This body has no legal obligations to report doctors to their employing authorities. The Medical Council of Ireland now also has a Health Committee that is similar to its GMC counterpart.

SUMMARY

1. The prevalence of abnormal stress reactions among doctors is high and estimates vary between 27% and 55%. Most studies have used screening schedules and few have carried out diagnostic interviews.
2. Risk factors are related largely to the administrative and resource aspects of practice although dealing with suffering has also been described as placing doctors at risk.
3. Violence is an ever increasing problem for general practitioners, particularly those in inner cities where up to 63% have been the subject of physical attack or verbal abuse in the previous year.
4. Doctors have an increased risk of suicide when compared with other professionals and this is accounted for by the increased risk among female doctors. General practitioners are among those at particualr risk.

REFERENCES

Anon (1994). News: Doctors are more miserable than ever, says report. *British Medical Journal*, **309**, 1529.

Caplan, R.P. (1994). Stress, anxiety and depression in hospital consultants, general practitioners and senior health service managers. *British Medical Journal*, **309**, 1261–1263.

Coomber, S., Todd, C., Park, G. *et al.* (2002). Stress in UK intensive care unit doctors. *British Journal of Anaesthesia*, **89**, 873–811.

Forsythe, M., Calnan, M. and Wall, B. (1999). Doctors as patients: postal suurvey examining consultants' and general practitioners' adherence to guidelines. *British Medical Journal*, **319**, 605–608.

Hawton, K., Clements, A., Sakarovitch, S., Simkin, S. and Deeks, J.J. (2001). Suicide in doctors: a study of risk according to gender, seniority and specialty in medical practitioners in England and Wales, 1979–1995. *Journal of Epidemiological and Community Psychiatry*, **55**, 296–300.

Hobbs, F.D.R. (1991). Violence in general practice: a survey of general practitioners' views. *British Medical Journal*, **302**, 329–332.

Lindeman, S., Laara, E., Hakko, H., and Lonnqvist, J. (1996). A systematic review on gender-specific suicide mortality in medical doctors. *British Journal of Psychiatry*, **168**, 274–279.

Ramirez, A.J., Graham, J., Richards, M.A., Cull, A. and Gregory, W.M. (1996). Mental health of hospital consultants: the effects of stress and satisfaction at work. *Lancet*, **347**, 724–728.

Redfield-Jamison, K. (1995). *An Unquiet Mind: A Memoir of Moods and Madness*. A.A.Knopf, New York.

Tyssen, R., Vaglum, P., Gronvold, N. and Ekberg, O. (2001). Suicidal ideation among medical students and young physicians; a nationwide prospective study of prevalence and predictors. *Journal of Affective Disorders*, **64**, 69–79.

Wall, T.D., Bolden, R.I., Borrill, C.S. *et al.* (1997). Minor psychiatric disorder in NHS Trust staff.: Occupational and gender differences. *British Journal of Psychiatry*, **171**, 519–523.

Weinberg, A. and Creed, F. (2000). Stress and psychiatric disorder in healthcare professionals and hospital staff. *Lancet*, **355**, 533–537.

FURTHER READING

Redfield-Jamison, K. (1995). *An Unquiet Mind: A Memoir of Moods and Madness*. A.A. Knopf, New York.

Tillett, R. (2003). The patient within – psychopathology in the helping professions. *Advances in Psychiatric Treatment*, **9**, 272–279.

USEFUL CONTACTS

The General Medical Council
178–202 Great Portland Street
London W1N 6JE
Tel: 0845 357 8001
Email: gmc@gmc-uk.org
Website: www.gmc-uk.org

The Irish Medical Council
Portobello Court
Lower Rathmines Road
Dublin 6
Ireland

The Sick Doctors' Scheme
c/o The Irish Medical Organisation
10 Fitzwilliam Place
Dublin 2
Ireland

National Counselling Service for Sick Doctors
Website: www.ncssd.org.uk

21

Herbal Remedies

The general public is increasingly interested in alternatives to conventional medicines in the treatment of all illnesses, including psychiatric disorders. A recent study from the United States found that 16.5% of householders responding to a telephone survey had used complementary or alternative therapies in the previous 12 months and of these over 20% met the criteria for one or more psychiatric disorders (Unutzer *et al.*, 2000). Clearly, psychiatrists and general practitioners need to be aware of the evidence base for the effectiveness of these preparations and also of their likely side-effects and interactions with conventional medicines.

A few have been examined scientifically and these are described below.

KAVA

This is the extract of a Polynesian plant, *Piper methysticum*, and is used in religious ceremonies and recreationally in the South Pacific. It is ingested in beverage form or by chewing. Early double blind studies suggest that it may be superior to placebo and equivalent to benzodiazepines in the treatment of anxiety. In addition the incidence of side-effects is reported to be very low with probably little risk of dependence. However, these studies are few in number, the diagnostic criteria for anxiety were non-specific and there is no clear information on optimal dosage. In addition the duration of treatment was no longer than a few months and so firm information on the dependence potential is lacking.

A recent study that did specify the criteria for anxiety (generalised anxiety disorder) compared it against placebo in a randomly assigned double blind trial lasting 4 weeks. Recognised measures of anxiety such as the Hospital Anxiety Depression rating scale were used as well as self-evaluation. Both groups showed some improvement, a phenomenon that is repeatedly reported in placebo controlled trials. However, kava was not superior to placebo (Connor and Davidson, 2002). A Cochrane review examining six studies found that patients receiving kava extract did improve significantly more than those on placebo. The report concluded that kava was effective and safe but for no longer than 6 months as further studies into its long-term efficacy and safety are required (Pittler and Ernst, 2004). As well as being used as an anxiolytic it also has muscle relaxant and hypnotic properties. It is mildly intoxicating and there have also been reports of its abuse, the latter causing scaly skin lesions, known as kavaism. It interacts with alcohol, antidepressants and analgesics and should not be used in pregnancy or when breastfeeding.

SAINT JOHN'S WORT

Also known as hypericum, this is perhaps the most commonly used herbal remedy for psychological disorders. A number of randomly allocated, placebo-controlled trials have demonstrated its effectiveness for short-term use against comparator drugs and its superiority to placebo in mild to moderate depression illness (Cochrane review). A recent study failed to confirm its effectiveness in treating depression (Shelton *et al.*, 2001) and further studies are required over longer observational periods and against standard antidepressants. A further problem is that the doses of comparator drugs tend to be lower than those recommended and there are few studies against the SSRIs.

St John's Wort suffers from a lag period of 2–4 weeks before the onset of symptom relief and a full therapeutic response can take up to 12 weeks. Side effects are much less common than with standard antidepressants, the main ones being gastrointestinal, allergic and either tiredness or restlessness. There is a case report of sub-acute polyneuropathy and a photosensitivity rash co-occurring.

As St John's Wort can increase the activity of cytochrome P450 the possibility of interactions with drugs metabolised using this system exists. It is recommended that concomitant use with warfarin, other antidepressants, digoxin, anticonvulsants, oral contraceptives, other antidepressants and anti-migraine drugs be avoided where possible although a total embargo is probably not necessary. An oral dose of 900 mg per day is suggested.

OMEGA-3 OIL

Fish oils contain the fatty acids eicosapentaeonic acid (EPA) and docosahexaenoic acid (DHA) and these act by maintaining the neuronal membrane structure and in the production of prostaglandins and leukotrienes. It has been suggested that EPA might help in the treatment of depression in those who do not respond to standard antidepressants. It is based on the belief that there is an abnormality in CNS omega-3 fatty acids in those with depression and some studies have found that these patients also have low blood levels. A recent placebo-controlled study found significant reduction in symptoms compared with the control group (Peet and Horrobin, 2002) when treated with 1 g daily. Case reports and prospective studies suggest that it might be helpful in residual schizophrenia, particularly in patients responding poorly to clozapine, but further studies are required (Taylor *et al.*, 2003).

VALEPOTRIATES (VALERIAN EXTRACT)

This substance has been suggested as being a potential anxiolytic and has recently been examined in a pilot study comparing placebo, diazepam and valerian extract (Andreatini *et al.*, 2002). Using a random allocation following a placebo wash-out period, 36 out-patients meeting DSM criteria for generalised anxiety disorder were randomised to one of the three treatments for 4 weeks. Diazepam and valerian extract showed a significant reduction in the cognitive aspects of anxiety but valerian did not impact on other features such as physical symptoms. This small study, while preliminary, does suggest that valerian extract might have an effect on the psychic component of anxiety. Clearly larger studies are required.

GINSENG

A herbal remedy that is widely recommended for treatment of fatigue and to ward off adverse reactions to stress is Siberian ginseng. Used for several millenia in China, it only became popular in the West in the 1950s. It has been widely used by Russian athletes to improve stamina and it is often prescribed by Russian doctors to improve general health, much as doctors prescribe tonics in Britain and Ireland. A recent study from the University of Iowa, USA, (Hartz *et al.*, 2004) compared Siberian ginseng against placebo in a group of patients with chronic fatigue and found that only those with less severe fatigue showed a positive response. As this was the first trial to examine ginseng the authors recommend further studies.

Although the evidence for the efficacy of herbal remedies is patchy there are also indicators that some are worthy of further scientific examination.

REFERENCES

Andreatini, R., Sartori, V.A., Seabra, M.L. and Leite, J.R. (2002). Effects of valepotriates (valerian extract) in generalised anxiety disorder: a randomised placebo-controlled pilot study. *Phytotherapy Research*, **16**, 650–654.

Connor, K.M. and Davidson, J.R. (2002). A placebo-controlled study of kava-kava in generalised anxiety disorder. *International Journal of Clinical Psychopharmacology*, **17**, 185–188.

Hartz, A.J., Bentler, S., Noyes, R. *et al.* (2004). Randomised controlled trial of Siberian ginseng for chronic fatigue. *Psychological Medicine*, **34**, 51–61.

Peet, M. and Horrobin, D.F. (2002). A dose ranging study of the effects of ethyl-eicosapen-taenoate in patients with ongoing depression despite adequate treatment with standard drugs. *Archives of General Psychiatry*, **59**, 913–919.

Pittler, M.H. and Ernst, E. (2004). Kava extract for treating anxiety (Cochrane Review). *The Cochrane Library*, Issue 1. Wiley, Chichester.

Shelton, R.C., Keller, M.B., Glenberg, A. et al. (2001). Effectiveness of St John's Wort in major depression: a randomised controlled trial. *Journal of the American Medical Association*, **285**, 1978–1986.

Taylor, D., Paton, C. and Kerwin, R. (2003). Fish Oils in Schizophrenia. In *The Maudsley 2003 Prescribing Guidelines, 7th edition*. Martin Dunitz, London.

Unutzer, J., Klap, R., Strum, R. et al. (2000). Mental disorders and the use of alternative medicine; results from a national survey. *American Journal of Psychiatry*, **157**, 1851–1857.

FURTHER READING

Ernst, E., Pittler, M.H., Stevinson, C. *et al.* (2001). *The Desktop Guide to Complementary and Alternative Medicine*. Harcourt, London.

Index